Africanizing Oncology

NEW AFRICAN HISTORIES

SERIES EDITORS: JEAN ALLMAN, ALLEN ISAACMAN, AND DEREK R. PETERSON

David William Cohen and E. S. Atieno Odhiambo, *The Risks of Knowledge*

Belinda Bozzoli, *Theatres of Struggle and the End of Apartheid*

Gary Kynoch, *We Are Fighting the World*

Stephanie Newell, *The Forger's Tale*

Jacob A. Tropp, *Natures of Colonial Change*

Jan Bender Shetler, *Imagining Serengeti*

Cheikh Anta Babou, *Fighting the Greater Jihad*

Marc Epprecht, *Heterosexual Africa?*

Marissa J. Moorman, *Intonations*

Karen E. Flint, *Healing Traditions*

Derek R. Peterson and Giacomo Macola, editors, *Recasting the Past*

Moses E. Ochonu, *Colonial Meltdown*

Emily S. Burrill, Richard L. Roberts, and Elizabeth Thornberry, editors, *Domestic Violence and the Law in Colonial and Postcolonial Africa*

Daniel R. Magaziner, *The Law and the Prophets*

Emily Lynn Osborn, *Our New Husbands Are Here*

Robert Trent Vinson, *The Americans Are Coming!*

James R. Brennan, *Taifa*

Benjamin N. Lawrance and Richard L. Roberts, editors, *Trafficking in Slavery's Wake*

David M. Gordon, *Invisible Agents*

Allen F. Isaacman and Barbara S. Isaacman, *Dams, Displacement, and the Delusion of Development*

Stephanie Newell, *The Power to Name*

Gibril R. Cole, *The Krio of West Africa*

Matthew M. Heaton, *Black Skin, White Coats*

Meredith Terretta, *Nation of Outlaws, State of Violence*

Paolo Israel, *In Step with the Times*

Michelle R. Moyd, *Violent Intermediaries*

Abosede A. George, *Making Modern Girls*

Alicia C. Decker, *In Idi Amin's Shadow*

Rachel Jean-Baptiste, *Conjugal Rights*

Shobana Shankar, *Who Shall Enter Paradise?*

Emily S. Burrill, *States of Marriage*

Todd Cleveland, *Diamonds in the Rough*

Carina E. Ray, *Crossing the Color Line*

Sarah Van Beurden, *Authentically African*

Giacomo Macola, *The Gun in Central Africa*

Lynn Schler, *Nation on Board*

Julie MacArthur, *Cartography and the Political Imagination*

Abou B. Bamba, *African Miracle, African Mirage*

Daniel Magaziner, *The Art of Life in South Africa*

Paul Ocobock, *An Uncertain Age*

Keren Weitzberg, *We Do Not Have Borders*

Nuno Domingos, *Football and Colonialism*

Jeffrey S. Ahlman, *Living with Nkrumahism*

Bianca Murillo, *Market Encounters*

Laura Fair, *Reel Pleasures*

Thomas F. McDow, *Buying Time*

Jon Soske, *Internal Frontiers*

Elizabeth W. Giorgis, *Modernist Art in Ethiopia*

Matthew V. Bender, *Water Brings No Harm*

David Morton, *Age of Concrete*

Marissa J. Moorman, *Powerful Frequencies*

Ndubueze L. Mbah, *Emergent Masculinities*

Judith A. Byfield, *The Great Upheaval*

Patricia Hayes and Gary Minkley, editors, *Ambivalent*

Mari K. Webel, *The Politics of Disease Control*

Kara Moskowitz, *Seeing Like a Citizen*

Jacob Dlamini, *Safari Nation*

Alice Wiemers, *Village Work*

Cheikh Anta Babou, *The Muridiyya on the Move*

Laura Ann Twagira, *Embodied Engineering*

Marissa Mika, *Africanizing Oncology*

Holly Hanson, *To Speak and Be Heard*

Saheed Aderinto, *Animality and Colonial Subjecthood in Africa*

Paul S. Landau, *Spear*

Africanizing Oncology

Creativity, Crisis, and Cancer in Uganda

Marissa Mika

OHIO UNIVERSITY PRESS

ATHENS, OHIO

Ohio University Press, Athens, Ohio 45701
ohioswallow.com
© 2021 by Ohio University Press
All rights reserved

Printed in the United States of America
Ohio University Press books are printed on acid-free paper ∞ ™

First paperback edition published 2022
Paperback ISBN: 978-0-8214-2509-1

Library of Congress Cataloging-in-Publication Data
Names: Mika, Marissa, 1981– author.
Title: Africanizing oncology : creativity, crisis, and cancer in Uganda / Marissa Mika.
Description: Athens, Ohio : Ohio University Press, 2021. | Series: New African histo-
ries | Includes bibliographical references and index.
Identifiers: LCCN 2021011141 (print) | LCCN 2021011142 (ebook) | ISBN
9780821424650 (hardcover) | ISBN 9780821447512 (pdf)
Subjects: LCSH: Uganda Cancer Institute. | Cancer—Hospitals—Uganda. |
Oncology—Uganda. | Medical policy—Uganda.
Classification: LCC RC279.U33 M55 2021 (print) | LCC RC279.U33 (ebook) | DDC
616.99/40096761—dc23
LC record available at https://lccn.loc.gov/2021011141
LC ebook record available at https://lccn.loc.gov/2021011142

For Aram and Shauna

"I know that the ones who love us will miss us."

Contents

Illustrations

Acknowledgments

My deepest gratitude extends to the staff, patients, and patient caretakers of the Uganda Cancer Institute (UCI). Thank you for welcoming me as a historian and ethnographer. Thank you for generously engaging with an outsider during times of great duress and quiet moments of quotidian life. To protect privacy, the names of patients and caretakers are not recorded here, but they are not forgotten.

In 2010, Dr. Jackson Orem agreed to meet with me after a phone call and a brief letter of introduction. Over the years, he has become a dear friend and mentor. He is also an extraordinary advocate for cancer research and care in Uganda. Thanks to Jackson for everything, especially entrusting me with reconstructing the history of this institution. And many thanks to Irene Nassozi for scheduling meetings and helping me on the ground with never-ending paperwork. The past directors of the UCI were astonishingly generous. Dr. John Ziegler mailed me archives and photographs, spent hours on the phone patiently answering questions, and welcomed me to his homes in California. John's humility, as well as his appreciation and respect for Uganda, helped to shape my own analysis and attempts to write with care. Professor Charles Olweny shaped this research profoundly by keeping the doors of the UCI open throughout the Idi Amin era. I thank him for his work as an oncologist, advocate, and historian. Dr. Edward Katongole-Mbidde generously took time away from his obligations as the director of the Uganda Virus Institute to meet with me and to attend the UCI's first History Symposium in 2014. His singular dedication to the Institute for four decades, and his commitment to the maintenance of high standards in the face of extreme difficulty and scarcity, is nothing less than remarkable. The UCI's current deputy director, Dr. Victoria Walusansa, also deserves special mention for welcoming me to the day-to-day activities of the wards. Other former and current Institute oncologists helped to shape the context for this project in important ways. Dr. Chuck Vogel shared his memoirs. Dr. Robert Comis offered his memories of working at the UCI in the 1970s just as Amin took over. Dr. Avrum Bluming sent photographs he personally took of Idi Amin. The late and esteemed Dr. Richard Morrow kindly shared his memories of taking blood samples in up-country fieldwork.

Dr. Joyce Balagadde Kambugu and the entire Lymphoma Treatment Center staff made large components of the ethnographic research at the UCI happen. I thank them all, particularly Allen, Susan, Mariam, Rose, Harriet, Misty, Collins, and Primrose. A special thanks to Dr. Geriga, Dr. Nixon Nyonzima, and Dr. Grace for their work in softening the edges of bone marrow aspirates, tending to emergencies, and answering questions from concerned parents and ethnographers alike. The families who pass through the Lymphoma Treatment Center in search of care and relief are lucky to have such dedicated staff on the wards. *Weebale kujanjaba.*

Late-tumor oncologist, master interpreter, and dedicated teacher Dr. Fred Okuku spent many hours of casual conversation regaling me with stories of the UCI's history and the general dilemmas of practicing oncology in East Africa and the United States. Without Fred, this would be a very different book. Thank you for all you do. Dr. Noleb Mugisha understood the contemporary and historical logic of this project immediately. I thank him for his ready willingness to be a sounding board on matters ranging from tracking down past historical actors to purchasing a car in Kampala. Dr. Abrahams Omoding taught me much about HIV medicine, oncology, and the possibilities of providing comfort at the end of life. Dr. Innocent Mutyaba and Irene Nassozi both made interviews with Burkitt's lymphoma caretakers possible.

Sister Mary Kalinaki kindly and freely shared the past of the UCI and suggested many others to meet with along the way. Mr. Nsalabwa and I drove around Kampala and deep into the village to meet his colleagues with memories of the past. I thank Mr. Nsalabawa, Mr. Tom Tomusange, Mr. Aloysius Kisuule, and Sister Simensen for conversation and tea on verandahs and in sitting rooms. Mr. Ephraim Katende brought us together, and I thank him for his tireless work behind the scenes to schedule interviews and interactions with colleagues of the past. He is a true *mzee* (gentleman) in every way. Mr. Alex removed the padlock from the door of the inactive records room and facilitated access to forty-five years of the UCI's archives. I am grateful to him and the rest of the records staff for their cooperation. Thanks also to Christine Namulindwa for supporting many aspects of the research at the UCI over the years.

In Seattle, Dr. Corey Casper graciously welcomed me at the Fred Hutchinson Cancer Research Center. I thank him and the rest of his team, especially Mary Engel, Erica Sessle, Jason Barrett, Katie Maggard, and James Farrenberger. Thanks especially to Jen Ashe for dealing with one scheduling headache after another. The local Hutch–UCI program staff, especially Mariam, Annet Nakagenda, and Andrew Okot, made me feel welcome. Dr. Warren Phipps provided deep contextualization on a number of levels, from memories of old buildings to running the fabulous research-in-progress meetings—the ultimate incentive to get to the UCI by eight in the morning, traffic jam or rain notwithstanding. Isma Lubega was the quintessential fixer. There are, of course, many other people at the UCI and Fred Hutch who helped to shape this work and offered their time. I extend my warmest thanks to all of them.

At the main Mulago Hospital and Makerere College of Health Sciences, Susan Byekwaso wrote critical letters of introduction. Dr. Elly Katabira offered sage advice and steered me in the right direction. Dr. Alex Coutinho and Dr. David Serwadda both shared their memories of working as medical students and clinical officers at the UCI in the early 1980s. The entire pathology department, especially Professor Henry Wabinga and Chief Technician Mr. Ssempala filled in important gaps about the history of cancer registration in Uganda. Thanks to the ladies at the Dome Café for coffee, samosas, the space to write fieldnotes, and regular Luganda lessons. Trusted drivers Paul, James, Jimmy, and Kiiza kept me in one piece.

Esther Nakkazi and I first met at the Uganda House in 2009, and she has been pulling me out of traffic, offering wise counsel, and working as an intellectual collaborator and a trusted friend since then. Kampala would not be the same without you, Esther. Thanks for the journeys down Entebbe Road and the vibrant discussions over plates of *muchomo* (roasted goat). Dr. David Kyaddondo and Dr. Herbert Muyinda shared much as scholars and friends. Dr. Asiimwe Godfrey provided intellectual support and freely shared many of the challenges of being an academic in Uganda. Mr. Waalabyeki Magoba and Mr. Deo Kawalya took me on as a student of Luganda, leaving an indelible mark on this project. To all other Ugandan colleagues left unnamed here, I thank you for your hospitality and friendship.

This project was fundamentally shaped by the thought collective at the University of Pennsylvania's History and Sociology of Science Department. Many of the issues discussed here in this book about social health, biomedical technology transfer, and care from below came out of long and productive conversations with Steve Feierman over the past decade. Thank you, Steve, for your intellectual generosity and for reading every word, asking the hardest questions, and believing in this project. Robert Aronowitz's wise counsel, friendship, close reading, and thoughts on how to write about cancer with both empathy and clinical acumen made this a better book. Adriana Petryna's work on traveling experiments shaped early drafts of research questions. I thank her, too, for suggestions on how to move forward after nearly a year of writing in circles. In a prior life, I worked in applied global health, and it was Randall Packard who showed me that pursuing history as vocation was possible. His encouragement to examine the long history of biomedical research in Uganda sent me to Kampala and Mulago. Sara Berry first suggested that the UCI would be a compelling place to situate a research project and offered impeccable feedback over the years. Julie Livingston supported this work with great intellectual generosity and supplied copies of *Improvising Medicine* to colleagues in Uganda. Gabrielle Hecht's thinking on technology and politics shaped parts of the theoretical architecture of this book. Cori Hayden graciously welcomed me to the Center for Science, Technology, Medicine, and Society at UC Berkeley. I thank Holly Hanson for her friendship, for the generous sharing of her time and ideas, and for much-needed moral and emotional support in the field. Derek Peterson offered both practical and critical advice regarding archives and tools for thinking about the creative political work of the 1970s in Uganda.

For solidarity and support during fieldwork in Kampala, London, and Seattle, thank you to the following individuals: Angela Bailey, Anna Baral, Ashley Rockenbach, Christopher Conte, Claire Medard, Edgar Jack Taylor, Elizabeth Dyer, Emma Park, Erin Moore, Esther Nakkazi, Eve Meisho, George Willcoxon, Glenna Gordon, Henri Medard, Jacob Doherty, Janet Lewis, Jennifer Child, Jennifer Lee Johnson, Jeremy Dell, Johanna Crane, John Arndt, Jon Earle, Joslyn Meier, Julia Cummiskey, Kate Von Achen, Kathleen Vongsathorn, Katie Hickerson, Keshet Ronen, La Fontaine staff, Lindsey Ehrisman, Meg Winchester, Megan Swanson, Myroslava Tataryn, Natalie Bond, Nir Jacoby, Paul Reidy, Peter Hoesing, Sam Dubal, Sarah Lince, Stephanie Farquhar, Tyler Zoanni, Ursula Child, Valerie Golaz. Thanks to Andrea Stultiens and Rumanzi Canon of History in Progress Uganda for fresh ways of seeing old and new things.

This book is a bit road weary. It traveled first to London in the middle of Brexiting Britain and then to a new experiment in global health in rural Rwanda and then back to California in the middle of a global pandemic.

I am grateful for the time at the University College London and the University of Global Health Equity to have the necessary distance from the project to see that it was nearly finished. At UCL I was fortunate enough to work on a team on chronic disease in Africa sponsored by the Wellcome Trust. Thanks to Megan Vaughan and Tamar Garb at the Institute of Advanced Studies for challenging me to think beyond cancer and Uganda. Anna Marazuela-Kim, Carlo Caduff, Dora Vargha, Eliot Michaelson, Keren Weitzberg, João Rangel D'Almeida, Løchlann Jain, Sarah Hodges, Stephen Hughes, Thomas Small, and many others made London home for me. Daniel Peppiat, Emma Peel, Francesca Guarino, Naomi Absalom, and the entire Yoga Like Water Crew reminded me to breathe. In Rwanda, I thank my students at the University of Global Health Equity, who are some of the finest young physicians in training I know. Thanks to Abebe Bekele, Agnes Binagwaho, Akiiki Bitalabeho, Carla Tsampiras, Darlene Ineza, Eugene Richardson, Ishaan Desai, Ismail Rashid, Juliette Low Fleury, Kara Neil, Katie Letheren, Nolwazi Mkhwanazi, Olivia Clarke, Paul Farmer, Samson Opondo, Shrestha Singh, Solange Nakure, Theogene Ngirinshuti, and Woden Teachout for making the time at Butaro a singular experience. And thanks to all who practiced yoga with me on the Kagame Deck.

Thanks also to the following colleagues and friends for their support over the years: Alice Weimers, Alicia Decker, Anita Kurimay, Anna West, Anthony Darrouzet-Nardi, Aya Cook, Beth Linker, Betsey Brada, Bob Timberlake, Branwyn Polykett, Brian Horne, Bridget Gurtler, Cal Biruk, Carol Summers, Cathy Burns, Chisomo Kalinga, Claire Wendland, Corina Benner, Corrie Decker, Cynthia Houng, Damien Droney, Dana Simmons, D'Arcy Dewey, Darja Djordjevic, David Barnes, David Mandell, David Schoenbrun, Deanna Kerrigan, Deborah Thomas, Derek Newberry, Divine Fuh, Dwai Bannerjee, Elaine Salo, Elizabeth Hallowell, Elizabeth Lim, Eram Alam, Erica Dwyer, Erin Pettigrew, Ernestine de Voss Williams, Freyja Knapp, George Alvarez, Gina Senarighi, Harry Marks, Jamie Kudera, Jason Oakes, Jennifer Nehila, Jeremy Greene, Jerry Zee, Jessie Saenz, Joanna Radin, John Lum, John Tresch, Josh Garoon, Kate Dorsch, Kearsley Stewart, Keith Wailoo, Kent Ferguson, Knoah Piasek, Kristin Doughty, Lindsey Dillon, Lori Leonard, Lucas Mueller, Luke Messac, Lynn Thomas, Mari Webel, Mark Gardiner, Marlee Jo Tichenor, Massimo Mazzotti, Matt Doucleff, Matthew Kruer, Michael D'Arcy, Michal Engelman, Michaeleen Doucleff, Michelle Yu, Mike Light, Mike Rahfaldt, Nana Qureshi, Nancy Hunt, Neil Kodesh, Noelle Sullivan, Noémi Toussignant, Patricia Johnson,

Patricia Kingori, Pier Larson, Projit Mukherjee, Rachel Elder, Rachel Meyer, Raphaelle Rabanes, Robin Scheffler, Robyn D'Avignon, Rosanna Dent, Ruth Cowan, Ruth Prince, Scott Zeger, Shannon Cram, Simukai Chigudu, Stefanie Graeter, Sunita Puri, Susan Levine, Susan Lindee, Susan Reynolds Whyte, Talia Konkle, Tamar Novick, Tara Dosumu Diener, Tauriq Jenkins, Trevor Getz, and Wenzel Geissler. Thanks to all who impacted this work but remain unnamed. Your acts of kindness and thoughtful questions are not forgotten and made things better. And thank you, the reader, for taking the time to pick up this book.

Many institutions provided time and space for this project over the years including the University of Pennsylvania, the University of California Berkeley, the University of Cape Town, Johns Hopkins University, University College London, and the University of Global Health Equity. Thanks to audiences who offered valuable feedback at workshops and colloquia, including those at Stanford University, Massachusetts Institute of Technology, Yale University, UC Berkeley, UC Davis, UC Riverside, University of Wisconsin–Madison, Washington University in St. Louis, University of Michigan, Oxford University, Cambridge University, University College London, King's College London, University of Manchester, University of Warwick, University of Exeter, University of Oslo, the British Institute in East Africa, the University of Global Health Equity, and the University of Witwatersrand. Financial support for the research in this book came from a Benjamin Franklin Graduate Fellowship from the University of Pennsylvania, an International Dissertation Research Fellowship sponsored by the Social Science Research Council, a Dissertation Fieldwork Grant and Engaged Anthropology Grant from the Wenner Gren Foundation, a Penfield Dissertation Research Fellowship, and the Helfand Fund from the University of Pennsylvania, among others.

Working with colleagues at Ohio University Press has been an absolute delight. I thank Derek Peterson, Jean Allman, Allen Isaacman, and Carina Ray for close reading, astute editorial feedback, and enthusiasm and care for the UCI's story. Sally Welch, Ricky Huard, and Tyler Balli, as well as the teams in book production, copy editing, and design, have been a pleasure to work with. Thanks to Audra Wolfe for providing exceedingly helpful advice on how to move from dissertation to book. I greatly appreciate the careful and thoughtful feedback of two anonymous reviewers who read the manuscript in a middle of a pandemic and made it better.

Aram and Shauna Mika taught me early on that the world was far bigger than Santa Barbara, California. I am forever grateful for that lesson.

It is a profound sadness to me that Aram Mika unexpectedly passed away in 2005 and was therefore unable to see how this project unfolded or that it even began. With cheer and enthusiasm Shauna Mika has supported work that takes me six thousand miles away from California. I thank her and Rick Callison for their ongoing, joy-filled support. Eric Mika's refreshing yet sardonic take on the world keeps me honest. He graciously attended several boring academic events on the East Coast over the years, providing much needed comic relief. Mic Hansen, cancer survivor, read many of the chapters here and also paid a visit to London in 2012 when family time was sorely needed. Patricia and Wallace Mandell offered encouragement at every juncture as did the rest of the Mandell family. Joe, Alex, Austin, and Susan Blanks offered hospitality in East Texas that facilitated writing and relaxation. I am thankful also for the kinship of the Damore family, Annie and Mill Peaks, and Brian and Alice Burke.

There is too much to say about the ways in which Hunter Blanks supported me and this work over the years. He endured multiple transcontinental moves, months of separation, and mediocre Skype connections. He line edited copy, fetched me at the airport, ferried books on the Tube, cooked memorable dinners, set up the projector for *Doctor Who* nights, and picked up coffee for morning redwood hikes. Thank you for making so many places home, be it Kampala, Baltimore, Philadelphia, London, Butaro, Kigali, Cape Town, Oakland, or Berkeley. I am excited for the next adventure together.

Lastly, but definitely not least, the Uganda National Council of Science and Technology, the UCI, and the Makerere School of Public Health granted permission to do this research. This book is not an official statement of the Uganda Cancer Institute, the Fred Hutchinson Cancer Research Center, or the Ugandan government. While many engaged with this project and provided substantial feedback on many of the chapters here, the errors, omissions, and interpretations are my own.

Abbreviations

FHCRC   Fred Hutchinson Cancer Research Center (also Fred Hutch)

IAEA   International Atomic Energy Agency

LTC   Lymphoma Treatment Center

NCI   National Cancer Institute

STC   Solid Tumor Center

UCI   Uganda Cancer Institute (also the Institute)

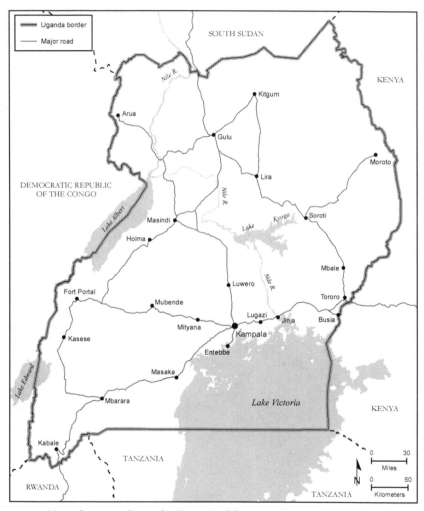

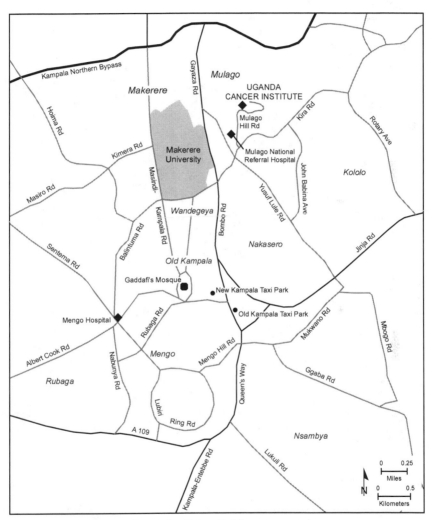

MAP 2. Kampala. Map drawn by Brian Balsley.

Prelude

A Week in the Life of the Uganda Cancer Institute

PRESENT-DAY KAMPALA is expanding at a breakneck pace. New buildings are mushrooming across the city on a daily basis. There is a booming middle class, and more cars on the road means punishing traffic. There is occasional tear gas during political protests and slum clearing in the name of beautification. But if you squint hard enough through the pollution and dust that settles on the city in between rainy seasons, you can still see remnants of a colonial garden city. This was a city designed in the 1960s with a maximum of three hundred thousand residents in mind, not the 1.5 million people who today call greater Kampala home.[1] If you see baby goats butting heads on the side of the road or tall stalks of silvery green maize being grown in the middle of town, it's a reminder that Kampala is a city where the pastoral and the urban meet.

Today, if you stand at the top of Makerere Hill, home to the oldest university in East Africa, to the south you would see Kololo Hill and Nakasero Hill, with their posh suburbs and government establishments. Farther to the east, Kamwokya is a rough working-class neighborhood being rapidly gentrified by malls and NGOs alike. If you buy groceries at the new and shiny Nakumatt housed in the Acacia Mall, you will see not only a photo of President Yoweri Museveni at the checkout counter but also a portrait of the current *kabaka* (king of Buganda), Ronald Mutebi, a reminder that Buganda kingdom is still celebrated. Standing at Makerere, if you look toward the east, past the valley of Wandegeya with its bustling clothing shops, food vendors, and auto repair garages, you will see a sprawling concrete building with a powder-blue roof and smaller, older facilities dotting the hill. This is Mulago Hospital, located on the hill that bears the same name.

Many patients, patient caretakers, physicians, nurses, social workers, and the like arrive at Mulago Hospital every morning via *matatu* (a minibus taxi that is also a ubiquitous form of transport in much of East Africa), footing, or increasingly by personal car. Plenty also arrive by *boda boda* (motorcycle taxis), often carrying large plastic bins and bed rolls, meticulously balanced along with an infant or child on the back of the motorcycle. Fewer come to Mulago Hospital via ambulance, although every morning, if timed properly, one can see the morning commute's motorcycle accident victims being taken into the "casualty ward" (what Americans would consider to be an "emergency room"), on the ground floor of Mulago Hospital. Accident victims are unceremoniously pulled by the ankles from dark blue police truck beds, thrust into a wheelchair, then wheeled to the casualty reception area to have their limbs cast back together or to be given blood.[2] Or in more serious cases, they are delivered to the morgue.[3]

Mulago National Referral Hospital is the teaching hospital of Makerere University's College of Health Sciences. Founded in 1913 as a small venereal disease treatment facility, the hospital has expanded over the past century to include multiple free-standing wards built between the 1920s and 1950s and a larger "new" Mulago Hospital that was opened in 1962. In its present-day incarnation, Mulago Hospital Complex includes a sprawling public teaching and referral hospital with over a thousand beds, a public health school, and a medical school. As the government's flagship hospital, Mulago receives the difficult cases from the national referral hospital system and also serves the urban poor in the greater Kampala area. It is a site of convergence for people across the country seeking care. For many decades, patients have come to Mulago for relief from mild ailments such as malaria or dysentery. Many have also come to Mulago for relief from less quotidian illnesses and misfortunes, including cancer. These patients are directed to the Uganda Cancer Institute (UCI), which stands at the very top of Mulago Hill.

On Monday mornings at the UCI, by the main entrance to the Lymphoma Treatment Center (LTC), approximately forty to sixty outpatients sit quietly on hard wooden benches, lab request papers crinkling in palms. You can hear the quiet sipping of steaming hot *chai* (tea). The silence is only periodically broken by Mr. D, the lab technician, wearing his white coat and glasses and a warm smile, calling out for a *mzee* (an elderly gentleman) to get his blood drawn. Mr. D is all business as he says, "Come inside, please. Come inside." Mr. D used to work down at a laboratory in lower Mulago where he would arrive late to work and leave early. Here at the UCI, he comes to work early and stays late. For him, this daily ritual of drawing blood and then running the vials through the newly acquired complete blood count machine allows him to keep an intimate connection between the samples he tests and the people he serves. He does not want to let the patients down.

After the adults have disbanded from the waiting area, children will line up to have new IV cannula lines inserted into their hands for chemotherapy treatments. Taking a seat on the hard wooden chair in the entry area, which doubles as a procedures room, some feign bravery and others melt into puddles of sobs as the nurse pulls out a latex glove that she will tie around the spindly arm to pull up a vein. Screams, whimpers, and cries of "*Omusawo!*" (meaning "doctor" or "medical person") fill the space, as do the consoling murmurs of the nursing staff: "Sorry, sorry, sorry."

Plates, cups, and forks clatter and clang around 1 p.m., and families shuffle outside to the kitchen area to line up for *posho* (a thick porridge, usually made from maize) and beans—the one free meal of the day. Patients and caretakers hum and chatter in various languages—Luganda, Acholi, Ateso, Runyankole, Lugbara, Lusoga, and even a smattering of Swahili swell and amplify in the line-up, eagerly talking in anticipation of eating. And then, an eerie silence falls, a deadly calm as people carry their lunches out to the verandahs and eat without saying a word. All you can hear are the children slurping at their fingers as they tear into the sticky hot posho. By the late afternoon, with chemotherapy finally administered through IV drips on the ward, the chorus of vomiting begins. Some children quietly retch into plastic buckets held out beneath them by their caretakers. Other kids go outside and into the bushes, heaving, choking, and sobbing. At 5 p.m., the buzz of car engines fires up in the parking lot adjacent to the LTC, as doctors and staff drive down the hill to meet the evening's jam. Wailing sobs sound through the adult ward of the LTC. Someone has just died. Sister H bursts into the nurse's room, asking loudly where all the death forms went. "I need them *kati kati* (now, now) so I can go home." Another Monday at the LTC draws to a close.

Tuesdays, the pace of work at the UCI is different. It's not an outpatient day, so the laboratories and outdoor waiting areas are slightly less congested. The major management meeting of the week happened on Monday, so you are more likely to hear the voice of a senior doctor outside of the Outpatient Center, politely demanding to know whether or not this patient or that patient has started on treatment now because treatment should have started yesterday. "Why is this patient not on treatment? Where are the biopsy results? This Burkitt's lymphoma is an *emergency*." Dr. Joyce Balagadde Kambugu, the newly appointed pediatric oncologist, intervenes and says, "We are taking care of it. The child is on the Burkitt's lymphoma project and will get special care and treatment."

On the wards, the sounds are largely those of teaching—major teaching ward rounds happen on Tuesdays at the UCI. They start anywhere between 9 and 11 a.m., and they can go until five o'clock in the evening, depending on how late they started and how many patients there are to see. On the Solid Tumor Center, which caters mainly to adults with a variety of solid tumors ranging from liver cancer to Kaposi's sarcoma to breast cancer to prostate cancer to malignant melanomas, patients are packed tightly into every nook and cranny of the space, and beds are jammed against one another and make a perimeter along the wall of the building that used to be an enclosed porch. Here, the cancers are often fetid, florid, fulminating, and the rot stinks. On teaching ward rounds, medical students, a medical officer, the nursing sister, and I all crowd around Dr. Fred Okuku, as we move several inches from bed to bed.

As a student in secondary school, Okuku was fascinated by biology, and his favorite part of class was the frog dissection. He used to carefully dissect frogs and then attempt to stitch them back together, with the hope that he would at some point manage to reanimate them. Nothing fazes Okuku. And the more extreme and advanced the bodily state and cancer stage is, the more important the teaching lesson. An elderly woman's malignant melanoma engorged with blood and roughly the size of a cantaloupe is carefully shown on ward rounds as an example of a patient coming "late." Some medical students are engaged and drawn in, others curl their nostrils, barely able to contain their disgust as a woman's stage-four breast cancer rot wafts up after she exposes her wound to us on the ward. We have joked about how he is, for all intents and purposes, "the late-tumor oncologist."

Teaching rounds at the UCI are a form of triage, both in terms of engaging with patients who are in bad shape and plotting a course of palliation or salvage, but also in terms of bringing in more medical staff to manage the crowded wards. Medical students clerk, do patient intake, man the night shift, run down the hill for blood, and read complete blood counts. They do not administer chemotherapy. Two or three are usually "poached" from a ward in any given year and brought in as volunteer medical officers to learn how to do lumbar punctures and manage emergencies. Okuku's teaching rounds are not horror shows, but they do have the quality of a hazing ritual, as medical teaching rounds are in many other settings.

On any day of the week at the UCI—but especially Wednesdays—there is the sound of laughter. There is the laughter of Paul and Stevie, two adolescent boys who are currently being treated for leukemia and live on the LTC full-time even when they are "not on a bed." They take turns pushing one another in a shiny red wheelchair (recently donated by a Christian organization) up and down the patch of grass directly outside the ward. They collapse into hysterical giggles every time the chair comes to a complete halt. The "mamas," the ten or so women who cannot afford to travel between treatment cycles for their patients, congregate in the back kitchen area and erupt in full belly laughs when I kneel down on their sitting mats and greet them in Luganda, Acholi, and Lugbara. Wednesdays are the relaxed days at the UCI. They are days for early research-in-progress meetings in the board room at 8 a.m. They are days for catching up on writing and paperwork, for doing fast "business" ward rounds, and for giving politicians and research scientists tours of the facility. They are a moment of reprieve from the chaos of outpatient Thursdays and cancer-screening Fridays.

Mondays and Thursdays at the UCI are quite similar—patients congregate in the morning for their bloodwork information outside of the LTC, which houses the laboratory, and then proceed to limp, shuffle, walk, or be carried to a camouflage green, open-air army tent directly outside the Outpatient Ward, where they will wait until names are called for chemotherapy. If it is not a day for chemotherapy, but a day to see a senior doctor for evaluation, the patient may congregate inside the ward, waiting for the doctor, be it Dr. J, Dr. F, Dr. A, or Dr. N, to reach his or her name in the thick stack of forty patient files that each of the doctors is expected to power through on an outpatient clinic day.

In the public chemotherapy administration room, a breeze is mercifully blowing up from Lake Victoria this afternoon, as Sister J and her team work methodically to insert, push, and drip chemotherapy into IV hand needles as quickly as humanly possible. Sixty to ninety patients are waiting to receive their treatments so they can go to the bus park before the night falls—providing cover for pickpockets and thieves—all so they can make the treacherous two-hundred-plus-kilometer night bus ride home. It is hard to say what is worse—vomiting into a Kanga cloth the whole way as the bus races over potholes and dodges goats crossing the highway, the prospect of a head-on collision, or harassment from the state police at a nighttime roadblock as they look for bribes. Like the LTC ward on a chemotherapy afternoon, this administration room, with its six plastic chairs and shared IV poles, endures periods of eruptive retching, whimpers, and silence. About every two hours, one of the cleaners will be called to mop up a new mess of pink sickness heaved onto the white tile floor.

By Friday, the UCI buzzes with the anticipation of the weekend, which for the staff means most likely attending a wedding or wedding introduction ceremony on Saturday, and an all-day extravaganza of ecstatic prayer at church on Sunday, if Pentecostal or Born Again, or a more reserved morning service at Namirembe or Rubaga cathedrals, for the Protestants and Catholics, respectively. And on a Friday, as nurses shed their uniforms and put on their Kampala city outfits of fashionable dresses and suits, some Muslim headscarves appear, beautiful shimmery pinks and yellows, covering well-coiffed heads of cornrows or braids. During Ramadan, the Muslim nursing sisters fast even during the day shift, working without food and occasionally without water.

For the patients and their caretakers who are staying at the UCI for the weekend, a month, or a year, the prospect of wealthier Kampala relatives coming to check in on their extended family members over the weekend, and the good meal of fish or chicken or beef that will most likely accompany that visit, is met with great anticipation. The traffic on an early Friday evening in Kampala is cacophonous, eruptive, and temperamental. Prados packed to the brim with family members are heading out to burials in the villages. Several large Friday markets, particularly in Kamwokya and Nakawa, snarl traffic on Kira and Jinja roads. Traffic police trying to add a few extra shillings to their pockets for the weekend pull over matatus with officious smirks. And as you walk down from the top of the hill at the UCI, the sounds of honking car horns and the smell of corn being grilled on the side of the road greet you, reentering the city.

Introduction

THE UGANDA Cancer Institute (UCI) has served as "Africa's living laboratory" for producing knowledge about cancer in sub-Saharan Africa for over fifty years.[1] It began in 1967 as a joint venture between the American National Cancer Institute (NCI), the Makerere Department of Surgery, and the British Empire Cancer Campaign.[2] Established in one of Old Mulago Hospital's abandoned maternity wards and surgical theaters, the two original wards of the Institute, the Lymphoma Treatment Center (LTC) and Solid Tumor Center (STC), provided the infrastructure for chemotherapy clinical trials on cancers that were highly common in East Africa but rare in the United States, such as Burkitt's lymphoma and Kaposi's sarcoma.[3] When Idi Amin assumed power in Uganda in a military coup in 1971, the American staff left and put a Ugandan oncologist, Professor Charles Olweny, in charge of the facility.[4] Despite a decade of economic instability and political precarity, Ugandans continued to run clinical trials and remain embedded in international cancer research collaborations.

Olweny left the Institute in the early 1980s for personal safety reasons. The Institute could have closed, but again Ugandans decided to keep this site going. Throughout the 1980s, 1990s, and 2000s, Dr. Edward Katongole-Mbidde worked as the Institute's director and sole oncologist in the country, providing oncology services in a severely underfunded context.[5] Over the course of the HIV/AIDS epidemic, the Institute served in part as a palliative care facility for those living with HIV and cancer.[6] At the same time, Mbidde maintained high standards and expanded the Institute's research mission largely by focusing on HIV and the treatment of Kaposi's sarcoma, working with numerous international research partners.[7]

In the past decade, under the directorship of Dr. Jackson Orem, the UCI experienced a profound renaissance as well as a remarkable enlargement of scale and expansion of purpose. It shifted from a place where you were "sent to die" to a site where cancer services are provided as a public health good backed with funding from the Ministry of Health. The combination of more ministers of Parliament getting cancer and the visibility of a long-term partnership between the UCI and the Fred Hutchinson Cancer Research Center (FHCRC or the Fred Hutch) expanded oncology services at the Institute. Thanks to collaborations and newfound institutional autonomy from Mulago Hospital in 2009, drug stocks are more plentiful, more nurses are on the wards, and the number of Ugandan oncologists has increased from one in the year 2000 to twenty in the year 2020. The number of patients, everyone agrees, has also increased dramatically, crowding the two original wards—the LTC and the STC—which were never designed to provide comprehensive cancer care for Uganda's entire population. As a response, the Ugandan government recently completed a five-story inpatient cancer hospital.[8] A new research and outpatient treatment facility stands on the site of the LTC, built through a long-standing partnership with the Fred Hutch in Seattle. These investments in public oncology and cancer research infrastructure in Africa are distinctive. There are few other sites on the continent with the depth or breadth of publicly available cancer services.[9] The UCI now serves a population catchment of approximately forty million residents in the Great Lakes region of Africa.[10]

It is tempting to read the current investments by Americans at the UCI as a new scramble for African research subjects in the global health industry.[11] However, cancer is not a new epidemic in Uganda. It is a long-standing health dilemma that has been under the gaze of biomedical researchers intermittently for the past century. Furthermore, Ugandans at the UCI have long used collaborative medical research as a resource for expanding and consolidating cancer services for a broader public. Many international partners, starting with the British Empire Cancer Campaign and the NCI, have come to Uganda since the 1950s to study and treat cancers. But international collaborators come and go. It was and is ultimately Ugandans who keep experiments going and freezers operating. They provide care to patients on the wards of the UCI long after international colleagues leave, research results are published, and funding cycles end. A collective commitment to keeping things going explains the remarkable durability of this institution over the past fifty years. Rather than a case of unilateral extraction, cancer research in Uganda was and continues to be generative for creating and supporting long-lasting cancer care infrastructures for Ugandan publics.

The UCI's current slogan is "Research Is Our Resource." And to be sure, this slogan reflects the current terrain of biomedical care in Uganda, where global research projects on HIV and AIDS bring vital funding for buildings, health workers, and therapeutics. But it also speaks to the UCI's necessity, since its inception, to develop context-specific knowledge and knowledge workers. Research on the specific epidemiology of cancers in Uganda, such as their prevalence and survivability, is vital for national health-care planning and resource allocation. The pronounced synergies between infectious diseases and cancers in Burkitt's lymphoma, Kaposi's sarcoma, and liver cancer have long shaped research questions and collaborations. Over the fifty years of the Institute's history, research partnerships have brought resources for cancer care to Uganda. And in turn, research at the Uganda Cancer Institute generated vital knowledge about cancer relevant to both the African context and beyond.[12] Some examples: research at the UCI generated knowledge about the curability of cancer with cytotoxic agents alone in the 1960s and 1970s. In the 1980s and 1990s, large numbers of patients with HIV-related Kaposi's sarcoma provided an indispensable source of clinical material on neoplastic disease and AIDS. In the 2000s, with newfound interests in the relationship between infections and cancers, the Institute is once again an attractive site for cancer research.

Africanizing Oncology argues that Ugandans use research as a powerful resource for mobilizing and extending care, even if they do so in a highly unequal world. This historical-ethnography tells the story of how the UCI transformed from a small experimental chemotherapy clinical trials unit in the 1960s into a site of oncological excellence in present-day Uganda. The book examines the ways in which physician-researchers, especially Ugandans, refashioned the resources and oncological technologies brought through transnational cancer research partnerships to meet the needs of Ugandan cancer patients and their caretakers. The book ahead tells the stories of physicians, nurses, laboratory technicians, administrators, patients, families, visiting scientists, and even the occasional politician who have lived and died on the wards of the UCI over four generations from the 1950s onward. These four generations map roughly onto distinct periods in Uganda's history—colonial developmentalism (1940s–1950s), Ugandanization and independence (1960s), Idi Amin's dictatorship (1970s), civil war (early 1980s), structural adjustment (1980s–1990s), the HIV epidemic (1980s–present), and Museveni's National Resistance Movement government (1986–present). I show how physician-researchers exercise creativity in crisis, be it straddling the demands of treating late-stage tumors and remaining viable to the international oncology research complex, or negotiating with Idi Amin's state police. The first four chapters of the book discuss the history of cancer research and care in Uganda, beginning with colonial medical research on cancer. They trace the founding of the UCI in 1967 and the ways in which the Institute survived Idi Amin, civil war, and austerity. The last two chapters of the book consider the ways in which international partnerships and research initiatives, coupled with the increasing visibility of cancer in Uganda as a public health problem, are remaking this fifty-year-old site into something new.

Drawing from insights in science and technology studies, medical anthropology, and works on everyday life in contemporary Africa, *Africanizing Oncology* makes three core contributions to African health histories. The first core contribution focuses on the long history of how research, including its social and material technologies, shaped oncology services in Uganda. Many of oncology's treatment technologies originally came to Uganda through international research partnerships or as gifts. Cancer research and experiments have shaped the built and social infrastructure for public cancer care in Uganda over the past fifty years. Practitioners and patients harnessed and transformed these international research collaborations to serve Ugandan publics. I use the term *experimental infrastructure* to describe the constellation of physical facilities, research questions, care practices, data collection procedures, and human labor that makes research and care function on a day-to-day basis at the Uganda Cancer Institute. Efforts to maintain, repair, and transform these traveling oncological technologies can teach us much about what it means to keep biomedical care going in contemporary Uganda. The histories of how oncology traveled to Uganda and the development of the UCI's experimental infrastructure further our understanding of the dynamics between research, resources, and the role of experiments in shaping health care in East Africa.

While the UCI's cancer research is well cited in the biomedical literature, especially on Burkitt's lymphoma and Kaposi's sarcoma, East African oncological expertise remains largely invisible in the historiography of biomedicine in Africa and more popular general histories of cancer. *Africanizing Oncology* amplifies the critical contributions East Africans (and Ugandans in particular) made to understandings of the etiology of viruses and cancers, the curative potential of chemotherapy, and the necessity of palliative care for cancers associated with HIV. The UCI's history offers a necessary and long-overdue opportunity to situate Africans at the center rather than the periphery of biomedical knowledge production as researchers, physicians, administrators, patients, caretakers, and laboratory technicians. Rather than focusing on the ways in which the substances of African bodies and lives are turned into scientific research commodities or data points on a survival curve, *Africanizing Oncology* highlights the political, moral, and medical ambiguities African knowledge producers face.

Finally, by combining historical and anthropological approaches in telling stories about biomedicine in Africa (and beyond), this book makes a methodological argument for further integration of these disciplines in writing contemporary histories.[13] Hospital ethnographies offer an intimate look at these spaces of care as social worlds unto themselves, liminal places with deep existential concerns about the end of life, and complicated relationships between the public and the state. Historicizing the hospital allows for tracing the impact of political, economic, and scientific events on everyday life as they play out in a microcosm of the state. Oscillations of fortune, waxing and waning resources, and epidemics have all impacted the scale, quality, and scope of biomedical care in Uganda. But there are also powerful continuities, particularly at Mulago Hospital, Makerere Medical School, and the UCI, which have long been sites of biomedical research, medical professionalization, and specialist care. Combining history and ethnography allows us to take a longer view of the material stakes, creative practice, and lived experience of biomedicine in East Africa over the past fifty years.

THE BIOMEDICAL TURN IN AFRICAN HEALTH HISTORIES

The idea for this book began in 2006 during an interview with a South African epidemiologist. Commenting on the rise of global health interventions and researchers on the continent, he said, "We're carving up Africa again! But this time it's for HIV and AIDS research. If you want to study something interesting, study that!" This conversation ignited many questions regarding how histories of biomedical research in East Africa shaped the provision of biomedical care. In a context where accessing biomedicine was (and still is) often tethered to colonial experimentation and the extraction of bodily materials and knowledge, how did African health workers and physician-researchers in newly independent countries such as Uganda, working at a hospital like Mulago and a medical school like

Makerere, think about their work in the context of these complex inheritances? What were and continue to be the legacies of tethering experimentation and research to the provision of care?

In retrospect, the epidemiologist's comment was astute and prophetic, anticipating a biomedical turn in histories and ethnographies of health and healing in Africa over the past decade. In the 1970s, 1980s, and 1990s, historians and anthropologists turned their attention to the "social basis of health and healing in Africa" and created a rich corpus on a variety of topics, including therapeutic and healing traditions, illnesses of God and man, missionary medicine, colonialism and development's impact on environmental health, and the political economy of disease.[14] As Nancy Rose Hunt notes, the emergence of the HIV epidemic dramatically changed the conversation about health and healing in Africa in the late 1980s and into the 1990s.[15] The epidemic's impact on demography, gender relations, and livelihoods, as well as the rise of the antiretroviral techno-fix and its attendant disparities dramatically shaped the preoccupations of the field.[16] Furthermore, the West African Ebola epidemic between 2013 and 2015 put issues of global health securitization into relief.[17]

Newer scholarship written largely at academic institutions in the Global North on African health and healing engages with these emerging therapeutics, epidemics, and global health infrastructures by closely examining how biomedicine works in a variety of local contexts. New histories explore the complexities of biomedical professionalization, medical and scientific experimentation, and the legacies of colonialism in postcolonial medical practice.[18] These works join a growing number of ethnographies of global health in contemporary African contexts and beyond, many of which consider how experiments, humanitarian emergency, and epidemics shape access to biomedical care.[19] This scholarship highlights what African scholars, physicians, epidemiologists, public health professionals, nurses, data analysts, and policymakers have known for years—that biomedicine, experimentation, and extraction often go together.[20]

A recent trend in the anthropology of health in Africa is to examine the repercussions of structural adjustment and neoliberal reform on the provision of biomedicine in spaces that Paul Farmer would witheringly call "clinical deserts." A rich conceptual vocabulary, including "capacity," "African science," "improvisation," "triage," and "normal emergency," has emerged to describe what it means for health-care workers to provide meaningful (biomedical) care in postcolonial spaces that appear to be largely defined by absence and scarcity.[21] Building on critical conversations about imperial debris, work on the fate of postcolonial "African science" after independence emphasizes the material remains, colonial medical detritus, laboratories in a state of ruin, and the discarded stuff of biomedical and scientific research on the continent.[22] The approach is both aesthetically pleasing and a critical theoretical intervention to track the afterlives of colonial medical initiatives and their objects in Africa after independence.[23] But the emphasis on the remains of the past can also inadvertently reinforce a narrative of state failure, Afro-pessimism, and inevitable decline, mirroring Fred Cooper's argument that opportunities were profoundly foreclosed in the decades following African independence.[24] How might we move beyond accounts of failure, exploitation, technocratic bumbling, and untimely death in contemporary African health settings?

Nolwazi Mkhwanazi has argued that there is a "single story" that dominates much of the contemporary medical anthropology literature on Africa produced by scholars based largely in the Global North. Through careful reading, Mkhwanazi shows us that "stories that are not about the state's inadequacy in health provision, suspicion, and distrust, or thwarted local agency, are rare in medical anthropological studies of Africa."[25] I fully agree, and the approach that I offer here follows Mkhwanazi's lead in more deeply historicizing local knowledge and experience. By focusing on the creativity of Ugandan health and knowledge workers over periods of stability and moments of crisis, *Africanizing Oncology* moves beyond a thick description of coping with scarcity to tracking how scarcity itself ebbs and flows over time.[26]

WHEN ONCOLOGY TRAVELS

One of the core concerns of this book is how oncology became part of biomedical practice in Uganda. That is, how did Ugandans Africanize oncology? To answer this question, I draw from theoretical tools in the history of technology and theories of infrastructure. I argue that cancer research projects were and continue to be key means of transferring oncological tools to Uganda.[27] Oncology came to Uganda in such forms as technology transfer, gifts, international research collaborations, technocratic solutions, and pharmaceutical collaborations.[28] Nevertheless, Ugandan medical practitioners and cancer patients remade these oncological technologies to suit the local context, and they continue to do so today.[29] For example, when the UCI was founded in the 1960s, the American National Cancer Institute staff brought boxes of gloves, stockpiles of syringes, vials of cyclophosphamide, and massive amounts of gauze to set up their "hospital built from scratch."[30] But these material goods were not the only things they brought. They also brought a set of practices from their training in medical oncology from US hospitals—ward rounding, specific ways of writing up a chart, protocols for doing complete blood workups before deeming it safe to administer chemotherapy. Almost immediately, Ugandan patients and practitioners started to change these systems of care. Ugandans pushed expatriate oncologists to expand their definition of supportive care and to take travel, food, farming, and shelter seriously.[31] The fact that patients and families stayed at the wards for months at a time demanded that Americans rethink who counted as a patient. Within six months, the UCI was treating entire families (not just individual cancer patients) for malaria and parasites. They ensured that there was a big scoop of pungent, nutrient-rich greens on plates of local food for pediatric patients. They hired a schoolteacher for village children who would be missing school. They adapted the resources of research to accommodate the needs of childhood cancer care in the vernacular.[32]

Anthropologists Margaret Lock and Vinh-Kim Nguyen have argued that biomedicine is best understood as a constellation of technologies. They define technology broadly, accounting for both objects and practices: "No doubt what springs most readily to mind when thinking about biomedical technologies are machines such as mechanical ventilators, imaging technologies including X-ray machines and CT scans, as well as devices such as prosthetic limbs, cardiac pacemakers, tooth implants, and so on. However, our lives are filled with far more mundane biomedical devices and technologies including the basic physical examination, patient history-taking (including self-examination and self-history taking), administration of injections, and the prescription of medications."[33] Oncology, as an arena of biomedicine, can be thought of similarly as a constellation of technologies embedded in a broader system of care. In contemporary America, everything from cancer screening to pathology laboratory reagents and breast cancer awareness campaigns—and to pharmaceutical companies conducting cancer clinical trials—comprise oncology's technologies, regimes of research and care, and infrastructure. Løchlann Jain calls this tangle of markets, medical practitioners, politics, and patients *the cancer-corporate care nexus*.[34] In comparison to the United States, Europe, or indeed other parts of the Global South, oncological treatment and care infrastructure is relatively shallow and tethered to experiment and biomedical research. The UCI was not established with the intention of providing comprehensive oncology services to the Ugandan masses, even when the population was less than ten million.[35] It was originally an enclave established to do research on African bodies.[36] This history partially explains why, until the mid-2000s, the Uganda Cancer Institute was largely a chemotherapy experimentation and treatment facility rooted in the socio-technical practices of oncology as they were in the 1960s and 1970s. It also helps to explain why there was only one Ugandan oncologist, one Ugandan radiotherapy machine, and one central place for receiving cancer care in the country for much of the 1980s, 1990s, and early 2000s.

Throughout this book I use the concept of *experimental infrastructure* to describe the Uganda Cancer Institute. The materiality and practices of oncology, the built environment of the UCI, and the movement of patients, drugs, biopsies, and knowledge are all components of experimental infrastructure. Infrastructure allows for the largely uninhibited movement of stuff, or ideas, or people, or services both across spaces and across time. In the 1990s, scholars such as Susan Leigh Star focused their attention on infrastructures situated in the United States and Europe.[37] Classic examples of twentieth- and twenty-first-century infrastructure include roads, electricity grids, aviation, water and sewage, and the internet.[38] Coordinated social action, standardization, repair, maintenance, long-sighted planning, and technocratic expertise are all vital to keep infrastructures humming in the background of daily life. Paul Edwards says that "this notion of infrastructure as an invisible, smooth-functioning background 'works' only in the developed world. In the Global South (for lack of a better term), norms for infrastructure can be considerably different. Electric power and telephone services routine fail, often on a daily basis; highways may be clogged beyond utility or may not exist; computer networks operate (when they do) at a crawl."[39] Edwards notes, however, that living with an infrastructure constantly in the foreground and highly visible due to its unreliability is "equally modern" and a feature of everyday life in the Global South.[40] More recent works in the anthropology of infrastructure consider the ways in which chronic economic or political instability, the atrophy of expertise, the systematic cutting of financial resources for maintenance, and the impact and aftermath of disasters can all cripple infrastructure or render its problems sharply visible.[41]

In Uganda, many infrastructural investments such as roads and railways, electricity grids, telecommunication systems, education systems, and indeed biomedicine have historical roots in colonial conquest and later colonial development initiatives.[42] There is a thinness and a lack of redundancy (i.e., backup systems or engineering fail-safes) to many of these old colonial infrastructures—think of the lone highway that stretches from Mombasa to Kampala, the singular tertiary national referral hospital in Mulago, the first university on Makerere Hill. And there is a legacy of resource extraction knit into many colonial-era infrastructures—think of the routes of mobility that slaves conscripted during the ivory trade endured in East Africa, the grotesquely inadequate housing infrastructure that was built to facilitate mining in southern Africa, or indeed the bureaucratic systems established for the trade of coffee and cotton in Uganda.[43]

The development of biomedical infrastructure in much of sub-Saharan Africa was inextricably tied to colonial conquest and later on, development aid. From quinine to venereal disease treatments, early colonial health programs in much of sub-Saharan Africa involved experimentation on African bodies in small enclaves and catchments, akin to sites of global health treatment interventions today.[44] Over the past century, biomedical services for the Ugandan population were offered at Mulago Hill often via experiments and research on issues such as venereal disease, yaws, malnutrition, tropical maladies, and "diseases of civilization" such as heart disease and cancer.[45] One of the long-term legacies of the development of colonial medical infrastructure in East and Central Africa is that many public biomedical care infrastructures have not been seriously "modernized" since they were established in the 1960s. Particularly since structural adjustment and financial austerity were imposed on African countries as a condition of debt relief, medical services on the continent have atrophied.[46] Some would go as far as to say that there is no meaningful medical care in some sites on the continent.[47] This infrastructural atrophy poses real dilemmas for the contemporary, booming biomedical research enterprise and HIV treatment complex in eastern and southern Africa. Drugs can be imported, staff can be trained, and computers can be hooked up to speedy internet connections for a price. But the physical spaces where potential and often poor research subjects congregate for care are often worse for the wear. The political and logistical work of international medical research on human subjects often consists of creating new infrastructures for care that operate alongside crisis-ridden government health services. This is certainly the case at the Uganda Cancer Institute, where major investments from international partners and the Ugandan government alike over the past decade have led to an expansion of oncology infrastructure not seen in the country since the late 1960s and early 1970s.

Originally, I did not set out to write about cancer. But serendipity shifted the focus from the history of HIV/AIDS research in Uganda to the history of cancer research in Uganda. I first learned about the UCI while going through the papers of an American scientist at an archive in Philadelphia. I found a copy of the Institute's annual report from 1971, which documented a series of chemotherapy clinical trials underway in Idi Amin's Uganda. It was too interesting to ignore, and I began to look for traces of the UCI's past in historical and popular works on cancer in the United States, United Kingdom, and Uganda. In the 1960s and 1970s, the UCI made major contributions to global understandings of the power of chemotherapy drugs in treating pediatric cancers. In Siddhartha Mukherjee's biography of cancer, *The Emperor of All Maladies*, which focuses extensively on the history of pediatric chemotherapy research, these contributions of the UCI to the promises of chemotherapy were relegated to a footnote. It reads, "Many of these NCI-sponsored trials were carried out in Uganda, where Burkitt's lymphoma is endemic in children."[48] Thinking that the UCI's contributions would be more visible to historians of medicine in Africa, I looked to John Iliffe's *East African Doctors*, where the critical research conducted on cancer in Uganda in the 1960s and the contributions of Olweny and Professor Sebastian Kyalwazi were briefly highlighted. Based on these thin accounts, I expected the UCI to be a thing of the past. Instead, arriving at the top of Mulago Hill at the Institute for the first time in 2010, I found not a ruin but a bustling hospital.

Over the past decade of working on this book, cancer itself has emerged as a more politically and epidemiologically visible phenomenon to African public health authorities and global health specialists alike.[49] Publicly funded cancer wards are opening across the continent from Botswana to Kenya to Rwanda.[50] As Megan Vaughan, Julie Livingston, and Emily Mendenhall, among others, highlight, epidemics of noncommunicable chronic disease are reshaping African health futures.[51] This cancer burden occurs alongside a host of chronic ailments, including hypertension, heart disease, stroke, renal disease, kidney failure, diabetes, liver disease, and mental health issues. These chronic conditions join a high burden of infectious diseases, and epidemics of violence and injuries, creating a "quadruple disease burden" or a crisis of "syndemics."[52] While threads of causation have yet to be fully pulled apart, public health experts and lay observers agree that increasing urbanization, consumption, and affluence are rapidly contributing to the growing burden of noncommunicable diseases in the Global South.[53]

Growing attention to a cancer crisis in Africa operates alongside a growing "global oncology" research agenda in the Global North.[54] New tools for studying oncogenes and vaccine development have reanimated research on the causal relationships between viral infections and cancers. Infectious diseases are a necessary link in the causal chain for cancers such as Burkitt's lymphoma, which is associated with Epstein-Barr virus, Kaposi's sarcoma, which is caused by human herpes virus 8, certain kinds of liver cancer from long-term hepatitis B and C infections, and cervical cancer, which is linked to human papillomavirus.[55] The synergies between HIV/AIDS and cancers are particularly pronounced in southern and eastern Africa. As HIV-positive patients on antiretroviral therapy live longer, they are more vulnerable to developing infection-related cancers, particularly cervical cancer.[56] In Uganda, data from the Kampala Cancer Registry suggests that in the twenty-five years between 1991 and 2015, most cancer incidence rates increased in Uganda. Incidence rates of prostate cancer, breast cancer, and cervical cancer were all higher in 2010–2015 when compared to 1991–1995. Cases of Kaposi's sarcoma and non-Hodgkin's lymphoma, both cancers associated with HIV/AIDS, were on the rise in the 1990s and then declined in the late 2000s. According to colleagues at the Kampala Cancer Registry, these trends "reflect the changing lifestyles of this urban African population, as well as the consequences of the epidemic of HIV/AIDS and the availability of treatment with antiretroviral drugs. At the same time, it highlights the fact that the decreases in cancer of the cervix observed in high and upper-middle income countries are not a consequence of changes in lifestyle, but demand active intervention through screening (and, in the longer term, vaccination)."[57]

Academic monographs on cancer in Africa and elsewhere in the Global South generally remain scarce. The notable exceptions are Benson Mulemi's moving work on cancer in Kenya and Julie Livingston's portrait of the emerging cancer crisis in southern Africa. Livingston viscerally draws us into the human stakes of cancer treatments in a stripped-down setting where analgesics are few and oncologists are even fewer. Published in 2012, *Improvising Medicine* made the emerging cancer epidemic in Africa strikingly visible. But cancer is neither a single disease nor is the situation in Botswana generalizable to the diverse experiences of cancer and practices of oncology on the continent. The cancer ward of Princess Marina Hospital (PMH), which opened in 2001, offered a window into the emerging infection-related cancer epidemic in southern Africa where malignancies often present "without oncology."[58] The bodily experiences of cancer care at PMH, including the pain epidemic, botched surgeries, exploding tumors, and riotous vomiting, are certainly present on the wards of the UCI. But the UCI is a space where cancer research and care have long coexisted.

Oncology in Uganda grows out of a long-standing biomedical research culture, which began at Mengo Hospital and soon after at Mulago Hospital in the early 1900s. Research at these sites shaped much of the knowledge about the prevalence and treatment of cancer in East and Central Africa over the twentieth century. The Uganda Cancer Institute consists of multiple sedimentary layers of infrastructure, research legacies, and a culture of oncological practices that go back to the 1950s. Furthermore, those who practice oncology as specialist physicians in Uganda are, at this point, Ugandans. This has been the case since the 1970s. They are not expatriates like Dr. P fleeing the economic and political atrophy of Zimbabwe or South African specialists escaping the grind of Johannesburg. The physicians who practice oncology at the UCI are, for the most part, Ugandans who grew up in Uganda. Some cared for relatives at the height of the HIV epidemic and now pay the school fees of children whose parents did not survive. These Ugandan physicians could be practicing oncology anywhere, but they choose to remain in Uganda not only because they are deeply invested in furthering the well-being of the Ugandan public but also because it is home.

NEW DIRECTIONS IN UGANDAN HISTORIES

The research for this book occurred during a period of increased national reflection about Uganda's past. Since Uganda celebrated independence on October 9, 1962, with the lowering of the Union Jack at midnight, political struggles, prolonged periods of economic crisis, mercurial state-sponsored violence, and the challenges posed by the HIV/AIDS epidemic have all profoundly shaped political, social, and economic lives and livelihoods of Ugandans. The National Resistance Movement (NRM), which has been in power since 1986, brought relative economic prosperity and political stability to Uganda. NRM leaders in particular use this narrative about the transition from apocalyptic chaos to prosperity and growth as a justification for remaining in power in what Aili Tripp has dubbed a "hybrid regime."[59]

The celebration of fifty years of independence—the Golden Jubilee—created a public space for national discussions about the country's past and future. This was particularly evident in the news media. Starting on January 1, 2012, for example, both the *New Vision* and *Daily*

Monitor newspapers started a Golden Jubilee countdown, with every issue including a short history lesson starting from the 1700s and working its way up to the present. These stories highlighted the biographies of important Ugandan intellectuals, key moments in the history of precolonial kings and kingdoms, African land agreements with European colonial officials, stories of escaping police in the times of Idi Amin, and much more. The flurry of public storytelling was a marked departure in a context where there are few sites of public commemoration for Uganda as a nation. With the milestone of fifty years of independence, and nearly thirty years of NRM governance, Ugandan citizens are beginning to ask what is beyond the seemingly impenetrable smoky cloud of violence that obscured much of Uganda's past between 1962 and 1986, and more generally about the politics of erasure and memory in modern Ugandan history.[60] Historians of Uganda's past are benefitting from this turn to national reflection, thanks in part to an unprecedented transformation in the availability of documentary sources in the country.[61]

    Africanizing Oncology joins this new wave of contemporary histories of Uganda. But rather than using ethnicity or high politics or a single disease like HIV/AIDS to reconstruct the history of Uganda since independence, this book focuses on the history of the cancer hospital. Over the years, staff and patients alike at the UCI felt the reverberations of critical political, social, and economic events in Uganda.[62] The Institute itself was founded shortly after Milton Obote consolidated power by abolishing the historic kingdom of Buganda, among others, and declaring himself president in 1966.[63] While situated in central Uganda and the heart of Buganda, the UCI's mandate was national in scope and the patients it recruited for research trials and treated came from all over the country.[64] It is not insignificant that the UCI became a place where Obote's wife routinely took visitors and dignitaries to see the fine scientific work that Ugandans as well as Americans were conducting on cancer.[65] Amin's declaration of the expulsion of the Asian population in 1972 severely disrupted the everyday workings of the Institute as most expatriate staff left.[66] The violent punctuation of the Tanzanian War of Liberation in 1979 turned Mulago Hospital into a war hospital.[67] Institute staff dodged bullets to attend to night emergencies.[68] In Museveni's Uganda, the current renaissance at the UCI is in part a reflection of a broader culture of public-private partnerships, which dominate development initiatives in the country today. The UCI offers a unique vantage point for understanding how Ugandan health workers in particular navigate shifting relationships between politics and science.

ON METHODS AND AUDIENCE

This book draws upon research conducted in archives and institutions across three continents and combines historical and ethnographic methods. In summer 2010, I met with Dr. Jackson Orem for the first time and asked him if he would be interested in allowing a doctoral student to reconstruct the history of the Uganda Cancer Institute. I started shadowing work in the LTC's wards shortly thereafter. I returned to Uganda in summer 2011, worked as a historian-ethnographer in the country from January to October 2012, and made yearly shorter return trips of one to eight weeks from 2013 to 2020. Methodologically, I drew a great deal of inspiration from the turn toward "hospital ethnography," wherein a hospital or medical ward is used as a primary field site.[69] My original intention in triangulating ethnography with archival research and oral history was to inform a baseline of comparison for interviews with actors about the past. By understanding how chemotherapy was, for example, administered on the wards in 2012, I could provide a point of comparison in interviews with nurses about practices of working with cytotoxic agents in the 1960s, 1970s, and 1980s. The ethnographic research in and of itself wound up creating a vivid yet only partial account of a place that no longer exists. I treat these fieldnotes as an additional archive and as a collection of personal papers, observations, and photo snapshots from the UCI as it was in 2012. Both the places and the people depicted in these fieldnotes, and indeed Kampala itself, have changed dramatically in the space of just a few short years, and the differences have only become more pronounced as this book goes to press.

In addition to ethnographic fieldwork, I conducted approximately forty formal oral histories with prominent people in the history of cancer in Uganda, and about twenty interviews with patient caretakers to get a sense of some of their experiences of life on the wards. Interviews were conducted by me and Irene Nassozi with patient caretakers in June, July, and August 2012 in Luganda. I accompanied and listened to the interviews and asked follow-up questions in English, which were then translated. Irene Nassozi then wrote translations of the interviews verbatim in English. These interviews followed five months of intensive participant observation on the wards of the UCI, and most of the patient caretakers interviewed already knew me relatively well. We followed an informed-consent procedure approved by both a Ugandan university institutional review board (IRB) and an American university IRB.

Blending history and ethnography shaped decisions regarding identification and anonymization. The individuals and institutions named and identified in this book are already well established in the public historical record. Wherever possible I've used the public record as a point of reference in identifying individuals and institutions. If it was not already on the public record, or if it was not said to me specifically on the record, I erred on the side of caution and used my best judgment. In the consenting process for oral histories, individuals were given the option to remain anonymous or be publicly identified. Pseudonyms, in the form of a title followed by an initial, are used for contemporary medical staff. All names of patients are pseudonyms. Despite the use of anonymization and pseudonyms, some medical staff, patients, and patient caretakers may still be recognizable to those who know the UCI well.

Research in Uganda was complemented by archival research conducted in the United Kingdom and the United States, as well as interviews in Seattle with colleagues at the Fred Hutch. I worked extensively from the UCI's archives. This included patient records from the 1960s to the present, as well as old personnel files, logbooks marking the events of a night's shift on the wards, and old oncology journals, and home visit reports from epidemiology studies in the 1960s. There were also patient records written out on student exercise notebook paper in the 1980s and assembled with tiny strips of gauze—a signal of just how scarce materials were during Uganda's civil war in the early 1980s. The archive was in remarkably good shape given the years behind a padlock. As Dr. John Ziegler, the founding director of the UCI, said in email correspondence about these materials, "Uganda is extraordinary in that nothing is discarded. Offices are like museums."[70] I am grateful to the director, Dr. Jackson Orem, and deputy director, Dr. Victoria Walusansa, for granting me permission to work with these vital materials. And I am also grateful to the entire staff of the records department for kindly accommodating my work.

This book is but one component of a broader corpus of publicly engaged work at the UCI. Over the years, I have organized history workshops and research-in-progress presentations and also collaborated with the photographers Andrea Stultiens and Rumanzi Canon of History in Progress Uganda to document the changes at the Institute in real time. In 2017, to celebrate the fiftieth anniversary of the UCI's founding, we exhibited some of these images from both past and present at the Afriart Gallery in Kampala for the show and book launch of *Staying Alive: Documenting the Uganda Cancer Institute*.

Readers will engage with this book across multiple time zones, cultural contexts, and professional backgrounds. Many who read this account will no doubt be thousands of miles away from Kampala. They may never have had the misfortune of a cancer diagnosis or caring for someone with cancer. For other readers, the stories within will hit a deeply personal nerve. And some colleagues, especially in Uganda, may feel that this book dwells too much on broken things, the dark side of oncology and on those who died rather than the survivors. I have found over the years that many who work at the UCI are the first to acknowledge that the Institute can be a tough place. Still, I am well aware that it is a delicate matter when institutional challenges are described by a *muzungu* ("White person," or "the person who wanders") outsider, whether she be a journalist or a historian-ethnographer.[71] Despite my best efforts, there is no doubt some of the research and writing replicates knowledge-production asymmetries of the White expatriate colonial and postcolonial physician-researchers I discuss in this book. During a particularly hard day of fieldwork, an American physician I knew urged, "Write your truth!" I have endeavored to do so in these pages. But truths can only tell part of the story. Charles Olweny's memoirs, oral histories with NCI expatriates such as John Ziegler, Denis Burkitt's autobiography, and countless medical journal articles all offer counterweights to my narrative and interpretations of the past. The book intentionally ends in 2015 with the opening of the UCI–Fred Hutch Cancer Center and the new government-sponsored facilities at the UCI. Much has changed since then, including fully equipping the new UCI hospital, procuring new radiotherapy machines, building new radiotherapy bunkers, and expanding training and research programs at the UCI.

Other readers may decide I dwell too much on the good deeds of Ugandan doctors and too little on the suffering of strangers.[72] I am reluctant to minimize the great bravery (the very definition of heroism) involved in keeping the UCI open in the 1970s, or downplay the choice to come back to war-frayed Uganda after studying in the UK in the 1980s. Nor do I want to discount the bravery of patients to show up for medical appointments and endure harsh treatments, or the courage of a parent to prioritize a child over a marriage that then dissolves. At the same time, I am mindful of Mkhwanazi's critique of "single stories" about African health contexts, especially single stories that are overly celebratory. She says, "Drawing on the narrative of the state's lack of or inadequate involvement in the provision of health care, medical professionals working in Africa are conventionally presented as working tirelessly and selflessly under impossible conditions in the service of humanity."[73] There is plenty of tireless labor at the UCI every day, but I think of the medical professionals in this book differently. Drawing inspiration from historians of health and healing in Africa who have highlighted the pivotal role of public healers in maintaining social and political order in precolonial Africa and then actively, vocally, powerfully leading resistance against colonial powers, I see the work of Ugandan medical practitioners at the Institute as an example of what we could call "postcolonial public healing."[74] Mitigating malignancies relies on care, political networks, hospitality, and shrewdness. In particular, I see the Ugandan directors of the Institute—Charles Olweny, Edward Katongole-Mbidde, and Jackson Orem—serving the social, moral, and political function of upholding the health of the public by actively navigating Uganda's political scene in a quest for securing oncology goods and engaging in research. They are physician-intellectuals. My attention to the courage and care of Ugandan health workers and knowledge makers is intentional. But my intentions are not whiggish. African histories of medicine and the practice of oncology itself demand holding healing and harming in the same frame.[75] This is not a story of linear progress but one of multiple and overlapping cycles of creativity and crisis, repair and destruction, and hope and despair. And there is so much to learn from how Ugandan physician-intellectuals, fieldworkers savvy in forging friendships, resilient patients, and invested caretakers keep things going: be they buildings, bodies, experiments, kitchens, therapeutics, blood banks, or optimism.

1 ᔚ The African Lymphoma

IN 1957 the physician Dr. Hugh Trowell asked Dr. Denis Burkitt to examine a pediatric patient for a surgical consultation. The boy was a five-year-old with massive swellings in all four quadrants of his jaw. Jaw swellings were not uncommon, and children often came to Mulago Hospital with this sort of complaint, their jaw swelling either from infections or single tumors. But a swelling distributed in all four quadrants of the jaw simultaneously was, Burkitt and Trowell agreed, quite rare. A few weeks later, Burkitt visited Jinja District Hospital and saw another young boy with jaw swellings in all four quadrants. Burkitt and colleagues convinced the patient's family to come to Mulago Hospital. At Mulago, Burkitt examined the boy and found similar tumors in all four jaw quadrants. Going back through old case records, Burkitt found that patients with this distinct jaw tumor often had other tumor deposits throughout their bodies, suggesting that this was a multicentric tumor. Burkitt thought that perhaps this was a new discovery, an East African oddity he had uncovered.[1]

Burkitt took his notes, photographs, and tissue samples of these patients to Dr. J. N. P. Davies in the pathology department. Davies looked through the materials. Lymphosarcomas were, according to Davies, known "to be common in both children and adults since 1948."[2] Davies informed Burkitt that he and his colleagues were well aware of the tumor and researching unusual pediatric and adult jaw tumors. These colleagues included Dr. Pritham Sing, Dr. J. Cook, Dr. A. G. Davies, and Dr. Gillian Jacobs. Working in concert, the cancer registrar, the pathology laboratory, and the radiography department conducted research on the tumor and published a report on jaw tumors for the *East African Medical Journal* a year before Burkitt's consultation.[3] In 1956, Jacobs, a pathologist, identified the childhood tumor as a lymphosarcoma. The Makerere-based Cancer Research Committee presented its collective research efforts on jaw tumors to the Colonial Medical Research Council and International Cancer Congress in London in the 1950s.[4] In 1951 Davies had invited Burkitt to be on the newly formed Cancer Research Committee at Makerere Medical School. At the time, Burkitt was dismissive of the whole enterprise. As Davies would later recall, "Mr. Burkitt, who had been a school friend of mine, promised all the assistance he could give but thought I was wasting time, as he could assure me as a surgeon that there was not enough cancer in Kampala to make it worth investigating. So he did not become a member of the committee."[5] Burkitt was "rather crestfallen" when he found that Davies and colleagues were already working on this tumor.[6] Cancer was, it turned out, worth investigating.

This chapter offers a schematic history of cancer research in Uganda before the founding of the Lymphoma Treatment Center (LTC) at the Uganda Cancer Institute (UCI) in 1967. I focus on the history of two forms of knowledge making about cancer in Uganda in the 1950s and 1960s. One form of knowledge making revolved around cancer pathology, surveillance, and disease registration, which was spearheaded by Davies. Cancer research was made possible by sedimentary layers of cancer case records from Mengo Hospital, the demand for locally specific knowledge about Uganda's disease patterns (which facilitated medical education at Makerere), and the concentration of patients and expertise circulating through Mulago Hospital. The other form of knowledge making revolved around the jaw tumor that would eventually be named Burkitt's lymphoma. This was both a field- and hospital-based endeavor that involved describing and documenting the tumor, mapping the tumor across the African continent, and conducting early experiments in chemotherapy with donated drugs from cancer centers in the United States and United Kingdom. Cancer experiments during this period were not conducted as randomized controlled trials. They were clinical and observational studies informed by treatment dose standards from cancer protocols in US and UK metropolitan spaces and then applied to individual cancer patients on the wards of Mulago.

The historical record available in oral histories, personal correspondence, memoirs, and medical publications is largely silent on how colonial medical men such as Burkitt understood and interpreted the ethical, racial, paternalistic, or imperial dimensions of their medical careers and actions in cancer research in Uganda. The record is also largely silent on how pediatric patients and their families understood cancer research and care at Mulago. Instead, the record is brimming with mundane safari adventure stories, clinical discoveries, and the challenges of scaling medical care and education in Uganda.[7] Today, at the UCI and in international cancer research circles alike, Burkitt is framed as a powerfully observant surgeon who changed the course of cancer care by showing that some forms of cancer could be treated with chemotherapy alone.[8] But there is ambivalence as well as admiration. Reflecting on Burkitt's lymphoma research conducted in Uganda in the 1950s and 1960s, a Ugandan colleague commented to me that this was the sort of "heroic medicine" that just simply would not be approved by Mulago Hospital's institutional review board in the twenty-first century.[9] Nevertheless, I avoid casting a retroactive twenty-first-century bioethical gaze and sensibility onto Burkitt's lymphoma research and care in Uganda in the 1950s and 1960s.[10] Instead, this account offers a thick description of cancer research and care practices before efforts to Africanize oncology began at the UCI. In particular, it situates Burkitt's lymphoma research within the broader context of medical education, clinical care, and biomedical research in Uganda between the end of World War II and the 1960s.

MAKING CANCER IN UGANDA VISIBLE

Cancer research at Makerere Medical School began with observations at the pathology lab and on the autopsy table at Mulago Hospital in the 1940s and 1950s, largely under the direction of the pathologist Davies.[11] Like many others working at Makerere at the time, Davies came to Uganda through the Colonial Medical Service.[12] Davies recalls that "it was shortly after D-Day that Dilly (my wife) and I heard that we had a chance for going to Uganda" with the British Colonial Medical Service.[13] During World War II, Davies had taught at the University of Bristol Medical School, and his wife worked as a nurse at the British Royal Infirmary's operating theater. Both were excited about the opportunity to leave the United Kingdom. But neither knew much about Uganda, having originally expressed a preference for going to Malaya, nor much about tropical medicine. As a remedy, Davies requested that he attend the University of Edinburgh for a diploma in tropical medicine before leaving for East Africa. Arriving in Scotland in early October 1944, the Davieses were greeted by the first snowfall. The courses themselves were very unevenly taught. As he said, "It was wartime, the staff had been over-worked and were tired and I found the teaching generally disappointing. . . . While even in 1944 the ex-Indian Army Officer who taught Tropical Medicine seemed not to have heard of Sulphonamides, treated Dysentery with Bacteriophages and said he did not believe in Statistics."[14] Upon completion of the course, they returned to the milder rains of Bristol and prepared for the trip to Uganda. Owing to a combination of wartime scarcity in the UK and a general paucity of supplies in Kampala, the Davieses took out a four-hundred-pound loan from Lloyds Bank and did preparatory shopping in London just off of Regent Street at "the famous tropical outfitters, Griffith's McAlister [sic]."[15] As Davies recalled, "Everything they advised us to purchase turned out to be really needed and served us well. The exception was a large solar topee which I bought, in a metal case, the case was useful for years, the sun helmet I never wore but gave it to an African assistant who found it useful when he rode to work on his bicycle."[16] The Davieses celebrated one last Christmas in Bristol, and then set off for Uganda via steamer out of Liverpool early in 1945.

For many Colonial Medical Service officers, going to East Africa during and after World War II was not just an opportunity for what they saw as a grand adventure or a chance to do God's work, as individuals such as Burkitt and others reiterated so often in their accounts.[17] Given the level of wartime scarcity and material deprivation in the United Kingdom, colonial medical work offered an opportunity to have a relatively high standard of living with house help and a garden.[18] There was a social life at the club for the colonial medical officer and his wife to enjoy strong drinks, banter, and tennis. The surgical theater itself was often downright dramatic, with extreme injuries to repair and scrotums filled with liters of fluid to drain.[19] In other words, the combination of perks usually only afforded to proper gentlemen of the English countryside, puzzling medical maladies, and the rush of the wartime hospital without the war was a fulfilling prospect for these colonial medical officers. Indeed, it was a welcome alternative to staying on a damp island and eating yet another can of beans in dingy, bombed-out 1940s London.[20]

Davies arrived in Kampala later that year over land and sea to assume his post on Mulago Hill. Kampala was a cosmopolitan city where lifestyles, habits of dress, patterns of cultivation, and power were visibly written into the landscape. And hospitals themselves were an important cosmopolitan zone within Kampala. Davies wrote in 1958:

The hospitals deal with all local cases of serious disease, but are also besieged by hordes of patients, whose complaints vary from the trivial to the rapidly lethal. While most of these patients are local, others may come vast distances, from ocean to ocean and from the Sahara Desert to South Africa. Hausa, Zulu, and Somali figure in the hospital records, and notable linguistic difficulties may be encountered in dealing with far-travelled patients. Pressure on beds is extreme; there are no radiotherapeutic services of any sort, and patients beyond hope of cure or relief have to be discharged to their own homes or to the care of friends.[21]

This cosmopolitan concentration of patients at Mulago created an "abundance of clinical material" that Davies and many others at the teaching hospital worked with as they engaged in research projects on diseases common in East Africa.[22] Much of the research conducted at Mulago from the 1940s onward was characterized by the desire to articulate the specific disease ecology of East Africa and also to consider the ways rapid urbanization and changing patterns of food and material goods consumption reshape patterns of illness. This agenda had a political edge. In describing the style of medical research at Makerere in the 1960s, historian John Iliffe argues that these individuals belonged to a "generation of researchers [who] set out to demonstrate that in so far as East Africa's disease patterns differed from those elsewhere, the reasons were generally economic or environmental rather than ethnic or cultural."[23]

When Davies arrived at Mulago, his supervisor gave him the task of developing the pathology education program at Makerere Medical School. The attitudes of British colonial medical officers varied widely toward the African medical students they were charged to teach and train. Some teaching staff embraced the task, finding their students to be impressively smart, keenly attentive, and genuinely excited about biomedicine. Other teaching staff members were decidedly disparaging of their students and the task of educating East Africans, including Davies's supervisor.[24] Davies himself was enthusiastic about both the students and the practical challenges of tailoring medical education in the Ugandan context.[25] That the laboratory space and autopsy room were rather bare bones was to be expected. For Davies, the larger issue was an absence of readily available teaching materials. The pathology slides or organ samples you would find in a standard UK pathology teaching museum—with samples preserved in chemicals and stored in ghoulish jars—were simply unavailable. In addition, textbooks and medical journals were in short supply.[26] During the war, many of these materials were stolen for their paper and then used in the shops of Wandegeya to hold sugar and other sundries.[27] On the other hand, Mulago had an abundance of unusual patient material when compared to Bristol or Liverpool or Edinburgh. For example, one of the first cases Davies and his new group of African medical students collectively examined was a case of pulmonary tuberculosis that had also invaded the heart tissue. Davies assured his students that this was rare and probably the only case they would ever see. They went on to see several more cases of the exact same presentation in the ensuing months.[28] Teaching pathology at Makerere required new ways of documenting and disseminating information on the ways diseases presented themselves in East Africa. Given the need for teaching materials in real time, it did not make sense to write and then publish a full textbook that captured the specificity of pathology in greater Kampala. Davies and his students opted instead to write for and develop the *East African Medical Journal*. They wrote up interesting cases and published them as they went along. Through publishing detailed case histories and conditions, the *East African Medical Journal* became a key teaching tool.

After a series of negotiations, Davies was able to access old autopsy reports at Mulago Hospital, which allowed him to retrospectively evaluate the distribution of disease burdens in Uganda. Working with his wife after hours, he went through all of the old autopsy records and death reports to reconstruct the mortality patterns seen at hospitals around Kampala from the early 1900s to the late 1940s.[29] Part of this mortality data showed that not only were Africans dying of maladies associated with "diseases of the tropics" such as malaria, typhoid, and sleeping sickness but that they also suffered from cancer, heart disease, and other illnesses that were described at the time as "diseases of civilization."[30] A careful review suggested that the cancers found in autopsy reports rarely mapped onto cancer incidence and prevalence patterns in the United Kingdom. Dominating the cancer records of Africans were liver cancers, Kaposi's sarcoma, malignant melanoma, and a strange jaw cancer that appeared to be a sarcoma or lymphoma. The data available suggested that cancer, while present in Africa, looked quite different from cancer patterns seen in European hospitals.[31]

It was these observations, both the visceral encounters with tumors on the autopsy table and the wealth of found autopsy data, that inspired Davies and colleagues at Makerere Medical School to start an inquiry into the patterns and incidence of cancer in Uganda. This began as a retrospective study of cancer incidence in Kampala, drawing from inpatient records from Kampala hospitals from 1952 to 1953. The quality of the information from these hospital records was uneven. Omissions and missing staging information made it difficult to create a cancer registry. Davies and his colleagues at Makerere applied for money and support from the British Empire Cancer Campaign to establish a comprehensive cancer registry in Kampala, which began in 1954.[32] The Kampala Cancer Registry, modeled on other cancer registries across the British Empire, worked by going to medical and surgical departments across hospitals in and around greater Kampala. This registry data would then be cross-checked by a team who would check histology department records, obtain records of surgeries, request information from X-ray departments, and review hospital records. In 1956 Davies and colleagues hired a Ugandan social worker, Mr. Kayanda, who was responsible for interviewing patients both in the hospital and in the home. On these home visits, Kayanda would arrive with a form to fill out, which would offer detailed information about how to find the patient and their home in the future. Recording these personal details was not always straightforward.[33] As Davies recalled: "The *name*, or details of its spelling, may be given and recorded differently at various times, as on repeated admissions to the same hospital or on admission to different hospitals. Partial recording may cause difficulty as well when one patient attended three hospitals and was biopsied three times, once as 'Kosia,' once as 'Kolo,' and the third time as 'Kosia Kolo.'"[34] In addition to varying the spelling of names, Kayanda and colleagues also found that patients would sometimes offer up a different name, such as the name of a fellow resident of the village. In some cases, during Kayanda's follow-up visits, he would meet individuals who had the name, housing compound, and material possessions of the patient, only to later discover that this individual was in fact the deceased patient's relative.[35]

In 1964, the *British Medical Journal* published a two-part series on cancer in Uganda from 1897 to 1956. The study compared two data sets of case records—one from Mengo Hospital, the old Church Missionary Society hospital founded by Sir Albert Cook in the late 1890s, and the other from the more recently established Kampala Cancer Registry, founded by Davies and colleagues at Mulago in 1951. The study aimed to answer two questions: "How common was cancer in the past? And were the varieties of cancers the same as we have recorded in recent years?" Davies continued:

> The study starts at a time when everything imported into
> Uganda was carried by headload and when the first doctor to study
> and treat disease in the African population had walked the great
> distance from the coast. It began in reed huts. It ended in days

of concrete and chromium, of radioisotopes and autoanalysers brought in by modern railways or jet aircraft. Our study covers a period from almost the Iron Age to Rocketry.

We have found that the ratio of cancers to total admissions at Mengo Hospital has remained remarkably stable over six decades. The ratios are low, as low as those which in the past were used to support the idea that cancer was a rare disease of 'primitive peoples.' Yet out of such ratios in recent years it has been possible to construct incidence rates based on annual registrations which in the younger age-groups are comparable with those of Norway.[36]

"Cancer in an African Community, 1897–1956" painted an evocative picture of both the profound changes in Uganda over a sixty-year period and also an equally profound continuity over time. Diagnostic tools, medical infrastructure, railways, imported goods from clothing to soap, new legal structures, and bureaucratic machinery all proliferated throughout central Uganda from the time of the Mailo land agreement to the Buganda riots in 1949 to the eve of independence in the late 1950s. At the same time, cancer patterns themselves did not change much, nor did improvements in the tools available for detection and diagnosis dramatically alter the epidemiological profile of cancer in Kampala and the surrounding milieu.

BURKITT'S LYMPHOMA RESEARCH

Given the time and care that Davies and colleagues were already investing in cancer research at Mulago Hospital, it is perhaps not surprising that Davies was irritated with Burkitt's jaw tumor "discovery." And in the decades to come, the Cancer Research Committee's collaborative labor, scientific contributions, and centrality in identifying and researching this pediatric jaw tumor in the late 1940s and 1950s would fade from the foreground of accounts of Burkitt's lymphoma history. Instead, scientific articles would champion Burkitt as a medical pioneer whose keen and simple observational prowess changed the course of cancer chemotherapy in 1957.[37] Part of this is simply about ownership of the story. Davies left Kampala in the early 1960s after his wife died unexpectedly, while Burkitt stayed in Uganda and continued to do cancer research until 1967, staking a greater visible claim to the cancer.[38] Part of this is also about the simplistic appeal of celebratory narratives that tell of medical discovery and up-country safaris, perhaps best captured by Bernard Glemser's account of Burkitt's work, published in the United States as *Mr. Burkitt and Africa* and in the United Kingdom as *The Long Safari*.[39] And part of it is about the ability to tell a good story. In both his lectures and his writing, Burkitt was attuned to the drama of the curative spectacle of treating this jaw tumor and the exploratory texture of his far-reaching travels.[40] At the same time, in his memoirs Burkitt highlighted that he neither worked alone nor unraveled the full complexities of the tumor. He said, "I have been given the opportunity to make tracks through the bush, but it has fallen to others with more knowledge and equipment to develop these into eventual highways, serving the needs of many. It has been thus with the tumor with which I became associated . . . in which my simple observations were to be converted into a massive highway over which numerous research workers would pass, each improving the surface and widening the track."[41] Many of these research workers would later pass through the UCI.

From 1957 onward, Burkitt cultivated an obsession with this unusual tumor. Building on the work of the Cancer Research Committee and collaborating with Davies and others, he investigated the clinical presentation, geographical distribution, and pathological features of the tumor with the sort of zeal one associates with imperial explorers.[42] Aiming for maximum visibility within the British medical research establishment, Burkitt submitted the paper "A Sarcoma Involving the Jaws in African Children" to the *British Journal of Surgery*.[43] Photographs taken by Burkitt documented the consequences of these malignancies with a disquieting (and to my mind, invasive) level of detail. The publication included images of swollen jaws, loosening teeth, and eyes bulging out of the sockets of Ugandan children without any attention to privacy or anonymity.[44] When "A Sarcoma" was published in 1958, Burkitt's hope that the article and the "discovery" of this sarcoma would make a major impact fell flat. It garnered little attention or recognition from the British surgical community or from East African medical researchers.[45]

Nevertheless, Burkitt, Davies, and other colleagues within the pathology department and the broader medical and surgical community at Makerere Medical School continued their line of inquiry, focusing on a few avenues of further research from observations, which were documented in the 1958 article. The major observations were as follows. Firstly, this tumor grew very rapidly, sometimes doubling in size over a twenty-four-hour period.[46] Secondly, the tumor itself was highly responsive to nitrogen mustard. Treatment with chemotherapeutic agents alone in a context where there was no radiotherapy proved to induce temporary remissions. Thirdly, the tumor had a unique geographic distribution, which was suggestive of environmental factors, possibly a viral infection spread by an insect vector.[47] Mapping the distribution of Burkitt's lymphoma, Burkitt worked with A. J. Haddow, director of the East African Virus Research Institute in Entebbe. They concluded that the geographic distribution of the lymphoma across Africa corresponded with altitudes below five thousand feet and areas with more than twenty inches of rainfall a year, that is, environments where mosquitoes thrived, and insect-vector-driven diseases were common.[48]

At least initially, collecting information about the geographic distribution of Burkitt's lymphoma was done largely through armchair explorations in Kampala. Burkitt created a one-page sheet of information on the tumor, which included descriptions of clinical presentation and photographs of patients, which was then sent out widely to missionary and colonial hospital networks across the African continent.[49] Medical staff wrote back, either saying that they had indeed seen this tumor with some frequency or that it was rarely seen at all. Those who wrote back saying they encountered the tumor with some frequency were geographically distributed across "tropical" Africa, corresponding with wet conditions, warm temperatures, and plenty of malaria. This eventually became known as "the lymphoma belt," which included West Africa south of the Sahara, Central Africa sandwiched between the Sahara and the borders of southern Angola and (what was then) Rhodesia, East Africa, and a dangling tail south and down Mozambique into the northern part of Natal.[50]

Fieldwork in the form of a "tumor safari" accompanied this desk work in mapping the jaw tumor. In 1961, Burkitt and two medical missionary friends and colleagues, Ted Williams and Cliff Nelson, packed a newly purchased used Ford station wagon. They loaded a primus stove, folding chairs, and camp beds. They appended spare tires and a six-gallon receptacle of fuel onto the roof rack. They brought documentary materials—an audio recorder, a typewriter, and a moving-pictures camera. Williams installed a metal box in the car to store passports, money, and important documents in case of thieves. And Burkitt packed a large booklet of case photographs of the lymphoma to share with the fifty-eight missionary and colonial hospitals they were to visit over the course of a ten-week journey.[51]

The planning for this "long tumor safari" took about two years. Crafting research questions, developing a travel itinerary, contacting hospitals in advance, and applying for multiple small infusions of cash to procure the car and cover basic expenses on the road all went into shaping the expedition. The overarching research agenda behind the road trip was to determine the eastern and southern border of the lymphoma belt: that is, at what elevation and at what levels of humidity was Burkitt's lymphoma rare? And at what elevation and levels of humidity were Burkitt's lymphoma common? The working hypothesis was that some environmental factor facilitated carcinogenesis, or that Burkitt's lymphoma was caused by an infectious agent such as a virus transmitted through a mosquito vector. They hoped that mapping the southeastern perimeter of the lymphoma belt would help to determine whether altitude, temperature, rainfall, or some combination of the two was at play in shaping tumor incidence. This line of thinking about the interplay between the environment, insect vectors, and disease prevalence was similar to research already being done on yellow fever at the Uganda Virus Research Institute.[52]

Burkitt kept a diary over the ten weeks of traveling across Tanzania, Northern Rhodesia, and Nyasaland into Mozambique, then into South Africa via Swaziland, back up through Southern Rhodesia into Northern Rhodesia, and finally back to the shores of Lake Victoria around Kisumu. The diary itself is peppered with accounts of lunches: delicious sandwiches prepared by wives or the staff of hotel kitchens or cans of simple beans harkening back to rationing times in the army. The car is also prominently featured in the account, with plenty of bad roads and close calls with an empty gas tank. To pass the time in the car, Burkitt, Williams, and Nelson would sing church hymnals and look for wildlife on the horizon. And they stopped off at Victoria Falls, where "the sight is so awe-inspiring that it nearly hypnotizes you. To think that the giant spectacle of ever moving cascades of water has continued unchecked since it first awed Livingstone and for eons of times before."[53] The reference to Livingstone is not incidental. On the tumor safari, Burkitt took a copy of David Livingstone's travel diaries from his explorations of Central Africa in the mid-1800s and would read those entries at the end of the day's long drives by hurricane lamp or bare light bulb.[54]

These moments on the road were punctuated by visits to hospitals. Upon arriving at the hospital of the day, they would greet the medical officer in charge, introduce the work, share the photograph book, see if there were any patients of interest on the wards, and then ask to go through patient records. When they were satisfied with their data collection, they would either camp or go to a hotel or guesthouse to relax and make notes for the rest of the day. A typical diary entry from these downtimes would read: "Sitting on the verandah of a rather third-class hotel at Shinyanga [in Tanzania]. After a very profitable morning when I found records of no less than 21 cases of the tumor that has been interesting us, more than we found in the whole of Northern and Southern Rhodesia."[55]

Upon returning to Kampala after the tumor safari, Burkitt wrote up the results and submitted them to the *British Journal of Cancer*. As he recalled, "It must have been a most unusual article for such a journal but it was accepted without question and aroused considerable interest."[56] The key findings of the article were as follows:

1. In Uganda, Kenya and Tanganyika, the tumor can apparently occur anywhere except in areas over 5000 ft. above sea level.
2. In the Federation of the Rhodesias and Nyasaland, the condition is found only in the river valleys and on the lake shore.
3. The condition is widely recognized throughout the central lain of Mozambique as far south as the southern tip.
4. It is virtually unknown in South Africa.
5. It is virtually unknown in Ruanda-Urundi.[57]

The findings suggested that the altitude cutoff for the tumor was above five thousand feet. However, places below five thousand feet with temperatures that dropped below sixty degrees, such as South Africa, had very few if any cases of the tumor. From this expansive survey of the geography of the tumor, Burkitt, drawing from conversations with Davies, suggested that the tumor was dependent on temperature, implying vector transmission.[58]

Looking back on these research questions and the orientation of the tumor safari, the cancer specialist Dr. Ian Magrath, who would later work at the UCI, remarked that these "were very simple studies" that "laid the foundation of our present-day knowledge of the factors that appear to predispose BL [Burkitt's lymphoma]."[59] He also noted that Burkitt's epidemiological work and the lymphoma itself demonstrated the potential to "learn from the sometimes remarkable variability in the patterns of cancer that occur in different geographical regions—often related to different local patterns of infection which, incidentally, provide potential targets for the simultaneous prevention of both the chronic infection and the cancer or cancers related to it. Denis Burkitt showed what could be achieved with extremely limited resources over 50 years ago, and this too should be recognized as one of his achievements—the demonstration that valuable research can be done, even in countries with limited resources."[60]

In his reminiscences, Burkitt celebrated what he saw as the financial thriftiness and enterprising adventurism of the tumor safari. Reflecting on this period, Burkitt noted that he had been involved in three different kinds of lymphoma research: "Experimental, which is the concept and is mostly laboratory based. Observational, which can be clinical or epidemiological, and had been the foundation on which our work was based. And then recreational, which our safaris appeared to be. They certainly were recreational, but also profoundly fruitful, partly I am sure because they were enjoyable. The quality of any work as a drudgery is likely to be inferior to that undertaken as a consuming interest. A sense of humor is an essential ingredient to oil the wheels of any enterprise in Africa."[61]

INTERNATIONAL CIRCUITS OF CHEMOTHERAPY TREATMENTS

In the three years between the publication of the sarcoma paper in 1958 and the tumor safari in 1961, Burkitt and colleagues also put considerable time and energy into understanding the histopathology and clinical presentation of this lymphoma. This knowledge and news of the "discovery" of Burkitt's lymphoma circulated beyond East Africa in medical journals and landed on the desks of US-based cancer chemotherapists such as Dr. Joe Burchenal and Dr. Daniel Karnofsky at Sloan Kettering and Dr. Paul Carbone at the National Cancer Institute (NCI).[62] Since the 1940s, American cancer researchers had experimented with cytotoxic drug therapies, particularly focusing on pediatric leukemia, where it appeared that chemotherapy treatments would bring about temporary cancer remissions. This led researchers on a quest for permanent cures for cancer with cytotoxic drugs alone.[63] By the early 1960s, there was increasing interest in combining different cytotoxic agents, and in 1961, the NCI launched their flagship VAMP trial for leukemia that capitalized on combination drug therapy—vincristine, amethopterin (methotrexate), 6-MP (mercaptopurine), and prednisone. As Mukherjee writes: "A child with leukemia was already stretched to the brittle limits of survival, hanging on to life by a bare physiological thread. People at the NCI would often casually talk of chemotherapy as the 'poison of the month.' If four poisons of the month were simultaneously pumped daily into a three or six year old child, there was virtually no guarantee that he or she could survive even the first dose of this regimen, let alone survive week after week."[64] Patients who participated in the VAMP trials initially had astonishing remissions. The vast majority of patients eventually succumbed to leukemia, which persisted in their central nervous systems, although a few did survive.[65]

Burchenal had the opportunity to visit Nairobi in January 1960 with a team from Sloan Kettering to meet with the surgeon Dr. Peter Clifford, who ran a small on-site cancer treatment ward. Burchenal also visited Kampala and met with Burkitt. Reflecting on that visit, Burchenal said: "I thought I had seen all childhood tumors in Memorial Hospital during the past twelve or fourteen years, but I had never seen anything like these tumors."[66] Discussing the treatment options available at Mulago Hospital where surgery proved ineffectual and there was no radiotherapy, Burchenal suggested that Burkitt try treating patients with methotrexate left over from the Kenya visit. The doses of drugs Burkitt was giving were lower (and therefore less intense) than what would be standard practice on the pediatric wards of Sloan Kettering.[67] This was due in part to scarcity. The material resources to provide supportive care at Mulago were considerably lower, and the human resources of designated nurses available to monitor the side effects of chemotherapy, such as renal function or sepsis, were just not available.[68] The drugs Burkitt used were part of the standard of care at the time for common pediatric cancers in the United States and the United Kingdom. What was different about the Ugandan context was the absence of radiotherapy, minimal supportive care, and concentration of chemotherapist expertise. In contrast to VAMP, the results of chemotherapy used on Burkitt's lymphoma were hopeful. Children were often only receiving one dose of a single cytotoxic agent and then going into full long-term remissions. For example, according to preliminary follow-up data on Burkitt's lymphoma published in 1965, of the sixty-three Burkitt's lymphoma patients treated with cyclophosphamide at Mulago Hospital between 1960 and 1963, nineteen were living in 1965 with full remissions, twenty-eight were lost to follow-up, and sixteen had passed away.[69] The material circumstances of biomedical care at Mulago made these early Burkitt's lymphoma remissions all the more impressive.[70]

Despite the promise of cytotoxic drugs to create Burkitt's lymphoma tumor regressions and long-term remissions, the data coming out of Mulago Hospital had a major empirical hole. There were so many patients who were lost to follow-up that it was difficult to say, using the statistical standards of the day, whether or not these results were due to chance or bona fide therapeutic efficacy.[71] The vast majority of Burkitt's lymphoma patients were from rural up-country villages. Neither the patients nor the parents spoke much English, and Burkitt did not speak much of the forty or so languages commonly spoken across the country. As he remembered, "It was not uncommon for a child under treatment to be removed from hospital by her mother in the middle of the night."[72] During Burkitt's tumor safari with colleagues throughout East and Central Africa, he looked for signs of the lymphoma at various government and mission hospitals. He did not spend time engaging with Central and East Africans themselves in the context of meeting with village chiefs or seeking out local healers who may have treated tumors with a variety of herbs or prayers. Burkitt's gaze was a biomedical one. His medical networks were muzungu networks. Although medical contemporaries praised Burkitt for his powers of keen observation over the years and commemorated him for making clinical problems in tropical Africa visible, the village life of the patients and families he engaged with remained starkly invisible to him. When patients "vanished," he lacked the social resources to do much other than mark these patients as "lost to follow up."

Occasionally patients with Burkitt's lymphoma surfaced in the United States. For example, in June 1965, while interning at Memorial Sloan Kettering in New York City, a young oncologist named Dr. John Ziegler admitted a sixteen-year-old girl from Connecticut with a lymphosarcoma. Ziegler remembered, "During internship I actually admitted a young girl with Burkitt's lymphoma and discussed this case with the senior staff there because this was a new disease — not previously understood very well — that responded dramatically to chemotherapy." The clinical presentation and histopathology appeared to be much like Burkitt's lymphoma. Drawing on dosage and treatment practices from East Africa, particularly Burkitt's work at Mulago Hospital, Ziegler and colleagues treated the girl with a dose of cyclophosphamide, and "two days later a striking decrease in the size of the left breast was noted and there was a 50% reduction in the size of the abdominal mass. Four days later the breasts were normal in size and no tumor could be palpated. . . . The patient was discharged feeling well on July 10, with no medications, and in apparent complete remission."[73] These initial results were similar to data coming out of Mulago Hospital and elsewhere in East Africa, where colleagues reported similar tumor-melting effects from the drugs.[74] But less than a month later, the Connecticut girl was back at Sloan Kettering with "recurrent swelling of the breasts and was treated with irradiation and a short course of cyclophosphamide given orally. . . . The patient suffered progressive deterioration marked by pancytopenia, paraplegia due to spinal cord compression, and terminal respiratory distress unresponsive to supportive measures. She died on September 8 [1965] following a grand mal seizure."[75]

Although this patient died, her condition made a major impression on Ziegler. After his internship, Ziegler joined Carbone's working group at the NCI's Public Health Service with a major interest in chemotherapy and Burkitt's lymphoma. Carbone's group at the NCI was interested in understanding why African patients with Burkitt's lymphoma were more responsive to chemotherapy treatments than American patients with Burkitt's lymphoma. In particular, the group wanted to determine whether this evidence was simply anecdotal or if it would withstand a serious clinical trial. NCI staff in Bethesda pondered the question of how to ethically generate medical data on the survival of African children with Burkitt's lymphoma that would be relevant to cancer researchers in the United States. Of the options available, Kampala had the local contacts, medical facilities, and patient populations best suited to establishing a chemotherapy research center.

As Ziegler remembered:

> Paul had just returned from a visit to Uganda, which also included Kenya, Uganda, and Nigeria, and he stopped at a number of centers talking to people who had been involved with treatment of Burkitt's lymphoma. In Nairobi he met Peter Clifford, a head and neck surgeon. In Kampala he met Sebastian Kyalwazi, a Ugandan surgeon, and Denis Burkitt who was just preparing to leave at the time. He also spoke with Sir Ian McAdam, the head of surgery where most of these tumors were being treated. Paul also went to Ibadan, Nigeria, and visited with Professor Ngu, who was a surgeon also treating Burkitt's lymphoma.[76]

Carbone asked Ziegler if he would be interested in running the day-to-day operations of this soon-to-be-established unit. As Ziegler remembered, "I don't think he knew very much about me [at first] and I think I knew even less about what they were doing, but as we talked we hit it off just fine, and I said sure let me talk it over with my wife and we said okay, let's do this."[77]

In January 1967, Carbone and Ziegler attended a conference on "Cancer in Africa" in Nairobi.[78] It was "sort of a perfect storm of really good people coming together" to discuss a variety of cancers endemic in Africa, including Burkitt's lymphoma, Kaposi's sarcoma, hepatocellular carcinoma, esophageal cancer, and others that "were very much indigenous" on the continent. When the conference closed in Nairobi, Ziegler, Burkitt, Carbone, Dr. Richard Morrow, Dr. Angus McCray, and Dr. Malcolm Pike piled into a car and drove from Nairobi to Kampala, via Lake Nakuru. "By the time we got back to Kampala we were the best of friends."[79] And in meetings with Dr. Ian McAdam, Dr. Denis Wright, and a new cadre of African physicians, there was right away a kind of camaraderie, an acceptance, and a willingness to make this happen. Thinking back now in various research settings that I've seen, you could imagine people would be very threatened and say no this is our turf and all these muzungus in Uganda [shouldn't be here]. Other people might say what are you going to offer? Is this going to make us better or is this going to threaten my career? So what you ended up with is this perfect collection of like-minded people and somehow not a one of them was threatened or pushed back.[80]

While Uganda was "rich" in cancer patient material, Mulago Hospital was not particularly well resourced for running clinical trials or providing expansive supportive care for patients on the wards or a dedicated follow-up care infrastructure in the 1950s and 1960s. The absence of a dedicated experimental infrastructure during this period meant that cancer research and care initiatives were scattered across case records in Mengo Hospital, surgical wards at Mulago Hospital, and on autopsy tables and pathology lectures at Makerere Medical School. At the same time, similar hospital sites in Nairobi in Kenya and Accra in Ghana did not offer the same alchemy of personalities, ongoing cancer research programs, or foundations such as those laid by Burkitt, Davies, Kyalwazi, McAdam, and others.[81] Leadership at the NCI understood that in order to conduct serious research on the long-term impact of chemotherapy on Burkitt's lymphoma remissions, they needed to do more than transfer drug technologies. To conduct systemic clinical trials on Burkitt's lymphoma, the built and human infrastructure to facilitate the movement of patients, drug therapies, statistics, funds, and knowledge in cancer research would need to be actively made. They would need to create an entire cancer hospital. Six months later, Ziegler and his family flew to Kampala to begin work setting up the LTC.

2 ✒ A Hospital Built from Scratch

IN JULY 1967, John and Audrey Ziegler stepped off the plane at Entebbe Airport with their children. It was warm but not sticky, as the family arrived in the middle of the dry season. Their clothes, books, photographs, and other worldly possessions were stuffed into suitcases. Ziegler also brought "boxes and boxes of stuff. Mainly drugs, syringes, and needles, and gauze pads, and just about anything that I could think of that you would possibly need in a hospital."[1] They made their way up the Entebbe-Kampala road, a slender twenty-mile, two-lane thoroughfare that snaked past Lake Victoria's beaches, swamps, and banana gardens before finally arriving in Kampala. In contrast to the brick-and-mortar look of New York or Washington, DC, Kampala was a verdant garden city. It was lush, green, and full of trees, with houses tucked away behind gardens on several rolling hills.[2] The family settled in at a colleague's home on Makerere Hill, and a few days later the work began on a new cancer research center.

Ziegler came to Kampala under the auspices of the National Cancer Institute (NCI) with the task of establishing a small cancer chemotherapy clinical trials research unit. The Lymphoma Treatment Center (LTC) would examine the long-term survival outcomes of treating Burkitt's lymphoma.[3] A collaborative project between the Ugandan Ministry of Health, the Makerere Medical School's Department of Surgery, the NCI, and the British Empire Cancer Campaign, the LTC was not intended to provide comprehensive cancer care for the Ugandan population. Rather, the vision was to create and disseminate knowledge about cancer survival and differences in disease patterns and etiology between Africa and the United States.[4]

Up until 1967, cancer research and treatment at Mulago Hospital lacked a dedicated ward or free-standing facility and was instead distributed across surgery, pediatrics, pathology, and general medicine. This absence of centralized staff, dedicated space, and comprehensive treatment systems made it challenging to administer chemotherapy protocols or manage Burkitt's lymphoma clinical trials.[5] The Ugandan government allocated an abandoned maternity ward from the "Old" Mulago Hospital to serve as the new LTC. The gift of the maternity unit shifted these decentralized dynamics and made it possible to create an experimental infrastructure for cancer research in Uganda.

Ziegler recalled that the building gifted to the LTC "was in horrible shape. Rat infested and everything needed a lot of work."[6] The task of equipping and refurbishing the shell of the donated building, with a collapsed roof, peeling paint, and plenty of rat excrement on the floors, fell largely on a longtime Mulago Hospital administrator, Mr. Hilary Martins, whom the NCI hired to run the day-to-day administration of the new unit. Part of the Goan community, Martins had extensive networks with many of the Asian-run businesses in town and ample experience furnishing and equipping hospital wards.[7] Ziegler, Martins, and other colleagues spent most of the summer of 1967 outfitting the unit and tracking down patients. Outfitting the unit took on an organic and iterative quality. "We realized we needed beds and bed curtains for privacy. And we needed some furniture and a table and chairs and a dining room for feeding people. So over the summer we put this together and it was entirely ad hoc. We said what about this? What about that? So we would jump into the car and get what we needed and would haul it back and set it up."[8] By the time the unit was completed eight weeks later, the Uganda Cancer Institute comprised the LTC's wards, a pharmacy, a laboratory for doing both basic blood counts and more experimental techniques, a dining room, a kitchen, cleaned-up bathrooms, and offices. The LTC also established relationships with the pathology department for biopsy processing and the medical imaging department for taking photographs of patients.

In order to fill the wards, Ziegler and colleagues did a two-week driving tour of the country, looking for Burkitt's lymphoma patients. They visited mission and government hospitals from Hoima to Arua to Gulu to Soroti, "all around in a big circle . . . and showed them pictures of Burkitt's lymphoma and said if you have patients with this condition and want to send them to Kampala for treatment this is the place to send them."[9] They handed out maps to the LTC and offered to pay for a bus to transport patients to Kampala. "At the end of the safari we had put the word out and put in on the radio as well."[10] Reflecting on this startup hospital years later, Ziegler said:

> We walked into an empty room and turned it into a hospital. It was all done in a resource-poor country where you have to hire all the nurses, hire all the floor-keepers, organize the food, organize the pharmacy, organize the lab, bring in beds and bedclothes and pillows, everything. Plus develop a major research lab. We had to build a hematology unit and a clinical chemistry unit, and all of this just sort of came together. It was a lot of fun. . . . It was building a hospital from scratch, really.[11]

In many ways, Ziegler's turn of phrase about the Uganda Cancer Institute (UCI) being a cancer hospital built from scratch describes the situation at the top of Mulago Hill in the late 1960s with finesse. Not only did the staff recruit Burkitt's lymphoma patients from Uganda's mission and district hospital and bring them to Mulago Hill on buses, but they also refurbished and tailored the physical spaces of this former maternity ward to pediatric cancer research. In addition, the research protocols for conducting chemotherapy clinical trials had to be developed and then approved by Makerere's newly formed research ethics committee.[12] Ziegler's comment echoes a sentiment shared by other Ugandan and expatriate staff who established the UCI. Much like Burkitt, they saw themselves as medical pioneers, actively building cancer research and care practices "from scratch."[13] At the same time, Ziegler and his American, Ugandan, and British colleagues built the UCI on the foundation of roughly fifty years of evidence generated by missionary and government medical physicians and researchers on the patterns, distribution, and prevalence of cancer in the area surrounding Kampala, not to mention a decade's worth of Burkitt's lymphoma research.[14]

One of the core arguments of this book is that oncology developed at the UCI through the importation of technologies for cancer care and research from the Global North, particularly the American NCI. These technologies and treatment systems were in turn transformed and refashioned by the immediate needs of Ugandan pediatric patients and their families, the material realities of practicing biomedicine in East Africa, and the political demands of Africanizing the medical profession in

Uganda in the 1960s. The American NCI staff who established the UCI in partnership with Makerere's Department of Surgery and the British Empire Cancer Campaign took the material and social circumstances of Burkitt's lymphoma patients and their families seriously.[15] Colleagues who established the UCI recognized that catering to the medical care and socioeconomic requirements of families, rather than just treating individual pediatric patients in an experimental vacuum on the wards, was necessary for the technologies and systems of cancer research to function. Part of this is likely a reflection of the research questions themselves, which shifted the gaze from the cancer epidemiology and geographical pathology to evaluating Burkitt's lymphoma treatment and survival outcomes. These questions required developing long-term relationships with cancer patients and their families.[16]

I also think that taking the families of patients seriously was a reflection of the idealism and pragmatic orientation of those who founded and worked at the UCI itself. In cancer care and research in the 1950s, a culture of British colonial medicine dominated, shaped by the demands of World War II scarcity, colonial developmentalist policies, White paternalism, and the adventurous orientation of medical missionaries.[17] In the 1960s, decolonization and the rise of American imperialism shifted the pool of expatriate physicians drawn to working in East African cancer research. The largely American group of expatriate oncologists who came to Uganda in the late 1960s and early 1970s brought a fresh set of sensibilities shaped by working at flagship cancer research centers which celebrated efforts to save cancer patients who were terminally ill.[18] They brought new forms of idealistic politics shaped by the social transformations echoing through the United States as well as the personal and political desire to do anything but serve in the Vietnam War.[19] The British physicians who chose to stay on in Uganda after 1962 had strong political commitments to training African medical specialists.[20] Young, enthusiastic, and dedicated Ugandan physicians who worked at the UCI saw themselves as medical pioneers and national leaders. The chapter that follows discusses how oncologists, patient outreach workers, nurses, X-ray department staff, cooks, hospital administrators, patient caretakers, and most importantly patients themselves created not only a hospital from scratch but also an infrastructure for cancer research that combined and reconfigured oncological tools from Bethesda, tumor safaris from Burkitt, and the caretaking realities of families in Buganda and beyond.

The source material draws on oral histories conducted by me as well as those found in repositories in libraries in the United States and the

United Kingdom.[21] These sources are complemented by the UCI's administrative records from this period, published medical journal articles, personal photograph collections, patient records, and comparisons with contemporary ethnographic observations on the wards. The historical and archival asymmetries of this period— where the healthy are speaking, and the ill are silent—leave a number of unanswered questions about patient experience and the lived reality of what it meant to be a patient on the wards. It is also worth noting that all of the oral histories were conducted at least twenty but in some cases over forty years after the opening of the LTC. Invariably, the oral sources share reminiscences of the "good old days," before Idi Amin, HIV/AIDS, war, and structural adjustment. It may be tempting to dismiss these memories as wistful exaggerations or professional tall tales. However, operating budget figures, staff-to-patient ratios, patient survival data, and scholarly outputs in medical journals from this period all suggest a time of experimental productivity and quality care, even within the resource constraints of East African biomedical practice.[22]

OPENING THE LTC

Burkitt and his fellow British colonial medical officers conducted cancer research during a decade of transitions, both within the institution of Mulago itself (as the doors of the new hospital opened) and as Uganda became independent in 1962. Uganda's political transition in the early 1960s raised numerous questions about how to effectively hand over colonial institutions to a talented and rising class of civil servants, educators, and medical personnel. Decolonization signaled the end of indefinite contracts for British colonial medical officers. Burkitt was aware that he would, in all likelihood, be asked to resign from the Colonial Medical Service due to "increasing pressures for Africanization of the medical services."[23] Notes from his diary in June 1962 read, "Not really worried. The Lord will open the way."[24] Ian McAdam suggested that Burkitt apply to the Medical Research Council and have the work in geographical pathology continue to be funded. "Discussed it with Olive and prayed about it. The idea is probably to provide an opening for an African. Olive felt 1 Samuel 10 was in the form of guidance [The verse reads 'Then Samuel took a flask of olive oil and poured it on Saul's head and kissed him, saying, "Has not the Lord anointed you ruler over his inheritance?"'] the following day I wrote 'Feeling at peace over Ian's suggestion.'"[25]

In the wake of national independence in 1962, Ugandan leaders and British physicians, many of whom were former colonial medical officers, sought to ensure that Africans took over positions of leadership within Mulago Hospital and Makerere Medical School.[26] This political ethos of Africanization, I would suggest, encouraged the American and British to think about the UCI not as a short-term initiative but as a long-term investment in treating East African cancer patients and expanding Ugandan biomedical expertise. The coprincipal investigators at the UCI, Professor Sebastian Kyalwazi and Sir Ian McAdam, both symbolically and practically encapsulated this ethic of Africanization.

Kyalwazi, was one of the first Ugandans (and East Africans) to qualify as a formal surgeon in Edinburgh as a fellow at the Royal College of Surgeons and was particularly interested in Kaposi's sarcoma and chemotherapy research at Mulago.[27] Over the course of the 1960s, he climbed the ranks of Makerere Medical School's surgery department—he was appointed as a lecturer (the British equivalent of an assistant professor in the United States) in the department in 1968 and assumed the chairmanship of the department in 1973. He kept the Department of Surgery going at Makerere in the 1970s. He died of cancer in 1992. I made several unsuccessful attempts to contact his family and tried to track down his personal papers over the course of fieldwork in 2012. McAdam, professor of surgery at Makerere Medical School, was committed to building the international reputation of the medical school but also to training the first generation of East African surgeons as part of a broader vision of Africanizing medical research and care in Uganda and more generally across East Africa.[28] McAdam was also a character on the larger stage of Uganda's politics in the 1960s. As noted in his obituary, "There can be few surgeons who have had to deal with a major head wound sustained by their country's president (Obote) after a failed coup and operate in a theatre full of excited soldiers with automatic weapons [in 1969]."[29] McAdam, who was head of Makerere's Department of Surgery and also a great supporter of the Institute, enacted this ethic of training, mentoring, and handing over responsibilities both at the hospital and also in everyday life. His home in Kololo was often turned into an informal medical education salon, with Ugandan medical students and colleagues discussing the latest strange surgical cases, often with beers and photographs from the medical imaging department in hand.[30] Together, McAdam and Kyalwazi offered hospitality to their American collaborators, even as they sought to ensure that Africans took over positions of leadership within Mulago Hospital and Makerere Medical School.[31]

When the LTC opened officially on August 4, 1967, foreign dignitaries and local politicians alike came to see the opening of this small joint research endeavor to study "certain types of cancer common in Africa and of theoretical and practical interests to US scientists."[32] McAdam welcomed colleagues and visitors:

> This Unit which is being opened today has the unique opportunity of adding a vital chapter in the fight against cancer. The first objective is to provide the best available treatment for patients suffering from malignant lymphoma. On this foundation the research staff will investigate some of the fundamental problems concerned with cancer—the aetiology of Burkitt's tumour, the host response to cancer and the dramatic remissions (I am not saying cures) which have resulted from treatment with chemotherapeutic agents. Answers to some of these problems would be of benefit to the whole human race. Is it too imaginative to see this building the workroom of a future Nobel Prize winner? The Ministry of Health has provided the building and the National Institutes of Health in the United States have generously given the money to renovate the building, to equip it, and pay the salaries of the staff, which includes a Consultant Chemotherapist.
>
> We now have an ideal environment in which the research team of Makerere and Government Consultants can work. Your presence here, Mr. Minister, is an indication of Government support.[33]

After the speeches, the Ugandan health minister officially opened the LTC by bestowing a commemorative dedication plaque to the building, honoring Burkitt and his contributions to Burkitt's lymphoma research in Uganda.[34] On the tour of the new ward, it was Kyalwazi who engaged with patients and examined them at their bedsides. Burkitt looked on, his hands neatly folded across his camera.[35] His medical officer contract with the Ugandan government had already expired.

The LTC opened about a year after Milton Obote abolished the kingdoms and took full control of the Ugandan government. It was an extreme move to address political troubles around the geographic and social cleavages that had dominated the Ugandan protectorate from the early 1900s onward.[36] In a sociopolitical context where cleavages between the north and the central, southern, and eastern regions of recently independent Uganda often dominated, the UCI was remarkably national in scope. It was understood that the Institute had to reach out beyond central Uganda and engage with patients and families across the country. Epidemiologically, this was necessary, as many of the Burkitt's lymphoma patients were concentrated in the northern and eastern regions of the country.[37] There was also political value in the geographic reach of the Institute. By researching cancers found to be important in East Africa as a whole and not narrowly limiting the site's activities to Kampala and the surrounding area, this site transcended some of the rifts between northern and southern Uganda and the high politics of Buganda and the State House.[38] Although the support and nursing staff at the UCI were primarily Baganda, and, at the time, predominantly Catholic, these fieldworkers, administrators, and nurses learned languages, expanded the offerings of the kitchen to meet different dietary tastes, and rendered the city navigable to a largely rural patient and caretaker population who had little reason to leave their farms.[39] This isn't to say that Institute staff were blind to differences across the country. Difference mattered. The ethnicity and geographic location of patients and their family caretakers were carefully noted on "face sheets" in the patient files as the first entry. Nevertheless, on the wards, cancer subsumed other kinds of identities, whether it was the illness identity of being a cancer patient, cancer survivor, or caretaker of someone with cancer. The Institute was at once strikingly heterogeneous but also unified, mainly due to the common cause of researching and studying cancers.

CARING FOR WHOLE FAMILIES, NOT JUST INDIVIDUAL PATIENTS

In a photograph of an everyday scene at Mulago Hospital, taken by Ziegler in the late 1960s or early 1970s, women sit under the shade provided by a corridor walkway, holding small children or infants in their arms. Kids cluster together or swing around the pole supporting the awning. Laundry is laid out on the grass to dry. Woven bags hold food and other sundries. Today, if you walk through the open corridors of Mulago Hospital, you'll see a very similar dynamic where caretakers and children dominate the scene. Pediatric patients are accompanied not only by a parent but also siblings and additional family members. On pediatric wards, parents, especially mothers, are expected to provide the bulk of day-to-day care: feeding, changing bed linens, monitoring bathroom needs, and generally providing comfort—soothing the nerves as well as the fevers of patients.[40] This is a health-care context where the family serves as health insurance, nursing care, chef, and laundromat. Mothers of pediatric patients in particular are often caught between the needs of a sick child and the one or three additional children who come to the hospital as well. These dynamics of intensive caregiving in East African hospital settings, as historians of health and medical anthropologists note, can often be invisible to expatriate medical practitioners and local public health officials alike.[41]

These caretaking demands became obvious to Ziegler and colleagues within the first six months of opening the LTC, as Burkitt's lymphoma patients started coming into the center for care and treatment. Ziegler and his American colleagues found that the relatively narrow mandate of the research site did not map onto the realities of the disease burden of cancer or the ways in which Ugandan families allocated resources and provided care to the ill. As Ziegler remembered:

> After the safari the patients started to flow in. We quickly realized two things. Number one was that not everybody had Burkitt's lymphoma. Some of them had other stuff but we couldn't literally turn them away. We ended up being a children's cancer ward, basically. And we saw rhabdosarcomas and neuroblastomas and Wilms' tumor, retinoblastoma. Every children's tumor came to us because nobody knew what to do with them. And so we began to see every childhood cancer that there was in the country that could travel.
>
> The other interesting thing was that these parents, mostly moms but a few dads also brought the rest of their children with them. So they brought little kiddies, usually packed on their backs, and we gave the moms mattresses to sleep on under the kiddies' beds. So very quickly [the ward] filled up with families. The kid would be in the bed and the mom would be under the bed and the rest of the family would be under the bed with her. And we fed them all and we took care of them all and of course when the little kids came in, many of them had malaria. They had hookworm. They had all of this other stuff so we ended up treating everybody, literally. If mom came in with a cough she would have X-rays and if she had TB we would give her treatment. Pretty soon it was just a general-purpose ward with a focus on childhood cancer.[42]

Ziegler and his American colleagues understood that they were working in a caregiving landscape where their pediatric patients were entangled in much larger family support networks than most of their pediatric patients in Bethesda.[43] They understood that if they had any hope of treating Burkitt's lymphoma patients and controlling for infections on the wards, they would have to treat entire families.

Chemotherapy trials can be brutally long, requiring patients and their families to stay in residence at the UCI for several days and sometimes weeks at a time to monitor tumor regression and also to manage the side effects of treatment regimens, which could bring kidney failure and immunosuppression. The material circumstances facing the caretakers of patients mattered, particularly the agrarian rhythms of farming that are readily disrupted by multiple cycles of chemotherapy. A poorly timed chemotherapy cycle could mean losing the opportunity to plant seeds in the growing season or harvest before crop rot which means losing vital income. Parents were also concerned about halting education for their sick children. To meet patient caretaker and patient concerns about school, the LTC hired a full-time primary school teacher. To address concerns about planting seasons and following up with the needs of the rural homestead, they offered bus vouchers for parents and patients to go back and forth between Kampala and the village. Recognizing that hunger could deter patients from staying on, the hospital also provided several generous meals a day to both patients and their families.[44] Consider the memories of one of the longtime administrators who started working at the UCI in the 1960s when she was still a teenager:

> In those days, we actually had a tailor on site who would
> sew patient clothes of different sizes. We had sheets and towels,
> all in a supply room with cubbies. Let me tell you how we used
> to feed the patients. We used to go around in the morning and
> take orders . . . this one wants fish, that one wants chicken. We
> would use our switch boards to make the call down to the surgery
> in Kololo, which would make the food and deliver it. We would
> give breakfast in the morning with porridge and milk and maybe
> a bun . . . and dinner too. Patients were allowed to have one care-
> taker with them, and they usually stayed around Mulago. If they
> were Karamojong and came without any clothes, we would go
> into town and get them secondhand clothes to wear.[45]

These may strike you as small gestures, but this was a markedly different culture of supportive care than what was to be found on the wards of Lower Mulago Hospital, where families and patients had to fend for themselves. Ziegler and colleagues appreciated something that historians of health and healing in Africa have long discussed—the role of the "therapy management group" in determining the course, duration, location, payment system, and caretaking burden involved in providing relief for ill family members.[46] And I would suggest that these social interventions at the LTC were just as vital to patient survival as administering fluids after a chemotherapy course.

Day-to-day activities at the Institute settled into predictable routines. Ziegler and colleagues would arrive at the Institute between 8:00 and 8:30 a.m. They would gather in the nurses' breakroom and would discuss any events that happened during the night shift over steaming cups of coffee and tea. Then, they would proceed to the ward round, laying hands on bodies, ordering blood counts, and marking tumor regression or growth. The wards were usually full, and so ward rounds would last until 11:00 or 11:30 a.m. Staff would then take a brief tea break and prepare patients for lumbar punctures and bone marrow aspirations as needed, as well as chemotherapy orders. To save time and also to spare the pediatric patients from the worst pain of a bone marrow aspirate, they autoclaved lumbar puncture and bone marrow needles together in the same bundled kit, administered a calming dose of Demerol, and then quickly drew spinal fluid while the child was held down. They would run the spinal fluid to the laboratory on site and, if necessary, administer methotrexate to mitigate central nervous system involvement for Burkitt's lymphoma. They averaged between five and six children an hour. After procedures there was a brief lunch break, and the afternoon was then devoted to seeing outpatients and running the general-purpose clinic for patient families and attending to the "lumps and bumps" referrals from Lower Mulago Hospital. Afternoons often also meant continuing education and teaching in the form of journal clubs, lectures, or rounding in the main hospital. By 4 p.m. on most days, activities would be finished. Doctors would go for a swim or off to play tennis, and then families would congregate for dinner. Patients would look forward to dinner and to another (one hoped) quiet night on the wards. These daily cycles of rounding, evaluation of patients' blood counts and liver functions, drug administration, downtime, outpatient care, education for both medical students and patients, and all-important meals formed the backbone of everyday life on the wards.[47]

Americans on staff brought a sense of urgency in the style of "Cornell medicine," which is Ziegler's gloss for tending to emergencies and providing care with swiftness and alacrity. Makeshift dialysis units, punishing night shifts, and hustling to get blood diagnostic workups done in a timely fashion was the norm, and in contrast to a style of medicine practiced in Lower Mulago, which was more crowded, more chaotic, and largely structured around clearing beds as quickly as possible. Within about six months of opening the center, Ziegler himself fell ill with a bad case of meningitis. British and Ugandan colleagues alike urged him to dial down the pace of tending to emergencies or risk burnout.[48]

It became clear over the course of 1967 that there were also a sizeable number of adults with interesting tumors, including Kaposi's sarcoma, hepatocellular carcinoma, and melanoma. The NCI provided the funds and staff for an additional ward to open—the Solid Tumor Center (STC)—run by Dr. Charles Vogel, another young American chemotherapist. In 1968 the STC opened in a former surgery building. Together, the LTC and STC made up the Institute. In contrast to New Mulago Hospital, which was designed with 850 beds in mind—but that often saw at least two hundred more "floor cases" at any given time in the 1960s—the scale of the operations at the Institute, with its forty beds, was appreciably smaller. Even with the general-purpose outpatient family clinic and the "lumps and bumps" policy of at least seeing all the referrals of cancer from the bottom of the hill, the emphasis was on Burkitt's lymphoma, Kaposi's sarcoma, hepatocellular carcinoma, and malignant melanoma. The need to create reliable data and standardized disease staging and blood workup protocols shaped a strong culture of diligent excellence at the Institute. But cultivating research excellence necessitated triage. They simply could not treat everything. From its inception, the raison d'être of the Institute was to engage in cancer research. It was never supposed to be the only cancer hospital in the country. These forty beds were never meant to care for Uganda's total cancer burden. Nevertheless, Ugandan patients and patient caretakers began to reshape the scope and mandate of the LTC shortly after the doors opened.

"MAKING FRIENDSHIP" AT THE LTC

Africanizing oncology required tailoring cancer research and care protocols to the realities of constrained medical resources at a place like Mulago. The systems and protocols created to support clinical trials at the LTC stand in marked contrast to the experiments conducted by Burkitt in the early 1960s. However, Burkitt's key research method, the tumor safari, provided a model for shaping a key aspect of the UCI's experimental infrastructure—the patient follow-up safari. Just as the needs of patients and their families shaped care on the wards, so too did patients and families shape Burkitt's lymphoma patient care and follow-up. Creating long-term cancer survival data was only possible through forming lasting relationships with patients and patient caretakers both at the urban referral hospital and in their largely rural village homes.[49]

The rigorous patient follow-up program at the UCI was developed by Mr. Aloysius Kisuule, a Ugandan clinical medical officer, and Dr. Richard Morrow, an American epidemiologist working for the World Health Organization.[50] Morrow came to Kampala with his family in 1966. His time there overlapped with Burkitt's for about two weeks, during which period Morrow charted a course of initial inquiry: What happened to the Burkitt's lymphoma patients that Kyalwazi and Burkitt had treated with a variety of cytotoxic drugs over the past decade? Were they still alive? Had they died or become debilitated? Were they still living with their parents in villages that spanned from Koboko in the farthest corner of West Nile bordering Zaire, or the bustling border town of Busia on the road from eastern Uganda to western Kenya? Uganda is characterized by extraordinary linguistic, ethnic, and geographical diversity, and Morrow faced a unique challenge in adapting routine methods of case finding in epidemiology to this heterogeneous landscape. In contrast to Burkitt, who relied almost entirely on European or African medical professionals, Anglophone linguistic networks (with the exception of Mozambique), and hospital records on his tumor safaris, Morrow would need to directly engage with villages and patient families to map survival patterns.[51]

Recognizing the cultural, social, and linguistic chasm between himself and patients and their families, Morrow did something both wise and ordinary—he asked his colleagues who they would recommend among Mulago's expanding number of Ugandan medical officers to act as a translator and case finder for the initial work of tracking down Burkitt's lymphoma patients long lost to follow-up. This was how he and Kisuule came to work together. Kisuule was a medical officer working in the pediatric ward at Mulago who also happened to know twenty of Uganda's thirty to forty languages, "including the northern ones, which were not Bantu."[52] Kisuule first worked in patient follow-up in the 1960s, and later served as the principal administrator of the Uganda Cancer Institute in the 1970s. On the wards, Kisuule was frequently brought in to translate, especially for patients who were coming from the north and not able to "hear" their own languages in the Bantu language of Luganda, which was commonly spoken by Ugandan nurses and part of the medical vocabulary the *bazungu* (White people) were able to pick up over time. The Americans who worked with Kisuule described his counseling of patients, linguistic ability, perseverance, and intrepidness as "truly extraordinary."[53]

Kisuule became interested in working as a medical officer early in life: "Right from birth I liked treating patients. [I had] that personal feeling that I would like to treat patients, to take care, especially of the children." After going through training as a clinical officer in Mbale Town, he was sent to Karamoja, which was (and in many ways still is) a socially isolated, remote part of Uganda, where most make their livelihood through cattle herding rather than banana planting. "It is the largest district mind you in Uganda. I was helped by learning Karamojong in six months. I was purely speaking Karamojong. Therefore, I didn't find problems with the Karamojong. Indeed, they were wild."[54] Kisuule's commitment to learning the language, of going out into villages for outreach on a regular basis, and building relationships with local political authorities enabled his clinical work during this time.

After four years in Karamoja, Kisuule applied for a transfer to Mulago Hospital and was posted to the pediatric outpatient section in Mulago, where his work was "purely clinical":

> You don't have any machines to help you. You are just look-ing at the patient, sensitizing him or her on your findings, what you are actually doing, and why you are doing it. That is clinical to me because we didn't have a laboratory. We didn't take blood from the fingers to find malaria parasites and so on. But you had it in your head, this clinical medicine enabling [you to decide] that this patient may be suffering from malaria, pneumonia, and so on.[55]

At Mulago, Kisuule developed a reputation for working well with patients and their families, engaging in his "purely clinical" style of education and interaction. When Morrow asked around for referrals to medical officers with linguistic acumen and an ability to interact well with families from all over Uganda, Kisuule immediately came to mind.

When Morrow and Kisuule started working together in 1966 and 1967, they had little to work with other than a list of patients from Burkitt and their accompanying "face sheets" of basic patient information that were routinely filled in on admission to Mulago Hospital. These sheets recorded names of patients and their relatives, age information, "tribe," diagnosis and date of admission, and where the patients were from.[56] Using this data, Kisuule set about tracking down patients who had been treated by Burkitt and Kyalwazi for follow-up interviews. Questionnaires would provide baseline demographic and survival data for Morrow to work with as an epidemiologist. Their research instrument of choice was the Volkswagen Beetle. As Kisuule recalls:

This patient follow up was more than 7 years. It was made up by experiences. Memory. Long drives. Mud going through the bush. . . . These long drives were very tiresome. Driving Volkswagen Beetles. They are really helpful. They can go through swamp.

Kampala to Gulu is 200 miles. Kampala to Fort Portal is 194. You can see. Fort Portal is in the West. Gulu is in the North East. Right up to Moroto is 336 miles from Kampala. From Moroto to Kaabong is 175. You can see. You can see Uganda.[57]

The geographic distribution of Burkitt's lymphoma across Uganda structured data collection for survival analysis in time-consuming ways. The system of roads functioned as the connective tissue linking major towns, but for the most part Uganda was still largely off the tarmac—and it still is today. Being a long-term patient at the UCI required travel to Kampala and thus familiarity with buses and an ability to navigate the city upon arrival. The long distances covered with the attendant challenges of mud, swamp, and fatigue for Kisuule and other UCI fieldworkers demanded patience and time. The long distances from Kampala and central Buganda also meant that the cultural, linguistic, and ethnic terrain encountered was quite different and variegated. Independence in Uganda in 1962 did not translate into a national project of smoothing over the heterogeneity of the country's agricultural, ethnic, and linguistic makeup. If anything, independence further entrenched cultural, linguistic, and ethnic divides between the northern part of the country and the rest of Uganda. Americans who worked in Uganda in the 1960s and 1970s remember these divisions as largely linguistic and cultural ones—the "Nilotic" speakers of the north and the "Bantu" speakers living below the dividing line of Karuma Falls. The Ugandans I interacted with from this period—mostly administrators and fieldworkers self-identifying as Baganda—remember these divides largely through the abolition of the kingdoms and the exile of the kabaka. For a Muganda such as Mr. Tom Tomusange, Obote's biggest political problem was that the president couldn't understand the importance of having a king because he was deprived of one in the north.

Despite the connectivity of roads, the networks of missionary and government hospitals, the movement of foodstuffs to the city, the circulation of daily newspapers, and the soundscape of radio across the country, fieldworkers from the UCI were inevitably strangers when they showed up in remote villages looking for patients. Kisuule remembered that on this long driving, on this tiresome driving, approaching patients was the problem because you were surrounded by them and the village chief along with his *askaris* (soldiers or guards) and so on.

To know who is this foreigner, though I'm an African. In Uganda, I was a foreigner in those areas. It took me time to get in and out and then to say please, can we see the patients? Can I be introduced to where his home is and taken there. And then they would say no no, he's actually doing something else. I would say no please, I am honest in my approach to you. . . . And then succeeding to get into that home and beginning interviews with these people, it took time.[58]

Taking time was part of Kisuule's "careful approach" to finding patients and conducting patient follow-up work. After gaining permissions and access from village chiefs to find and approach patients, Kisuule also had to ensure that family members understood his reasons for visiting the households of patients in order to fill out questionnaires and also in some cases to take blood for serum studies on the relationship between Burkitt's lymphoma and malaria. In these interactions, both the careful approach of taking one's time, and facility with language were critical in engaging with families and parents:

AK: I made headway in that area my friends. Mothers, mothers like children very much as you like yourselves so when you have a child from ward A from the labs you make friendship. And then you are using their own language. Idhi nade. You are in Lango. Wachano. You are in Luo. Maata. You are in Karamoja. And you go to the West. Muraho. You are in Rwanda.

This sort of thing. You are looking for the family, the sibling. You have made friendship with the mother first, therefore you are friends with the family.

MM: And friendships with the fathers?

AK: They are looking at what you are doing. They are listening to your words. They are dictating in mind what you are doing. Sort of investigating. Ahhh, they look at you suspiciously mostly for the whole day. If you have this method of going out soon you don't get what you want. You need time.[59]

Both up country in the village and on the wards of Mulago Hospital beyond the LTC, Kisuule understood how to take his time in establishing relationships. In my own experiences of conducting fieldwork in Uganda, I quickly discovered that it is considered rude to be in a hurry. Greetings are elaborate performances of interest and concern. A willingness to take your time and have a cup of tea, or to walk at a smooth and steady pace in town—these are all ways that people perform politeness. Kisuule and Morrow recognized this, and in their initial follow-up of patients who had been treated by Burkitt at Mulago in the 1950s and 1960s, they wrote: "We attribute our success to having a non-hurried approach, in particular to being willing to spend considerable time explaining what we were doing to people encountered in our searches. After this explanation information was often forthcoming that the informant either denied knowing beforehand or did not bother to remember."[60] Kisuule embodied a common sense in Uganda that transcended ethnic and regional variation. Part of this, of course, was through his linguistic acumen and his ability to speak fluidly across Uganda. But Kisuule also understood, in a sort of deep commonsensical way as well, the gendered and familial dynamics of everyday caregiving for sick children, which most usually fell on mothers or female kin, and the necessity of gaining approval for travel and treatment from fathers or other male heads of household. Kisuule's approach of engaging with mothers and "making friendship" through the work of socializing and quietly listening before approaching fathers with travel requests was time consuming, but necessary for ensuring that patients would actually come to the Institute (and keep coming back).

As a historian-ethnographer in 2012, it took several weeks of effort tapping into old UCI networks to find a working phone number for Kisuule and to arrange an interview. Riding with me in the RAV4 was Mr. Nsalabwa, the UCI's former X-ray technician. We stopped to pick up sugar, salt, and meat on the roadside before driving down an increasingly narrow dirt track into banana gardens. An elderly man with a gray beard and cloudy eyes was there, leaning on a cane, and he came out to greet us. We sat on a wooden bench inside his clinic's examination room and talked. Kisuule remembered the Americans as generous—salaries were much better at the UCI than they were in usual government posts—a real "incentive to the worker."[61] Issues of compensation aside, more than thirty years later, Kisuule's memories that remain of working with Morrow, Ziegler, and other Americans conjured paternal relations. Talking about the history of the UCI when we were taking a tour of the LTC in October 2012, he said, "It was through obedience and commitment that this place was built."[62] And it was largely through Kisuule's work in patient outreach and follow-up that Ziegler, Morrow, and others were able to turn clinical outcomes into meaningful survival data points.

THE MULTIPLE MEANINGS OF THE UCI

For the Ugandan physicians, medical students, and staff who worked at the UCI in the 1960s and early 1970s, research opportunities made the hospital at the top of the hill the best place for serious study. In contrast to Lower Mulago, where the work of a medical officer was largely relegated to pushing patients out of beds as quickly as possible, the UCI offered young medical officers and students an opportunity to learn how to conduct clinical trials and do the routine medical procedures needed to evaluate oncology patients. For Charles Olweny, as part of the inaugural master's-level medicine class, the Institute marked a place where he could engage in cutting-edge research for his master's thesis, rather than write an essay on typhoid fever.[63] For Institute staff, such as Tomusange, Kisuule, and Nsalabwa, the salaries were excellent, and standards were high. Decades later in interviews, Nsalabwa and Tomusange were especially keen in their recollections of the UCI's legendary parties that apparently flowed with beer and surged with dancing and music.[64]

For the Burkitt's lymphoma patients, many of them between the ages of five and ten, the LTC and the bone marrow procedures area in particular were dreaded places. One of Ziegler's first patients, whose cancer was cured by chemotherapy treatments alone and is today herself a medical doctor, was thirteen years old when she started treatment at the Institute. On at least one occasion, anticipating another round of chemotherapy, she told her attending physician that she was just going to head to town to pick up a few things in between her blood draws and her first drug dose of the day. She vanished from Mulago and only came back the next week to continue treatment.

For the young American physician Dr. Avrum Bluming, working at the Institute was, in his words, "fun" but also an opportunity to potentially cure cancer. In the United States, Bluming had given up on pediatric oncology after treating a child with retinoblastoma at the NCI who subsequently died because the drugs didn't work.[65] At the LTC, it was different: many of the kids actually got better and stayed better. As he remembered, it was an "incredibly empowering feeling."[66] Other American physicians like Dr. Robert Comis were similarly struck by the power of these drugs to induce remissions. Comis remembered treating one patient in particular whose tumor did in fact melt away over the course of a night shift after receiving drugs.[67]

For American researchers, there was also the excitement of being in a newly independent African country, of enjoying Kampala's excellent restaurants and beautiful weather, and of course, up-country drives. Vogel, who is remembered by his Ugandan colleagues as extremely social and outgoing, maintains that most of his closest American expatriate friends were actually CIA operatives, many of whom he played regularly with at the Kampala Rugby Club. He remembered:

> The Rugby Club and families and camp followers became our family's home away from home. Drank lots of beers, sang lots of songs and the club became one of the focal points of our family's social life. Once, a local former rugby player, a sergeant named Idi Amin stopped by to talk and joke around with us. . . . Amin must have been an imposing player standing well over 6 feet tall and weighing well over 200 pounds. I remember him as friendly, jovial and very sociable. Fortunately that was my only encounter with him during my four years in Uganda but certainly not my last encounter with members of his secret police during 1972 and 1973.[68]

Those who planned the LTC did not see it as a paternalistic gift from the British in the spirit of New Mulago Hospital nor as an exclusively nationalist project.[69] Rather, the colleagues who built the center saw it as a symbol of international cooperation and as a practical site for carrying out cutting-edge cancer research. From their perspective, they were building the space to potentially nurture a future Nobel Prize winner.[70] Looking back on the memories of the Ugandans who built this Institute, they may seem overly wistful about generous salaries, the abundance of meat and *matooke* (a large green banana), and the high standards of care. The memories of the Americans who built this experimental infrastructure fifty years ago may also seem overly sanguine, buoyed by a combination of therapeutic optimism, cheerful adventurism, and appreciation for the buzz of Kampala.[71] To understand this nostalgia, we must consider what happened next.

3 ❧ Africanizing Oncology in Idi Amin's Uganda

In November 1972, the Lasker Foundation recognized Uganda Cancer Institute (UCI) physician-researchers working on Burkitt's lymphoma. They were honored as part of the cohort of international cancer chemotherapists who demonstrated that chemotherapy drugs could bring about durable long-term remissions for leukemia, lymphomas, and other cancers.[1] The data on remissions in Ugandan Burkitt's lymphoma patients suggested that the cancer was potentially curable, either with cyclophosphamide or using combined chemotherapy treatments of cyclophosphamide, methotrexate, and vincristine.[2] Since 1955, the National Cancer Institute (NCI) had poured over $400 million into chemotherapy experiments in the United States and farther afield. As Mary Lasker put it, "A fairly large number of cancers can now be cured, or prolonged survival achieved, with drugs. . . . We now have an extra push in the form of more funds and the potentialities of immunotherapy. By and large, neither the public nor most of the medical profession is fully aware of what can be done. We are highlighting the progress that has been made and the men who have contributed outstandingly to it."[3] But while Lasker honorees were sipping on cocktails and exchanging stories at the awards ceremony in New York, the political situation in Kampala was rapidly deteriorating. Idi Amin came to power in 1971 in a military coup. When Amin declared an "economic war" in 1972 and announced the expulsion of Ugandan South Asians, whose community was largely responsible for trade and commerce, British and American research scientists working at the UCI started to contemplate leaving for their personal and familial safety and stability.[4]

A fierce debate ensued at the UCI. Should they close the unit and halt the research programs, including the necessary multiyear follow-up with patients to see if Burkitt's lymphoma could in fact be cured by chemotherapy treatments? Or should they keep the Institute open in a political climate where doctors, civil servants, and even vice chancellors were being put into the trunks of cars and murdered, never to be seen again?[5] The solution they saw was to accelerate the Africanization of leadership at the Institute and entrust day-to-day operations to one newly NCI-trained Ugandan oncologist, Dr. Charles Olweny. He and his team of Ugandan fieldworkers, technicians, nurses, and administrators would keep the UCI open and continue to run studies, provide care, and follow up with long-term survivors of Burkitt's who were scattered across Uganda. The NCI would provide drugs and additional financial support. Amid profound political and economic chaos, Ugandan researchers generated a decade's worth of knowledge about the relationship between chemotherapy treatments and Burkitt's survival.[6]

Throughout the 1970s, UCI staff continued to follow up with long-time Burkitt's lymphoma patients through ongoing patient outreach and site visits across the country. Out of a cohort of over two hundred patients, only about 6 percent were lost to follow-up in Idi Amin's Uganda.[7] In any long-term cohort study, losing 6 percent to follow-up would be quite remarkable. This success was all the more impressive in a context where, as historian John Iliffe puts it, "the near disintegration of the state in the 1970s and 1980s during General Amin's military tyranny and the prolonged succession struggle that followed" unraveled Ugandan health services.[8] Mulago Hospital was hit particularly hard during the 1970s, and institutional atrophy and infrastructural decline was highly visible. As Iliffe says: "Its [Mulago's] piped water supply broke down in 1974 for a decade. The mortuary's refrigeration system was out of action from 1975 and sewerage ceased to function at about the same period. . . . At that time [1978] not one of the hospital's twelve X-ray units was functioning. . . . Yet they kept the hospital functioning."[9] Further up Mulago Hill at the UCI, the situation was less dire. This is due in part to the small scale of the UCI itself but also to international financial support and national political interests. The international pipeline from the Americans at the NCI stocked the UCI with drugs and money for salaries until 1977, when the Ugandan government then took over and provided financial support. This drug supply and financing made it possible to maintain a high-level research profile at the Institute. Olweny and his colleagues published four to five scientific papers a year during the 1970s, mainly on the subject of combination chemotherapy trials for Burkitt's lymphoma, hepatocellular carcinoma, and Kaposi's sarcoma.[10] Cancer research continued to demand a high standard of everyday clinical care. Accounts from colleagues working during this period suggest that the wards of the UCI were usually full and patients were, for the most part, well fed.[11] Committed administrators, resourceful nurses, politically savvy physicians, and artful technicians demonstrated to Amin's government that they were engaged in cutting-edge research in Africa by and for Africans. In turn, Amin's government used the UCI as a showpiece of Africanized research for international visitors.[12] This is not to say that the UCI was somehow immune to the slow unraveling of the licit economy, food security, infrastructural stability, and personal safety in 1970s Uganda. Indeed, this slow deterioration made it increasingly difficult for African physician-researchers to remain at the center of international scientific networks as knowledge producers and oncologists rather than simply as intermediaries processing patient bodies for study and exchange.[13]

Mr. Aloysius Kisuule remembered the 1970s as "this political era, the deep years, where all progress was destroyed. All efforts were interfered with. Physically, morally, economically as such things."[14] Nevertheless, staff at the UCI kept practices and patients alive. The Amin years impacted cancer research and care in a variety of ways. It accelerated the Africanization of ownership of the Institute. Political and infrastructural instability made it increasingly difficult to be an equitable partner in research programs. At the same time, as the mystery of Burkitt's lymphoma survival was largely solved over the course of the 1970s, the significance of maintaining a Burkitt's lymphoma study cohort waned. This made it all the more challenging to make Uganda an attractive place for internationally sponsored cancer chemotherapy clinical trials. The UCI became increasingly reliant on the state rather than international scientific networks for patronage.

Taking these events into account, this chapter moves beyond the narrative of the "disintegrating state," as Iliffe puts it, an overly corrective championing of everyday agency that glosses over the violent stakes of this period, or a tale of irrevocable loss after the withdrawal of NCI funds from the UCI in 1977.[15] Instead, it examines how Ugandans navigated these challenges, tried to maintain a sense of normalcy, and retained a commitment to doing good work. In particular, I focus on the ways Ugandan staff maintained and repaired the Institute's experimental infrastructure in the 1970s. UCI staff worked to maintain patient safaris, ward-rounding practices, chemotherapy administration protocols, shipping contracts, salaries, and meal preparation. Theories of repair and maintenance allow us to think more explicitly about the relationships between medical research and the social and material technologies that made medical research possible. The 1970s at the UCI exemplified what science and technology studies scholar Steven J. Jackson has called "repair worlds." Jackson suggests that "we take erosion, breakdown, and decay, rather than novelty, growth, and progress, as our starting points [and take an approach that emphasizes] deep wonder and appreciation for the ongoing activities by which stability (such as it is) is maintained, the subtle arts of repair by which rich and robust lives are sustained against the weight of centrifugal odds, and how sociotechnical forms and infrastructures large and small, get not only broken but *restored*, one not-so-metaphoric brick at a time."[16] We will see that maintenance and repair, clever workarounds, and alternative routes can only go so far, though, in a context where infrastructures such as the market economy, electricity grid, and roads fall into crisis.

With regard to sources, I draw heavily upon the UCI's institutional records from this period. UCI staff wrote volumes of correspondence and patient follow-up reports that proved to be invaluable resources in reconstructing the 1970s. These archival records are complemented by oral histories, memoirs, and medical journals. These materials show that the lived experiences for medical staff and patients at the UCI in the 1970s varied widely. Some were forced into self-imposed exile in Uganda and feared talking about those events in oral histories decades later. They requested that the recordings be destroyed and that their private lives remain private. Others at the UCI were able to make international medical careers that reached far beyond the country. For many patient families, life continued on farms. People continued to grow starchy food staples and cook *matooke* (a large green banana). They kept chicken coops clean. They searched for the goat that chewed through her rope and got lost. Children still went to school. In Kampala, many directly benefited from the redistributions of the economic war. The photographer Deo Kyakulagira split his time between Makerere's Department of Medical Illustration and his new photography shop, the Central Art Studio.[17] At the Institute, life and death went on. As Olweny wrote in his memoir:

Life during the Amin era was not as bad as many depicted it. If you did your work and avoided confrontation with his soldiers you were safe. I did precisely that. I would leave my house in the morning, drop my kids off at school and collect them in the evening and we would be home in our safe haven by six in the evening. Amin did not have much to show the outside world. The Uganda Cancer Institute was one such show piece. He made sure that every Government guest visiting Uganda was brought to the Uganda Cancer Institute to show case how Ugandan institutions were running smoothly and efficiently. [Visitors from the World Health Organization] marveled the way this centre was functioning in the midst of chaos.[18]

It is estimated that between eighty thousand and three hundred thousand Ugandans lost their lives over the decade due to state-related violence.[19] But for the ten million or so Ugandans who survived the 1970s, whether civil servants, farmers, or mechanics, life in this decade was punctuated by two extreme events: the 1972 declaration of the economic war and the 1978 invasion or liberation of Uganda by the Tanzanian army. Over the eight years of Idi Amin's tenure, which culminated in the fall of Kampala and the retreat of Amin's army in 1979, most Ugandans were touched in some way by the violence and uncertainty of the period. Many also developed strategic ways to ensure survival in difficult economic and political times. A prime example of this was the *magendo* (illicit market) that grew into prominence over the 1970s.[20] Another example was the UCI itself.

FROM THE FIRST TO THE ONLY: "CHARLES IS THE INSTITUTE"

From its inception, the UCI's founders intended to hand over the facilities and day-to-day services at the Institute to an entirely Ugandan staff in the early 1970s.[21] "By 1972 or 1973, only one or two [advisors seconded by the National Institute of Health (NIH)] will be necessary, and by 1975 the Uganda Cancer Institute will be administered totally by Ugandan doctors."[22] Olweny was the first trainee of what was envisioned as a much broader oncology training fellowship program and one of the early beneficiaries of this ethic of "Ugandanization" at Makerere Medical School, as part of the inaugural class of the master's program in medicine. The master's program hinged upon original research, and Olweny initially proposed a project on the epidemiology of typhoid fever. Dr. William Parsons, the convener of the class, took a brief look at the proposal and said, "Charles, sorry. There is nothing new in typhoid fever. It will never make a difference. . . . Go and think again." Cancer, rather than tropical illnesses, was at the forefront of medical research and excitement at Makerere, and Parsons directed Olweny to the top of Mulago Hill to meet Ziegler. Olweny remembered, "So I went and met Dr. John Ziegler. And he said, 'Oh, you are the very kind of person we are looking for. Someone young. Someone enthusiastic. Someone who can move things forward and I've heard a lot about you.'"[23]

Olweny collaborated with Ziegler and the staff at the UCI to design a randomized controlled trial of the treatment of adult Hodgkin's disease with chemotherapy drugs. This was seen as particularly innovative in a setting where no radiotherapy treatments were available. Over a two-year period, Olweny worked at the Lymphoma Treatment Center (LTC) on a periodic basis, mixing and administering different cytotoxic drug combinations to adults with Hodgkin's disease, and doing patient follow-up.[24] The results published in the journal *Cancer* in 1971 were well received by the international scientific community, many of whom were surprised that 76 percent of the patients achieved full remission through chemotherapy treatments alone.[25] As Olweny remembered it, "As a result of my work on Hodgkin's disease both Ziegler and the late Paul Carbone and late Sebastian Kyalwazi said, 'You know what, we better start capacity building, and he's the right person.'"[26]

One of the main reasons Olweny was particularly promising as the future Ugandan leader of the Institute was his ability to run a randomized chemotherapy clinical trial smoothly. Olweny was a talented chemotherapist. Drug mixing requires careful attention to calculating doses by body surface area—a humane, careful approach to administering the drugs is necessary to avoid tissue necrosis—and one needs an eye for managing adverse side effects. But perhaps more importantly, like the oncologists at the NCI, Olweny was excited about the potentially curative effects of chemotherapy and about the prospect of doing research on cancer in Uganda that would be relevant to the broader scientific community in Africa from Lagos to Nairobi. Olweny's enthusiasm for the method of the clinical trial and an ability to publish independent research made him the preferred candidate for training in Bethesda at the NCI.

In 1972, Amin declared an economic war and decreed that people of Asian descent would have ninety days to leave the country.[27] At the heart of Amin's economic war decree was an agenda for the Africanization of the Ugandan economy. According to Amin, no longer would Ugandans be beholden either to colonial masters demanding cotton for cash cropping or to

Asian businessmen hiking up the prices of basic commodities. Ugandans would own the means of production and commerce.[28] At least that was the theory. Over the 1970s, the reality of the Africanization of the Ugandan economy was quite different. The formal national Ugandan economy functioned on a very low level as the East African economic community collapsed, while a second shadow economy, based largely on coffee growing, goods smuggling, and subsistence cropping, began to thrive.[29] Over time, for many the Africanization of the economy would make everyday life and survival contingent on the illicit.[30]

In August 1972, Olweny was halfway through the training program in oncology at the NCI in Bethesda when he was told over the phone, "Better come back now. If you don't, there will be nothing to return to."[31] While Olweny finished the last of his training and his family packed their bags, acting UCI director Dr. Charles Vogel and LTC director Dr. Ian Magrath worked to ensure that Olweny would have something to return to. "Mulago is in turmoil. The medical school is going to have enough on its hands simply trying to supply health care and a modicum of teaching to the students,"[32] Vogel wrote to Ziegler on October 16, 1972. Vogel continued:

> It's an incredibly good thing I returned [from travels outside Uganda]. There were rumors going as high as the Ministry that I would not return and that NIH was cutting aid. Kyalwazi was visibly moved by my return and the words of NIH support I brought with me. The Ambassador feels the UCI is one of the best things the US is doing in Uganda and with our goal of Ugandanization almost completed, the continued support is another example of US goodwill. My personal appearance here, as suspected was an invaluable shot in the arm for Ugandan-US relations.
>
> Professor Kibunamusoke . . . says he will place no obstacles in the path of our future plans for the institute. By this I assume he means that he will not call on Charles too heavily for routine Dept. of Medicine chores. He is fully aware that Charles is the Institute and the only hope for continuing support and expansion.[33]

Negotiating with the dean, Vogel and Ziegler were able to secure an appointment for Olweny in the Department of Medicine. This guaranteed housing and institutional status, but it also meant ongoing teaching and administrative duties within an increasingly stretched department. "We'll have to work, from within, to carve out his autonomy," noted Vogel.[34]

As a postscript, Vogel wrote: "Dr. Rwakihembo thanked me very much for our support during this time of need and reaffirmed the Ministry's intention of helping to keep the UCI going. He did mention practically however, that at the present time changes just seem to be happening often without the Ministry knowing in advance. E.g. the sudden expulsion of Prof. McAdam, Trussell and Dr. Barkham. I guess that is all for now. I shall try to get this into the pouch today."[35] McAdam's departure was due to a series of recommendation letters he wrote for his expelled Asian students and physicians at Mulago Hospital so they could take up further studies or medical positions elsewhere in the British Commonwealth. Amin's government caught wind of this work, and McAdam and his family were expelled from the country as well. They were given twenty-four hours. So they boarded up the house, shot the dogs, and tried to ensure the safety and financial support for the staff at the house in Kololo. To the best of my knowledge, McAdam did not return to Uganda during his life.[36]

Olweny reported for duty in Kampala in March 1973 and met with the head of the medicine department at Makerere, who said, "Charles, welcome back. You are going to run the Cancer Institute."[37] Olweny remembered, "I said, me? What do I know about this?" The medicine department head said, "Yes. You will run the cancer Institute. Don't you worry. Go and meet with Professor Kyalwazi." Kyalwazi met with Olweny that same week. "When we met, he held my arms and said, 'son, don't you worry. We are here to support you.' He did. He was there to support me. Every week, he came for ward rounds."[38] This moment echoes the experiences of many Ugandan physicians who remained at Mulago Hospital and Makerere Medical School in the 1970s. Circumstances in the 1970s recast these figures as the only Ugandan experts in their fields. They faced the herculean task of maintaining a national referral hospital and medical school in the midst of stock outs, political uncertainty, and mercurial violence. Much of this labor rested on the shoulders of newly trained specialist African physician-researchers like Olweny who were charged with keeping departments and units going almost entirely on their own.[39]

As the only practicing medical doctor with formal oncology training, Olweny realized that he needed to delegate labor on the wards wherever possible. Before Amin, medical doctors at the UCI were responsible for chemotherapy preparations and administration of drugs to patients. Olweny hired two chemotherapy nurses to take up these practices and invested his time in training nurses to be able to manage everyday drug complications. To make up for fewer physicians on the wards, Olweny also set up a research fellowship program for student health officers in their fourth year of training. The students were put in charge of emergencies and night duty on the wards.[40]

Olweny's experience as *the only* oncologist working in Uganda in the 1970s mirrors the experiences of many of the other physicians who survived purges and disappearances at Makerere Medical School. Professor Raphael Owor, who served as dean of the medical school for much of the 1970s, was also the only pathologist. He managed the pathology laboratory, taught tissue fixation methods, ran the cancer registry, and worked as an administrator. When I met Owor for an interview at his private laboratory in June 2012 and asked how he managed to keep a pathology laboratory up and running in the 1970s, he took me into his bench area and pointed to the microscope and to his temple. With these two things—some good optics and a sound mind—he noted, you could run a pathology service. As long as you were strategic and ordered formalin in bulk, you could keep a laboratory open.[41] Maintenance of basic equipment, strategic ordering of supplies, and stocking a handful of essentials that could be used either to treat a broad variety of medical conditions or run laboratory tests were indispensable to keeping the only oncology and pathology services in the country open.[42]

Ugandan physicians could have left the country and worked anywhere overseas. What compelled them to stay? Part of it was the paternalistic nature of medical education itself. Olweny, Owor, and others felt a strong filial duty to the mentors who had chosen them to lead the country as the first Ugandan experts in oncology, pathology, and other fields. Physicians were greatly obligated to their teachers and mentors, sometimes described as fathers, to keep units and facilities open and running under this process of accelerated Ugandanization. Medicine was also a way to keep the national interest at heart. They were committed to serving and caring for Uganda: the people, the patients, the landscape, the national project. The status as the only specialists made it all the more essential to stay on and keep things going in Uganda for Ugandans.

COHORT MAINTENANCE

When Olweny took over the day-to-day operations at the Institute in 1973, he inherited a broad spectrum of research activities. It was, as Olweny put it, "a lot of balls in the air."[43] Research at the Institute in the 1960s had already established the tumor's pathology, responsiveness to treatment, geographical distribution, and potential links to Epstein-Barr virus (EBV), making Burkitt's lymphoma a useful model for continued study on cancer therapeutics, etiology, and epidemiology.[44] In the 1970s, research at the Institute focused on three critical areas: (1) the long-term survival of patients treated for Burkitt's lymphoma; (2) better drug regimens to prevent tumor relapse and the involvement of the central nervous system; and (3) EBV, the environment, malaria, and their relationship to the development of Burkitt's lymphoma.[45]

Staff at the Institute maintained a cohort of approximately 109 long-term Burkitt's lymphoma survivors across Uganda.[46] These survivors were part of a larger cohort initiated in 1967 comprising 240 patients who were treated and studied from 1967 to 1977. During this time, 155 died either from complications of late-stage disease, illness relapse, or other causes. Sixteen patients were lost to follow-up.[47] Writing about these patients in a ten-year retrospective analysis of Burkitt's lymphoma survival in Uganda, Olweny et al. noted, "All attempts to trace them have been unsuccessful because they have crossed the national borders into neighboring Kenya, Rwanda, Sudan, Tanzania or Zaire. Most of these patients are probably still alive judging by remission status in excess of 1 year when last seen."[48]

Throughout the 1970s, patient follow-up was the essential research activity at the UCI. As Olweny remembered, "The UCI made its name not only because we were able to treat people well, but we were able to follow up everyone. And we knew what happened to *every* patient. . . . During those days they literally had to drive to West Nile. To Northern Uganda. To Eastern Uganda. To Karamoja. To trace these patients. And we traced everybody."[49] Patient follow-up was also the research project that could not be outsourced from Uganda and carried on with patient cohorts in the United States or the United Kingdom. Perhaps not surprisingly, a considerable amount of financial and human resources was put into these efforts. Maintaining the follow-up of this study population under Public Health Service contracts, the National Cancer Institute, and a grant from the National Research Council of Uganda was a sizeable chunk of change. For example, in the $142,871 total budget for the UCI for 1975–76, patient follow-up and fuel and vehicle maintenance totaled $25,000, or about half of the operation's budget not cordoned off for salaries.[50]

In the 1970s, staff at the UCI built upon the foundation of patient outreach and follow-up methods established by Dr. Richard Morrow and Kisuule in the 1960s.[51] After Amin's coup in 1971, the work of "making friendship" entailed more than the social awareness of fieldworkers to negotiate with reluctant families who feared blood taking, hair loss, or Kampala city life. Fearing violence occurring along geographical and ethnic identity lines, many villagers and families associated with long-term care at the LTC were reluctant to leave the daily work of cultivation on their farms to make the journey.[52] Patient follow-up relied on time, fuel, political savvy, financial support, functioning vehicles, and above all, patience with families and patients.

Consider the routine patient safari conducted by the Uganda Cancer Institute's administrator, Mr. Tom Tomusange, in June 1971, approximately six months after Idi Amin's January coup. Driving a Volkswagen Beetle, Tomusange went eastward, past the banana gardens, sugarcane fields, and tea bushes. He drove through Jinja, over the Owens Falls dam that harnesses the power of the Nile River for electricity, and into the flatter lands of eastern Uganda. This is where papyrus and swamps dominate the landscape, just until the road curves northward into the green hills of Tororo and Mbale Town at the foot of Mount Elgon: coffee cultivation country. Upon arriving in the east, "The car was producing queer noise from the engine, and so I took it to Mbale Prudential Garage who cleared the carbulator [sic]."[53] After solving his vehicle problems, Tomusange spent the next twelve days visiting village homesteads, mainly to meet with the families of young children with Burkitt's lymphoma who either needed to come back to the Institute or who were in danger of being "lost to follow up." He also hoped to track down the reasons for the deaths of several patients who had not survived their cancer treatments at the Institute.

Traveling up into the area surrounding Soroti, Tomusange found several families facing financial troubles. These parents were short on cash for travel and in need of bus warrants in order to make the journey to Kampala.[54] Patients were also doing well. Patients were doing so well that they were in school, feeling fine, and not all that interested in coming back to the hospital for follow-up exams.[55] We can see this from Tomusange's reports:

6.6.71 ATIM (TESO)

She was also overdue. She was quite well growing up and at school in primary V. Father had paid a visit to a relative in Jinja. Yet he never bothered to come along with Atim since Jinja was near Kampala! however I told the mother to see that father brings Atim to LTC when he comes back. And I gave them bus warrants.

7.6.71 Engemu (Teso)

Engemu was late too. Father reported that he had no money for transport to LTC. Engemu was at school where I went with father and asked the Headmaster to let off Engemu for about three days for a check up at LTC. Father was given bus warrants.[56]

Tomusange proceeded to Obote's home district, Lango. There, patient families had concerns about financial resources for going to the UCI and anxieties about the potential for violence on the road to Kampala. In the previous six months, stories of fighting in Kampala in the wake of Amin's coup and the violent targeting of soldiers and civilians from Lango and Acholi faithful to Obote by Amin's police forces and army circulated through northern Uganda.[57] These stories, as well as roadblocks and uncertain travel conditions between Lira and Kampala, led around nineteen patients to default. Tomusange's mission was to convince up-country patients that rumors about Kampala were nothing to be concerned about. Tomusange reports:

7.6.71 Ojede (Lango)

This was my first home to visit in Lango after the overthrow of Dr. M. Obote (a Lango by tribe). Naturally I was fearing to visit Lango after hearing of Guerilla recruits (Pro-Obote) going on in Lango. People on the way were quiet and some looked depressed and very much suspicious and to ask for directions to somebody's home, I had to explain clearly the reason why I want to visit that home. Others could pretend to be visitors in that village and tell you that they don't know the man you are looking for. But in the end you find out the very man you are looking for to be their neighbor. This is the sort of situation I faced in most homes I visited in Lango. Ojede was supposed to return to LTC on 5.10.70.
    Father of Ojede was at home. But Ojede was no longer staying with them. He was taken away by grandmother which was about 6 miles away. The father was open to me. He even told me that the rumour-mongers had told him that there was fighting in Kampala that is why he feared to return in time. I reassured him that Kampala was quite okay. He accepted to go with me to Grandmother and collect Ojede and then bring him to LTC. On our way to the grandmother he told me that his sisters had advised him not to return the child to LTC and had wanted him to even tell me that Ojede had died!

I foresaw that if Father stayed another night at his home, he was going to be advised strongly not bring Ojede back to LTC and thus I had to drive them to Soroti to catch a night Express to Kampala that very day.[58]

Amin's coup and the uncertainty that followed compounded the challenges of negotiating with families and maintaining friendship. Fear of violence, anxiety, misinformation, and "rumor mongering" shaped both sides of the negotiations with families, as we can see from the efforts to bring Ojede back to the LTC for a follow-up visit. On the one hand, Tomusange was quietly concerned about the potential violence of a guerrilla attack in Lango, and on the other, fear of violence in Kampala shaped an elaborate strategy on the part of Ojede's family to keep him off the bus.[59]

In addition to new fears of violence in Kampala, parents and caretakers had old anxieties and distaste for blood-taking procedures at the LTC during follow-up care. As Tomusange writes about Ocan on 9.6.71:

> Parents here are very difficult. They told me that too much blood is drawn from their boy whenever he comes to LTC. And thus disliked the idea of returning their boy to LTC. I explained to them that the doctors at LTC take blood from Ocan and other patients at LTC not for drinking or for sale as Ocan's parents through but for tests which guide the doctors in the sort of treatment to give to Ocan and then patients at the LTC. I reassured them that all the tests done are meant to benefit the patient like Ocan and not to hurt him. They asked me for bus warrants and I issued them some. Note: But on 12.6.71 I checked on this home but Ocan was still at home. I very much doubt whether he will turn up.[60]

This distaste for the physical act of blood taking and the anxieties about where that blood would eventually go after collection is not surprising. Indeed, it reinforces much of what we know about the combination of revulsion and rumors about blood draws in eastern Africa.[61] I think this encounter with Ocan's parents also suggests that families tired of the *repetition* of what they were being asked to do over the course of the 1970s—regular blood draws, frequent travel to Kampala, and constantly answering questions. It is one thing to go to a hospital to seek treatment. It is another thing to continue to go to the hospital over the course of a decade for relentless, repetitive follow-up and bloodletting.[62]

Other families did not want to return to Kampala because of the divide between city life and village life, especially with regard to everyday comportment and dress styles.[63] Consider the father in Lango who was "only interested in drinks and not in his daughter and he doesn't mind about dressing. He is always half naked. Fear of coming to Kampala half naked, makes him dislike the idea of bringing Akomo to LTC. And money given to him for transport back to LTC, is used on drinks. I then had to buy him a vest of three shillings plus shorts of four shillings and then returned Akomo to Centre."[64] Tomusange's patient outreach work took on the quality of convincing families of patients that not only is the medical care meant to "help" and ensure that patients get well and stay well but that Kampala was still safe and navigable, even for Ugandans living in Lango and Acholi in northern Uganda.[65] Tomusange's labor involved ongoing maintenance of vehicles, social relationships with patients and their families, and reliable maps of where patients lived, which were carefully marked on patient follow-up reports.[66] These efforts ultimately determined whether or not these patients would be included as data points in cancer survival charts, and in some cases, whether or not they would return to Kampala for another round of chemotherapy.

Even in the quietest of political times, a Muganda gentleman traveling by Volkswagen Beetle wearing a black suit, fashionable tie, shiny shoes, a freshly pressed handkerchief in his suit pocket, and Ugandan flag lapel pin was an odd occurrence for those living in rural villages in remote corners of Uganda.[67] He looked like an intelligence agent of the Ugandan government or a tax collector. Asking for the location of a specific village home of a child known to be disfigured and then miraculously cured by a visit to Kampala was a delicate business, as it could draw unwanted attention to the social standing and potential misfortunes or triumphs of the patient's family in the village. During these visits, Tomusange presented himself as an *omusawo*, (a medical man) of Mulago Hospital, ready to help with information and bus vouchers.[68] This medical persona allowed for strategic distance, both from being an arbiter of state bureaucracy or directly associated with unexplained illness and bodily misfortune. Being a biomedical man also granted Tomusange greater mobility. Soldiers at roadblocks were willing to let Tomusange through without a scratch largely because he was able to produce papers that showed he worked at the UCI.[69] "If you told them that you were doing medical work," Tomusange recalled, "the soldiers would let you move more freely throughout the country."[70]

The key social technology of follow-up, the patient safari, remained remarkably durable and consistent over the course of the 1970s. Notes from UCI fieldworker Gerald Angala from a trip to the northern region in 1974 are full of the usual car troubles and missing patients that Tomusange encountered after Amin's coup. Angala writes: "I took the whole morning of Saturday resting and checking on the car which by now was consuming a lot of oil and had dropped the left tail pipe which was trodded on by a following lorry. After correcting these minor things and having taken lunch I visited Obalo in the afternoon. The mother of Obalo had gone with him in West Nile so I had to return to Gulu."[71] Vehicle troubles with leaking oil and lost tailpipes were "minor things," nuisances on the road to be contended with. Convincing patients to come to the UCI well after the dust of the coup settled in Kampala was challenging. Parents were busy working, patients were doing well, and the rhythms of life and social reproduction carried on in the farms and *shambas* (farms) well beyond Kampala.

During his trip, Gerald followed up with several of the patients Tomusange had visited in 1971. Engemu, a longtime Burkitt's lymphoma survivor, was one such patient. Gerald writes:

29.7.74 ENGEMU BL

A long time surviver [sic]—now in PIII [Primary Three], slim and fairly healthy. Engemu, mother and sisters were at home when I visited them on the afternoon of Monday en route to LIRA. The mother had just had a new baby the previous week. The father had gone to ORUNGO some thirty miles away to bring home an EMURON (a witch doctor) to come and perform general cure of the whole family including the new born, because it was through his works that the mother of Engemu had the new baby, otherwise the family had lost hope in getting one! Engemu the mother stated could therefore not travel with me to Kampala before EMURON did his work on him![72]

Gerald negotiated with the family and attempted to convince the parents that Engemu's older sister could escort her brother to Kampala after the cleansing ceremony, but the family had other concerns. The sister needed to go to Soroti to sell millet and was not home when Gerald came to escort them to the bus park. The father needed to look after cattle and was reluctant to let Engemu travel to Kampala on his own for follow up because, as the father put it, "his I.Q. is not that good."[73]

While some families were welcoming life and going through ritual cleanses to protect themselves, other families on Gerald's trip were mourning the dead. Oyik, a Burkitt's lymphoma patient, "became very ill and was taken to Kitgum hospital. He was later removed from the hospital as a hopeless case and taken home."[74] Up toward the Sudanese border, Ocen passed away two months prior in a remote village about six miles south of the border. "After reaching the home and finding Ocen's grandmother, I was told he died some two months back. The poor old woman could of course not tell me the D.O.D. [date of death]."[75] Angala was eventually fired from the UCI for stealing supplies and general dishonesty. It is hard to know if he was writing exaggerated truths, pure fiction, or a genuine account in this report, but if we take his accounts at face value, they offer a picture of life outside of Kampala in the east and the north. Families engaged in the everyday work of making farms productive, selling cattle, and cleansing households.

RESEARCH AND CARE ON THE WARDS

On the wards of the UCI, studying central nervous system relapse and better drug regimens for Burkitt's patients required both chemotherapy drugs and food. This necessitated supportive care, which was cast in broad terms to include bus vouchers, translation services on the wards, and a place to sleep for family members. Administrators, nurses, and technical and service staff continued to uphold these everyday courtesies at the UCI in the Amin period, recognizing that these practices were just as important as cytotoxic drug regimens.[76] The UCI went to great lengths to ensure that the food-catering program at the Institute continued to operate not only for patients and their families but also for the staff. There were periodic shortages. Suppliers sometimes fell flat, leading to periods when it was "extremely difficult to run this Unit without soap, salt, sugar and cooking oil."[77]

Chemotherapy for continuing NCI trials came to the UCI via Entebbe Airport. These drugs, offered for free through the Cancer Therapy Evaluation Branch of the NCI in Bethesda, served as the primary treatments and shaped the care at the UCI in the 1970s.[78] The availability of these drugs in Kampala was unique when compared to hospital centers spanning from Nigeria to Zambia. In the 1970s, Olweny astutely saw that in addition to the NCI's drug supplies, he would be well served in reaching out to the broader global cytotoxic pharmaceutical market and offer up beds and bodies in exchange for much-needed therapies and financial support.[79]

For example, the UCI collaborated with Kenyatta Hospital's radio-therapy department to examine the effect of radiotherapy on Burkitt's lymphoma. Since some of the drugs themselves were unavailable in Kenya, Olweny arranged to ship vials of the drug from Kampala to Nairobi via Akamba buses as part of this clinical trial along with the UCI's pediatric patients to Nairobi for radiotherapy.[80] The staff member in charge of weekly shipments of drugs to Nairobi did not return to the office one afternoon. He had been arrested and taken to Nakasero Hill by Amin's state services, where he was interrogated and charged with smuggling Ugandan drugs out of the country and into Kenya. Olweny went to Nakasero to attempt to bring the staff member back to the Institute in one piece and was charged with "stealing the Ugandan nation's drugs." Telling this story years later, Olweny recalled that he patiently explained what a clinical trial was to state police and tried to convince the soldiers to let him and his procurement officer go.[81] The state police were also familiar with the Institute, some of them having visited the UCI previously, perhaps to get an X-ray or receive antimalarial treatment. So they finally agreed to let Olweny go.[82] "But your man will stay here and we will release him tomorrow. And they didn't go back on their word. They released him the next day. But in retrospect people say you must have been a fool. How could you have gone? They could have arrested you and you would never be seen again."[83] Decades later, when I asked UCI staff to recall the ways in which the politics of Amin's regime shaped their daily lives, most declined to comment. Some said they had simply forgotten everything. Others feared either for their own personal safety or the potential to disrupt the lives of others.[84] Olweny's story about the Akamba bus is one of the few stories of close encounters with the potential violence of the state in the 1970s that colleagues were inclined to share.[85]

It is perhaps in the space of the UCI laboratory where we can see most clearly how the general erosion of infrastructure in Uganda in the 1970s impacted medical research and care.[86] When Olweny assumed the day-to-day operations of the UCI in 1973, he also assumed the directorship of the laboratory, where tissue cultures, tumor marker assays, and chemotherapy mixing took place. From 1973 to 1975 or so, many of these laboratory procedures and research projects were kept "in house" in Uganda.[87] But disruptions of electricity supplies in particular took a toll on this work. Take the following example. In November 1975, Olweny wrote to the chief engineer at the Electricity Board to voice his complaints about frequent disconnections of power to the UCI:

I would like to point out that Uganda Cancer Institute is a hospital and as such we find it extremely difficult to render efficient services to our patients when power is disconnected for long periods without prior notice. Furthermore, we have a walk-in cold room where drugs are kept at −20 and a Revco refrigerator where valuable medical drugs, specimens and chemicals are stored, and it is now becoming virtually impossible to keep these drugs at the temperature recommended by the manufacturers. We have in the past relied on your prior notice and transferred some materials to other buildings, but of late no notice has been given to us and recently our patients even went without food as we had not made prior arrangements.[88]

This letter provides a glimpse into ongoing efforts to prevent ruptures, blackouts, and disruptions.

Harnessing electricity to keep freezers at appropriately chilly temperatures and keeping samples sheltered from the vagaries of the noonday equatorial sun during this period could not always depend on what Derek Peterson and Edgar Taylor have called "the politics of exhortation."[89] This was a common practice in 1970s Uganda, in which civil servants were consistently called upon to fix or jerry-rig services that were in a state of disrepair. When the Americans left the UCI in 1973, they made provisions with the National Cancer Institute to send backup tissue and serum samples to Bethesda to circumvent the threats of power outages, military upheavals, theft, or broken refrigerators that were not easily fixed.[90] Although the UCI had freezers and a cold room for storage, "anything could happen."[91] By 1975, as the electricity supply in Kampala became increasingly unreliable, it became clear that the decision to back up sample collections of the UCI in Bethesda was a prescient one. The politics of exhortation was not enough to keep the freezers running consistently. Already stretched by his duties on the wards, Olweny ultimately decided to end the laboratory's work in tissue culture and tumor-marker studies. Instead, the focus would be entirely on clinical research to tailor chemotherapy protocols and prevent central nervous system relapse in Burkitt's lymphoma patients.[92]

Although the UCI's in-house laboratory studies closed, the Institute continued to supply tumor tissues, sera, cell lines, and survival data to metropolitan cancer research centers.[93] The UCI also continued to send tissue cultures of Burkitt's lymphoma and Kaposi's sarcoma to the NIH for further research. Operating this tissue and serum bank was contingent on a set of preparation practices, supply chains, telegram operators, airports, quality control of the samples, and laboratory labor. This was a precise exercise, as instructions written by a technician at the Unit of Biological Carcinogenesis—a unit of the International Agency for Research on Cancer (IARC)—reminded staff in Kampala about gathering the tissue of Kaposi's sarcoma patients and a close relative: "IT IS OF ABSOLUTE IMPORTANCE THAT SPECIMENS ARE PLACED AS SOON AS THEY HAVE BEEN REMOVED ON CRUNSHED ICE AND SHIPPED TO PARIS. SERA ALSO SHOULD BE SENT ON CRUNSHED ICE OR FROZEN" (emphasis in original).[94] With periodic blackouts and power failures, acquiring "crunshed" ice was not always easy. There was room for improvisation within the IARC's shipping system. If no dry ice or regular ice was available, picnic bags were always an option: "Pack in a box, four previously frozen picnic bags on bottom of container, pack 10 to 12 cm of cotton above and place cardboard on top. Above place tubes, bottles, etc. previously wrapped in cotton."[95] Equipment and supplies were kept in the LTC's laboratory—sterile bottles, media and reagents, colored labels—and once a week, sometimes more often, the assistant administrator would accompany a driver to Entebbe to ensure that the samples were kept out of the sun until they made it onto the East African cargo plane to their next destination.[96]

The shipments out of the UCI were part of a major operation, one that was shaped increasingly by the scarcity of materials and the need to stretch out supplies as much as possible. A letter from the technician of Dr. George Klein's laboratory concerning the quality of the biopsy shipments from the UCI stages the conflict between the viability of the materials being shipped and the realities of stretching out vials and media: "It is very important that you don't put too big biopsies into small bottles and that you really fill the others up to the edge with medium. If you have a lot of material please put it into 2 or more bottles. And last, a very important thing. Be sure that the caps don't leak. Please use adhesive tape instead of scotch tape."[97] What the technician highlights as room for improvement is, I think, a reflection of the fact that laboratory workers did not always have access to different-sized bottles or the proper adhesive tape. These practices of conservation and contending with mismatched supplies were common across Mulago Hospital's campus. For example, in August 1976, the Department of Medical Illustration at the Medical School notified all members of school staff that the department was nearly out of printing paper and films and therefore would only be printing color and lantern slides of requested images.[98] Mr. Nsalabwa ordered X-ray films in bulk to keep the UCI X-ray department from shortages.[99] Cars would need repairs, and there would be no spare parts obtainable in Uganda.[100] Soap would be in such short supply that wives of civil servants, in an effort to conserve what little they had, would wash only the cuffs, collars, and armpits of their husband's shirts so they would be presentable at work.[101]

POLITICS AND SCIENCE UNDER IDI AMIN

In 1975 or 1976 (the exact year is unknown), Olweny took Amin on a tour of the LTC and the Solid Tumor Center, where nurses made beds and mixed chemotherapy, patients ate two meals a day, and student health officers did ward rounds and lumbar punctures. "This place does not smell!" Amin declared, his point of comparison being the wards of New Mulago Hospital, where services were already caving in under the pressure of shortages of necessary items—soaps, antibiotics, cleaning materials, staff.[102] Amin visited the UCI X-ray department, where Nsalabwa, the head radiographer, shook Amin's hand and showed him how they performed chest X-rays for every patient admitted to the Institute. The facilities were humble—the equipment hadn't been updated for several years. Nsalabwa, gregarious and also keen to capitalize on Amin's impression of the place, started to talk about the state of the equipment and hinted that it was old. Amin turned to Nsalabwa and said, "What do you need? A new machine? We will get you a new X-ray machine! Get this man a new X-ray machine!"[103] Miraculously, several months later, a new state-of-the-art X-ray machine arrived at the UCI, wrapped neatly in a large shipping box. However, the service contractors commissioned to set up the machine and calibrate it did not arrive. The machine was manufactured in the United Kingdom, and the company refused to send their technicians to set up the machine because of company policy to not send staff to Amin's Uganda. The machine sat for years in its unopened box. As Nsalabwa remembered, "They sold us the machine, but they refused to come in and install it. Because they wanted a white man to come and install it."[104] It was not set up until the Tanzanian invasion in Kampala in 1979, when the service contractors were given the go-ahead to travel and liberate the machine from its box.[105]

According to the memories of some Institute staff, Amin was so impressed with the Institute—this place that "did not smell"—that it was his preferred site at Mulago Hill for the medical care of his soldiers. Syringes for bloodwork, antimalarials that were not expired, and nurses who came on time were much easier to come by at the UCI than Mulago Hospital. Staff could not turn these soldiers away, nor could they do anything less than provide impeccable service, lest they become targets themselves of state-sanctioned violence. Amin either cast a blind eye to the NIH's financial pipeline to the Institute, or was unaware of it, as he routinely brought international visitors to the UCI to see Ugandan scientists working at a center of excellence throughout the 1970s.[106]

Amin's fondness for the UCI and its contributions to African science offered some immunity from the political violence and uncertainty that pervaded the atmosphere in Kampala. But this political support from the state provided a meager buffer against problems of scarcity and broken things that characterized everyday life in the 1970s. It became more challenging over the course of the decade to engage in the work of maintenance, either in the conduct of fieldwork with patients and their families in remote villages, or through the work of typewriters, signatures, time, and fuel to send letters throughout Kampala to keep the lights on.[107]

These issues were exacerbated when the NCI canceled its financial and administrative support of the UCI in 1977. The short version of the story is that the director of the NCI during the 1970s, Dr. Vince DeVita, decided that the research being produced out of the UCI no longer merited the expense and challenges of financing the Institute in an increasingly precarious economic and political situation in Uganda. Further, the UCI's efforts did not easily mesh with the rest of the agenda for Nixon's "War on Cancer."[108] Olweny was able to negotiate a standalone budget for the UCI under the Ministry of Health, ensuring that it did not get folded into the administrative crises of Mulago. He reached out to international partners willing to donate chemotherapy drugs, but work at the Institute greatly slowed after 1977. Without the support of outside funding, the financial and material limitations of the Ministry of Health made it increasingly difficult to pay the salaries of nurses or supply enough serum vials. And public infrastructure continued to deteriorate. Consider Tomusange's letter to the engineer in charge of telephone operations in Kampala, penned on October 17, 1977. Tomusange wrote:

> Dear Sir,
> Ref: Telephone 41232 at Makerere North House No. 3
>
> This is a residential Telephone for our Director Prof.
> C. L. M. Olweny. This telephone has been out of order for about two months. We have been contacting your department via telephone 997 almost daily but up to now 41232 is not working!
> Sir Uganda Cancer Institute is a hospital with over 40 patients and this doctor being the over all in charge, is bound to

be called any time for emergencies. His house is situated about two miles away from the hospital; and surely without a telephone we are bound to loose [*sic*] some lives! Please save us before such calamity takes place.

Sir we suggest that if this particular telephone is beyond repair, you give him a new telephone number, we are ready to pay for any extra service rendered.[109]

During the 1970s, Institute staff worked to keep politics out of science. An ethic of providing quality care in a context of extreme scarcity characterized the UCI's work. Drawing upon these experiences, Olweny became heavily involved with the World Health Organization's efforts to put together an essential drug list both for basic hospital care but also for oncology, a lasting contribution to increasing capacity of health systems.[110] He argued that with a strong painkiller, a multipurpose antibiotic, a deworming drug, and a handful of reliable cytotoxic drugs you could run a hospital as long as you had dedicated staff. This essential drug list and survival data are just two examples among many that illustrate how the Amin years brought creativity as well as destruction.

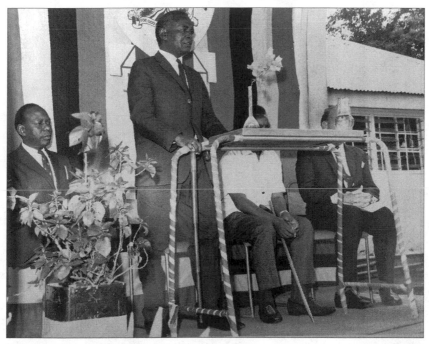

FIGURE 1. Opening the Uganda Cancer Institute. Photo courtesy of John Ziegler and Andrea Stultiens.

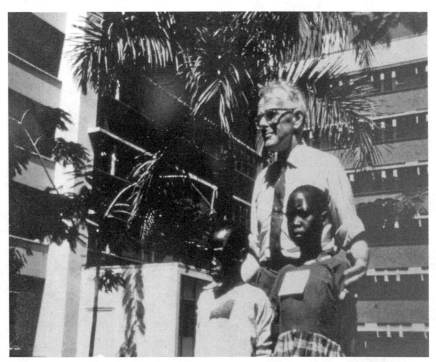

FIGURE 2. Denis Burkitt and patients. Photo courtesy of John Ziegler and Andrea Stultiens.

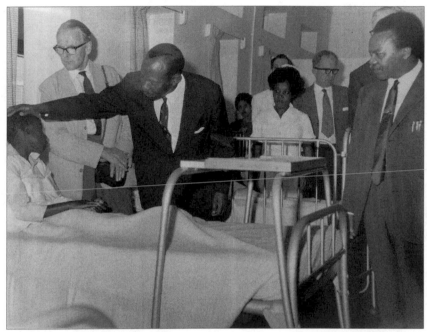

FIGURE 3. Sebastian Kyalwazi and patient. Photo courtesy of John Ziegler and Andrea Stultiens.

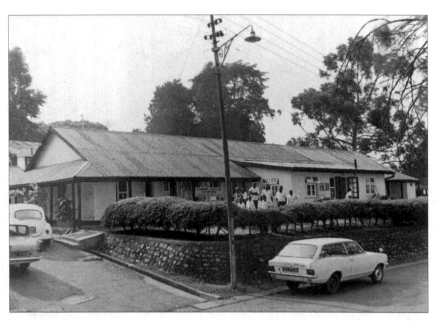

FIGURE 4. The Lymphoma Treatment Center. Photo courtesy of John Ziegler and Andrea Stultiens.

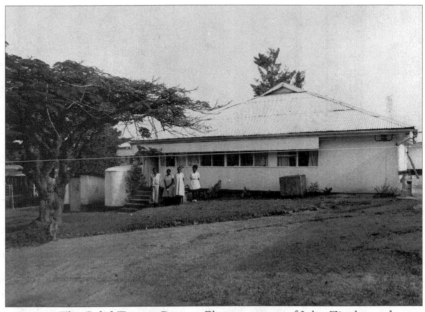

FIGURE 5. The Solid Tumor Center. Photo courtesy of John Ziegler and Andrea Stultiens.

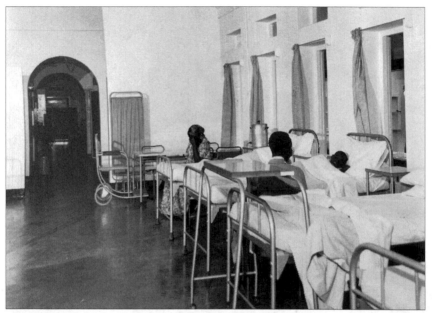

FIGURE 6. Inside the Lymphoma Treatment Center. Photo courtesy of John Ziegler and Andrea Stultiens.

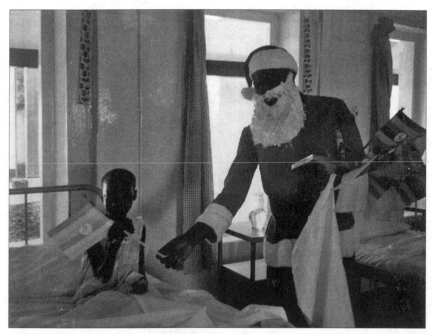

FIGURE 7. Christmas at the Lymphoma Treatment Center. Photo courtesy of John Ziegler and Andrea Stultiens.

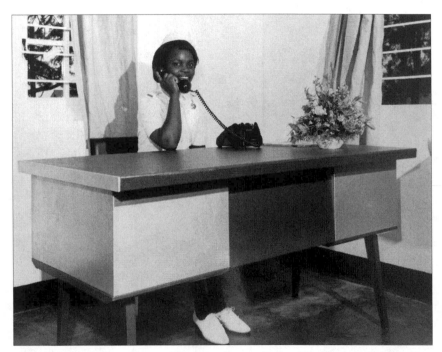

FIGURE 8. A warm welcome. Photo courtesy of John Ziegler and Andrea Stultiens.

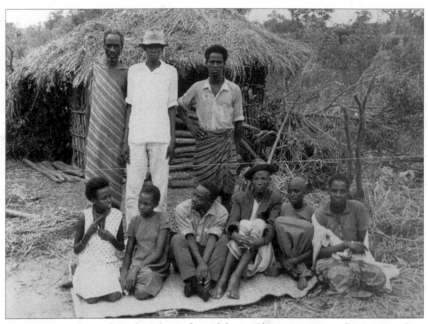

FIGURE 9. Fieldwork and making friendships. Photo courtesy of John Ziegler and Andrea Stultiens.

4 ⌇ Rocket Launchers and Toxic Drugs

On October 9, 1978, Idi Amin decided to invade northwestern Tanzania, annex the land bordering the north of the Kagera River, and preemptively stop the Tanzanian government, which was apparently plotting against him.[1] As Peter Nayenga notes, the invasion was meant to "divert attention from internal problems," including ongoing conflicts in the leadership of the military and the deteriorating economy.[2] Over the next several weeks, Tanzania made the decision to drive the Ugandan army out of the Kagera region. In the process of reclaiming Kagera, Tanzania opted to "liberate" Uganda by invading the country and fighting the Ugandan army until Amin had no choice but to back down and, in all likelihood, surrender his power and authority with the establishment of a new Ugandan government.

Although it was wracked by long-term shortages and infrastructural breakdown, Mulago became a war hospital in 1979. Physicians treated soldiers from both Amin's and Tanzania's armies. Civilians still came for care.[3] At the top of the hill at the Uganda Cancer Institute (UCI), the administration of chemotherapy and the treatment of patients continued. Olweny submitted manuscripts to the *Lancet* on the survival data for Burkitt's lymphoma patients who were followed from 1967 to 1977. In September 1979 the manuscript was formally accepted by the *Lancet*. The editor remarked that the publication "records an extraordinary achievement in the middle of chaos."[4] Student health officers stayed overnight in their small room on site in order to tend to emergencies. They remember dodging bullets at night in order to check in on patients whose immune systems were crashing or to manage a patient experiencing kidney failure.[5] In the midst of these disruptions, long-term cancer survivors still came to the wards for checkups to see whether or not their cancers were still in remission. One long-term survivor from the wards of the Lymphoma Treatment Center (LTC) who went on to work as a medical officer at the UCI came late for her annual checkup, "due to the war of liberation." In the last entry in her file, this patient signed off on her own bloodwork, a pause in the middle of chaos that many hoped would promise a new period of peace and stability in Uganda.[6]

With Obote's second presidency, the good fortune that had shielded the Institute from the worst of Uganda's politics under Idi Amin came to an end. Concerned about his personal safety and that of his family, Olweny left the directorship of the Institute and Uganda in the early 1980s.[7] His successor, Dr. Edward Katongole-Mbidde, inherited the UCI's two wards, a laboratory, the X-ray unit, a scientific legacy around combination chemotherapy clinical trials, and a dedicated staff. But in the mid-1980s, the UCI lost its institutional and financial autonomy and was formally absorbed by Mulago Hospital's administration and budget.[8] The Ministry of Health and Mulago Hospital did not prioritize cancer drugs in its budget or staffing needs for the UCI's forty beds. In the 1980s, 1990s, and 2000s staff remember getting a few scattershot shipments of drugs a year that were finished within a matter of weeks. Families were asked to shoulder the burden of purchasing chemotherapy treatments for their patients in need.[9]

The 1980s marked a significant break from the original founding purpose of the UCI, where chemotherapy trials and supportive cancer care were entangled with one another. When the Institute was folded into Mulago Hospital's bureaucracy, it transformed from being a research institution with beds for chemotherapy clinical trials to a palliative care triage unit.[10] The Institute's central purpose was to care for the hospital's unit for patients with late-stage cancers, who were often terminal and living with AIDS. Research efforts remained, especially regarding Kaposi's sarcoma, but these studies were no longer synonymous with the provision of potentially curative or at least remission-inducing cancer drugs.[11] The cancer chemotherapy clinical trial gave way to a research culture that focused on HIV/AIDS patients who found themselves at the Institute. Tissue samples from Kaposi's sarcoma patients were taken and analyzed in labs outside the country.[12] Some azidothymidine trials were hosted at the UCI, and cryptococcal meningitis and its treatment were investigated.[13] This is simply to say that by 1986, the UCI was no longer a place where research on the effects of chemotherapy on long-term cancer survival was at the top of the agenda. And in the absence of chemotherapy clinical trials, there was not enough financial and institutional support to guarantee a regularly available therapeutic arsenal.[14]

From its inception in 1967, chemotherapy, whether administering drugs, managing the side effects, or documenting whether or not the drugs led to durable cancer remissions, defined the purpose and presence of the UCI.[15] The harmful properties of the drugs could bring about nearly magical healing, which captured the imagination of a whole generation of Burkitt's lymphoma researchers.[16] The drugs were the principal therapeutic treatment for cancer in a place without radiotherapy technologies. Chemotherapy was an expensive commodity, only available through patronage from drug companies, the National Cancer Institute (NCI), the Ugandan state, or the pooling of family resources. Evaluating the effects of combination chemotherapy clinical trials and tracking the long-term survival of cancer patients was the research agenda that kept the UCI open and supported by external partners in the 1970s. Maintaining these studies was the key to accessing a steady supply of drugs in the 1970s, first through funds from the NCI and later through support from Amin's Ministry of Health.[17] But from the 1980s onward, civil war, structural adjustment, and HIV/AIDS all shaped the reconstruction of health services.[18] Revitalizing chemotherapy clinical trials research on cancer in Uganda was not a priority. The sporadic availability and frequent absence of drugs due to limited government drug procurement budgets, rather than the continuous presence of freely available chemotherapy thanks to sponsorship from NCI-sponsored clinical trials, defined work at the UCI from the early 1980s up until the late 2000s.

Coping with the limited availability of chemotherapy, what Olweny called the "armamentarium" of the medical oncologist, defined everyday practices of cancer care on the wards of the UCI in the 1980s, 1990s, and 2000s. Africanized oncology in this period can best be characterized as one of working with scarce resources. But this austerity cannot solely be attributed to policies of structural adjustment and the cost-sharing schemes of user fees, which the International Monetary Fund and World Bank imposed on African governments in the 1980s and 1990s. The violence and unrest from the war of liberation in 1979 and the prolonged civil war that followed shaped the revitalization of moribund health services in Uganda. The embodied experiences of the war also shaped everyday understandings of cancer care itself. Patients, nurses, and physicians all likened technologies of violence, particularly Soviet-manufactured rocket launchers called Katyusha that were used during the Tanzanian invasion, to the embodied effects of cancer treatments, especially chemotherapy. Many have criticized the valence of war and its metaphors to describe the experience of cancer in the Global North. From Susan Sontag to Audre Lorde to Løchlann Jain to many a palliative care physician, prominent thinkers have argued that reducing cancer to a battle where the patient is responsible for winning the war is its own form of discursive and literal violence.[19] I am not contesting that here but instead want to ask how we can interpret and engage with Ugandan vernacular understandings of cancer, the somatic and historical meanings of oncological technologies, and the legacies of 1979. By taking both the metaphors associated with cancer treatments and the materiality of these toxic treatments seriously, we add nuance and complexity to how families and biomedical caretakers adapted to conditions of profound scarcity after the hollowed state of Idi Amin and before the rise of global oncology.

THE LIBERATION WAR THAT DID NOT BRING PEACE

After the war of liberation, Olweny and colleagues imagined that they would transform the UCI into a center of oncology excellence in the country. In the early 1980s the World Health Organization planned to create three cancer centers in sub-Saharan Africa, and the UCI made a strong case that one of these centers should be in Uganda. Olweny envisioned a site that would continue to do cutting-edge research but also offer cancer care to the general population with the acquisition of a radiotherapy unit and a revamping of the pathology department. This required serious reinvestment in the Institute and the rehabilitation of Mulago's infrastructure and services as well.[20]

In October 1979, Olweny traveled to Washington, DC, on a mission to secure the funds to restore Makerere Medical School and Mulago Hospital. In the wake of the war of liberation, the remaining physicians and administrative staff of the Medical School and Mulago took stock of the fallout of eight years under Amin. The situation was dire:

> The health care services provided that once was the envy of
> most of Black Africa had almost become nonexistent. There was a

continuous brain drain throughout the 8 years and some of the departments within the faculty had to close down for lack of personnel. Recruitment became impossible. Laboratories could not offer even the simplest tests for lack of reagents. Drugs were constantly in short supply, and even life-saving drugs were more often than not out of stock. Equipment were never serviced and because of lack of spare parts the hospital workshop was turned into a graveyard for some very vital and expensive equipment. The linen was never replaced and because of soaring inflation some mattresses, sheets, [and] blankets, were carried away by petty thieves. The Faculty library stopped stocking new books and periodicals were never paid for. Research laboratories closed down for lack of proper supervision, chemicals, equipment and above all competent technical staff. This, briefly, was the state of affairs when the new regime moved in at the overthrow of dictator Amin.[21]

The deans of the medical school, the director of the hospital, and the Ministry of Health requested $4,625,000 in aid from the United States for immediate needs. New basic equipment needed to be ordered for nearly all of the wards to replace the old equipment that had either been broken or stolen. Drugs and vaccines were needed to stave off the threat of measles and polio epidemics. Many of the buildings were damaged during the war, and most were poorly maintained during Amin's period. These facilities needed electrical work, sewage systems, and basic repairs. On the manpower front, expatriate and Ugandan physicians who had fled Uganda in the 1970s needed to be given incentives to come back and restore the medical school's teaching program. The plan was to reinvigorate and establish partnerships with American medical schools. In addition to these immediate needs, $5,250,000 was requested for a variety of smaller but vital projects. The medical records room was in chaos. The blood bank had ceased to function and needed reagents and refrigerators. There were no working clocks on the walls. The intercom system had been decimated. Eighteen ambulances, thirty-six-bed trolleys, and twenty-four wheelchairs were needed for the movement of patients inside and outside of the hospital.[22]

Olweny also used this travel opportunity to highlight the importance of maintaining the UCI and renewing the vital connection between US-based institutions and the UCI. He was particularly anxious to resume the provision of chemotherapy drugs. The cost of the drugs, prohibitively expensive from currency devaluation, made it difficult to treat patients at the Institute. In the context of reconstruction, where basic medications like aspirin and materials like bedsheets were out of stock, making a case for prioritizing the purchase of cytotoxic drugs was a challenge. Olweny argued that the UCI was a touchstone of US-Uganda relations as a whole and a vital center of knowledge production. As the proposal noted, "The UCI has been a source of good will between the respective governments of Uganda and the USA. The cancer research program has added a great deal to Makerere's reputation on the academic map. Over the past 12 years, over 200 publications in international journals have been generated from the Institute."[23] Revitalizing the Institute would mean renewing and strengthening US–Ugandan relations. And maintaining the Institute depended on a steady supply of chemotherapy drugs and other tools of the medical oncology trade. As Olweny wrote, "The last 8 years have placed the Institute under considerable strain. Cancer chemotherapy drugs are extremely expensive and since radiotherapy facilities are not available the drugs are a must to the armamentarium of oncologists practicing in Uganda."[24]

Olweny received an emergency grant of $10,000 for vital chemotherapy drugs and other sundries. They purchased needles for bone marrow aspirates and chemotherapy administration as well as allopurinol tablets to prevent tumor lysis syndrome. In terms of chemotherapy, they procured $5,684 worth of methotrexate, $2,470 of cosmogen (dactinomycin), and $1,330 of mustagen (mechlorethamine). (These drugs are particularly suited to treating lymphomas and some childhood tumors like Wilms' tumor.)[25] On his visit to the United States and the United Kingdom, Olweny succeeded in making the rehabilitation of Mulago a central issue for foreign aid dollars and one that would have an immediate impact in Uganda. As he wrote, "The trip was fruitful, worthwhile, but tiring. It is hoped that the State Department will probably provide funds to enable the program to take off."[26] Renewing ties and exchanges with long-term expatriate physician friends of Uganda and those who had run away under Amin would be critical, and it would be necessary to show them proper hospitality, accommodation, and "all amenities including food and transport."[27]

Although Amin fled to exile in Saudi Arabia, the Tanzanian liberation of 1979 did not bring peace. Squabbles and power struggles regarding who would assume control of the country followed. And within a few months, Uganda's ousted leader, Milton Obote, returned to State House as president. From 1980 to 1986, a period of prolonged civil war and conflict between Milton Obote's second government and guerrilla forces of Yoweri Museveni's National Resistance Army devastated central Uganda.[28]

Meanwhile, Mbidde formally took over the leadership of the UCI.[29] His professionalism, accomplished intuition as a chemotherapist, and research abilities made him an obvious fit for training as the country's second oncologist. Arrangements had already been made in the early 1980s that Mbidde would pursue an overseas advanced training in medical oncology, with the expectation that he and Olweny would work together to ensure the smooth functioning of the unit while Olweny worked at the helm of Mulago Hospital and, eventually, the Ministry of Health. But given Olweny's quick decision to decamp from Uganda and work in Zambia (and later on, Zimbabwe, Canada, and Australia), this smooth handover did not occur. Decades later, as I was driving in my own RAV4 along Bombo Road by Mulago Hospital with some of the now elderly administrators who worked at the UCI during the early 1980s, they reminisced about that handover. They said they saw soldiers driving Olweny's red Volvo around town on joyrides after his departure. They joked that there was a more thorough handover of Olweny's possessions to the Ugandan state than there was of the administrative and institutional duties of the UCI. Uneasy laughter accompanied their memories of this period when they said, "With Olweny and Ziegler, there was a hand over. With Mbidde, there was no hand over."[30]

MBIDDE AND THE MUSEUM

At the history symposium held at the UCI in 2014, Mbidde shared his memories with an audience consisting of former and current UCI staff, Ugandan journalists, and other members of the public. We were unable to conduct a formal interview on that day as my copies of informed consent documentation with the official stamp from the institutional review board had been left in my file cabinet in the United States, and an unofficial copy was not sufficient. The following account draws from the public comments he shared at the history symposium. On that day, Mbidde recounted how he first came to the top of the hill when he was a medical student at Makerere and on his vacation between first and second year.[31] In March 1967, he had an opportunity to work with Dr. Richard Morrow, who was doing Burkitt's lymphoma epidemiology research at the time. It was Mbidde's first contact with the site. Over the next few years, Mbidde lived down the road from the UCI in medical student housing and used to see Dr. Chuck Vogel and Dr. John Ziegler coming and going up and down the hill from the Institute. He was fascinated by the work on the wards with cancer and oncology and also intrigued by the research opportunities. At the end of his third year of medical school he had the opportunity to apply for a studentship, which was extremely competitive. It turned out that they thought he was a fourth-year student because he seemed so impressive. Nonetheless, he was able to join and worked on the LTC side and never looked back. Like Olweny, Mbidde was heavily mentored by Ziegler, Vogel, Professor Sebastian Kyalwazi, Sir Ian McAdam, and others at the UCI. In his final year of medical school, Mbidde became involved with research on big spleens. He and colleagues were traveling sixty miles away into rural areas, collecting blood samples, and separating out sera and securing it in freezers for further study and transport. These two activities—on the wards and in the research capacity—cemented both a tireless work ethic within Mbidde and a commitment to patients. He described one evening preparing to leave the LTC that night after processing serum. Dr. Avrum Bluming had brought in a thirteen-year-old girl who desperately needed care. "Edward, you have to stay and work up this girl," said Bluming. And so he did.[32]

After this work he did an internship in New Mulago and later had an opportunity to rejoin the UCI as a medical officer. By the time Amin came on the scene, the manpower at the hospital had dropped to a third of its normal capacity. Mbidde joined the UCI in May 1974 and continued to work on the wards as a medical officer (special grade) after finishing his internal med master's. Mbidde was, for all intents and purposes, the deputy of the unit and worked closely with Olweny on the wards and in the lab. In the early 1980s Olweny left for good, leaving Mbidde as the only doctor in charge to maintain high standards in extremely difficult times. They were able to secure some lines of credit for drugs, but it was very hard to get staff, and patients found that mobility was difficult in these insecure times.[33]

In 1984 Mbidde went to Edinburgh for about three months of further training and then later received a World Health Organization fellowship for more formal training in medical oncology for a two-year fellowship in the United Kingdom. Meanwhile the situation in Uganda was no better. There was war and death. And Mbidde asked himself, "Should I come back?" Colleagues in the United Kingdom asked, "Are you sure you want to go back?" Mbidde said, "The people who paid me [to go to school] were the peasants. Am I going to abandon them?" Mbidde came back just as Museveni had taken over as president, and there was relative peace. Mbidde's work was to "try and put things together" to get drugs and other sundries. "I started from scratch, getting infrastructure, better drugs." And meanwhile, although Mbidde had health workers coming and going, most left or "disappeared." Of this team, it was Dr. Jackson Orem who, as a student health officer, ground his heels into the culture of the place and began working the overnight shift tending to emergencies.[34]

Mbidde was able to keep the Institute going into the 1980s, 1990s, and 2000s when resources had become so limited through maintaining high standards: "I wanted things [done] the right way." He used to arrive early and "could not go home until I finished my work." He had colleagues who would ask what was keeping him in his office at such late hours. "There's a lot of work for me to do," he would reply. Sometimes that would mean ward rounds at 9:30 p.m. He had an incredible team of nurses who were committed to patients and also to getting him what he wanted when he needed it ("I had my own systems," said Mbidde.) He could get a blood slide in ten minutes. He could get the results of a lumbar puncture immediately. These systems operated alongside a series of research partnerships mainly focused on HIV/AIDS. As early as 1987, collaborators were coming to the UCI to conduct HIV research. Fogarty, the National Institute of Health, University of California San Francisco, Case Western, Oxford University—they all came with research protocols for specimen collection, survey research, and clinical trials—but with just enough equipment to get the job done.[35]

Although the UCI became a triage unit operating under conditions of "normal emergency,"[36] the everyday practices of cancer care established in the 1960s at the Institute continued. Nursing procedures, ward-rounding practices, X-raying, and meticulous record keeping remained relatively intact. This was despite the fact that the drugs were rarely available, and the patient follow-up fieldwork, so critical to maintaining the Burkitt's lymphoma studies across the country in the 1970s, had long ended. As Ziegler, who returned in the early 1990s to work at the UCI as a lecturer at Makerere Medical School, noted in an oral history: "I've been back off and on since 1990 and the place is like a museum. It still runs exactly the way it used to run, and everything is still in place. Some of the nursing sisters who were there are still there, and Dr. Mbidde, of course who was trained by us and then went on to further oncology training in Britain, still runs the center very much in the same way. He's an extremely competent oncologist."[37] This "museum" was an exhibition of practices and procedures that had not changed dramatically since the 1960s. Although they often lacked the materials necessary to offer meaningful treatments for cancers that had been successfully treated at the Institute in its heyday, the site endured as the only publicly available cancer care in the country.

Staff relied on the infrastructures, routines, and practices that had been developed in the 1960s and maintained in the 1970s to conduct cancer research. These systems provided scaffolding for organizing works and days with professionalism and care. And nearly twenty years of collective oncological experience meant that knowledge about the course of cancer care and treatment, particularly for Burkitt's lymphoma and Kaposi's sarcoma, was quite high. Even if drugs were missing, gloves were rarely in stock, and blood was only to be found in the veins of relatives willing to donate, Mbidde and his team of nurses could still provide oncological practices and procedures. This does not mean, however, that the social and embodied meanings of oncological technologies remained static.

ROCKET LAUNCHERS AND TOXIC DRUGS

In the 1980s and 1990s on the UCI wards, the harsh effects of chemotherapy technologies were equated with the collective experience of violence during the war of liberation in 1979.[38] According to nurses and medical officers who worked on the UCI wards from 1986 to 1995 or so, chemotherapy treatments were called *saba saba* (translated in Swahili as "seven seven"). Colloquially, in Tanzania, *saba saba* refers to July 7, 1954, the day that the Tanganyikan African National Union political party was founded. In Luganda, *oku-saba* means "to ask." Among Protestants, *oku-saba* can also mean "to pray." *Saba saba* was the expression Kampala residents used to describe the Soviet rocket launchers used by Tanzanians and the sound these rockets made during the war of liberation in 1978 and 1979, an allusion to Tanzanian liberation and nationalism politics.

One of Uganda's only neonatologists, Dr. M, worked at the UCI from 1985 to 1993 as the medical officer in charge of the LTC. She imagined that she would become a pediatric oncologist, but irreconcilable differences with the Institute's leadership about the strategies of triage and rationing of drugs at the UCI led to her departure in the early 1990s. From Dr. M's desk at the private pediatric clinic she now runs in Rubaga (her "retirement" after creating a successful premature-baby survival program at Mulago), she shared her memories of working at the UCI in the 1980s and 1990s, recalling the relationship between chemotherapy and the war:

> When there was the war in Uganda, the Tanzanians, when they came for this liberation they had this big gun, which used to throw the bombs. And we called it *saba saba*. And so the patients had named this drug *saba saba*. The chemotherapy. It would hit them [snapping fingers]. The hair goes out [snapping

fingers]. The next day they are anemic. They are weak. Some would vomit when hit by the drug so they called it *saba saba.* Nobody told you? They would come for their *saba saba* and it would really hit them.[39]

As Dr. M recalled this story, she emphatically and rhythmically snapped her fingers to punctuate the way chemotherapy treatments violently hit the body. Administered through a push injection, the drugs feel like a thunderous clap. The blood counts crash. The eruptive vomiting comes. Eyebrows, eyelashes, pubic hair, and the hair on one's head comes out in clumps. For those living in Kampala during the time of the Tanzanian invasion, saba saba hit buildings, farming land, roads, and radio towers. Those who remember saba saba remember the rockets were different colors. Pinks, greens, blues, and smoky grays painted evening skies. Saba saba, when fired, would make a terrifying screeching noise. These rocket launchers, known as Katyushas, were a Soviet technology from World War II. Germans fighting on the Eastern Front called these rocket launchers "Stalin's organ" because of the particularly harsh sound they made.[40]

Bombing a targeted area with devastating effect and little precision—what Katyusha rockets are made for—can also be extended to describe the style of oncology practice at the UCI from the mid-1980s onward. The end of randomized trials and regular drug supplies meant that nurses and oncologists were left to bombard the body with whatever happened to be sporadically available. This practice worked directly against the logic and findings of approximately a decade and a half of research conducted at the Institute. As Dr. M remembered: "The drugs were never available. So most of the time we had to think of combinations. You would give a combination and one drug would be missing. These days at least I know they are available in the market. But those days, it was not in the country if it was not at the Institute."[41]

The shift from researching chemotherapy combinations and their effects to using whatever was available in the "armamentarium" of the oncologist that particular month or week to alleviate suffering was debated and contested in the period where the neonatologist worked at the UCI from 1986 to 1993. Most of the patients at the Solid Tumor Center (STC) came with fulminating AIDS-related Kaposi's sarcoma. Wound cleaning, fluid administration, providing comfort and palliative care to patients took up the majority of the nursing work on the STC side. The occasional patient would come with advanced-stage hepatocellular carcinoma, and there would be negotiations with pharmacies and families to try to put together the funds to purchase Adriamycin to debulk the tumor. On the LTC side, children with Burkitt's lymphoma still came to the wards, as did patients with leukemia and other kinds of lymphomas. HIV-positive children came to the wards with Kaposi's sarcoma. Their blood and biopsies were taken for ongoing research studies in collaboration with German scientists on pediatric Kaposi's sarcoma, but a treatment program was not part of the research agenda.[42]

Under these circumstances, "We would get a lot of terminal stage [patients] with huge tumors. I remember I would take a lot of risks. Dr. Mbidde would say you cannot put drugs in that one. And the patient would just die,"[43] Dr. M said. When she was able to act on her own, she often "took risks." At one point, a lymphoma patient with a huge abdominal tumor came to the LTC and "Mbidde said that one is going to die. But he was so uncomfortable. He was going to die anyway but maybe there is a 1% chance that we'll reduce the tumor a bit so he'll be more comfortable."[44] Dr. M had the patient sign a consent form saying that he understood that he was taking a highly toxic drug that might not have any benefit. His tumor significantly reduced over the course of several rounds of treatment before he eventually passed away. This sort of administration of chemotherapy at late stages of illness brought Dr. M into active conflict with other UCI staff who did not want her "taking risks with these patients"[45] and in the process squandering the scant supplies of drugs on patients who were going to die quickly of their cancer or from the complications of the drugs. The patchily available drugs needed to be saved for conditions that might actually bring about a "durable remission," like Burkitt's lymphoma patients who still came to the Institute for care. In 1993 Dr. M submitted her resignation and went on to specialize in pediatric neonatology. Today at her clinic, she still treats the families of some of the patients she treated for cancer in the 1980s and 1990s. The children with leukemia are long deceased, but she is still in touch with a few Burkitt's lymphoma patients in long-term recovery. They still remember arriving at the LTC clinic no later than seven in the morning to get their bloodwork done before treatment.

What does it *mean* that on the wards of the UCI chemotherapy treatments became synonymous with saba saba? It was a joke on the wards to a certain extent. Patients would come for their rounds of poisoning. After arriving early in the morning for bloodwork to ensure adequate white cell counts and functioning livers, patients would either be admitted to a bed and receive their drugs, or they would sit on a hard wooden chair in the "outpatient" areas of the STC and LTC, which doubled as reception and nursing break areas. "It's time for your saba saba!" was a moment of levity, as nurses would look for veins on the hands of patients to insert cannulas and then inject vincristine, cyclophosphamide, and methotrexate.[46]

Although I worked in interviews and on the wards to elicit greater reflection on what chemotherapy treatments such as saba saba meant for cancer patients and their care providers in the 1980s and 1990s at the UCI, the conversations stopped after confirming that cancer chemotherapy treatments were equated with rocket launchers and that the war of liberation continued and exacerbated instability and violence in everyday life in Kampala. In one such conversation about chemotherapy administration, one of the retired nursing sisters grabbed my left hand and said, "Oh! This is so nice!" I thought she was referring to my wedding rings, so I said, "Thank you! This one is for my engagement and this one is for my wedding," pointing out the simple band. "No, no, dear, I am admiring your veins. These are so nice." She peered through her glasses and pointed out the prominent blue veins on the tops of my hands. Apparently they are perfect for inserting a line for chemotherapy administration.[47] It was easier to discuss practices of administration than to speak directly about the experience of the war.

I think calling chemotherapy saba saba in the 1980s and 1990s was a way to talk about what it means to live through catastrophe and disorder. Chemotherapy as saba saba suggests a sudden, explosive moment of chaos. The body under the power of chemotherapy is ungovernable, eruptive, and impossible to rein in. But this is also a fleeting moment, a punctuated catastrophe, an episode of violence. Saba saba hits. And then it passes. I think calling chemotherapy saba saba provided an additional cue for patients. If they could survive the Tanzanian invasion, they could surely survive six rounds of poisoning. Cancer patients in the 1980s and 1990s survived a war. They lived through the years of misrule under Idi Amin. They could also survive cancer if they just held out through the "booms" of saba saba injections.

Calling chemotherapy treatments saba saba is historically contingent and an evocative analogy that connects the somatic experience of chemotherapy drugs to the exploding of bombs that destroyed villages, markets, and churches in 1979.[48] The analogy expresses the memories of the experiences of war, the circulation of healing and harming technologies, and practices of providing cancer care in the 1980s and 1990s. The analogy provides a way of characterizing the experiences of a generation of cancer patients and their biomedical care providers during a time of protracted war and violence brought about by the departure of Idi Amin in 1979.

TECHNOLOGIES OF HARMING: CHEMOTHERAPY AND KATYUSHAS

The broader history of the development of cancer chemotherapy is intimately intertwined with the history of chemical weapons research in World War I and World War II. Mustard gas (sulfur mustard) was developed as a tool of warfare. When bodies were exposed to mustard gas, within ten to twelve hours, their skin and mucosa would begin to painfully blister. Eyes burned. Lungs burned. Skin burned. Nausea, vomiting, and diarrhea occurred. Internal effects of exposure to mustard gas came afterward. Those who survived the initial physical symptoms of the gas would develop acute bone marrow suppression. That is, their bone marrow would cease to produce red and white blood cells, leaving the body vulnerable to infections due to immunosuppression and crashing fatigue from the lack of red blood cells and consequential anemia. Other tissues, especially lymphoid and testicular tissues, atrophied after exposure.[49]

Researchers initially assumed that mustard gas exposure was carcinogenic, but a decade later Berenblum and Riley-Smith published results showing that the application of mustard gas on tumors had an anticarcinogenic effect. World War II renewed both an interest in chemical warfare, as well as the long-term repercussions for soldiers. Researchers at a variety of medical and government institutions were called upon to investigate the relationship between mustard gas and its possible role in treating neoplasms. At Yale University, Gilman, Goodman, Philips, and Allen discovered the antitumor properties of nitrogen mustard in 1942, which were kept secret until after the end of World War II. Also at Yale in May 1942, Dr. Gustav E. Lindskog carried out a trial using nitrogen mustard treatments on a forty-eight-year-old man with X-ray-resistant lymphosarcoma who was in terminal stages of illness. The man experienced a temporary regression of his tumors after being given a daily dose of 0.1 nitrogen mustard mg/kg over a ten-day period. This patient showed astonishing tumor regression in the short term: "by the last day of treatment, all signs and symptoms of his disease were gone." He died after a relapse several months later.[50]

The military secrecy surrounding research on the effects of nitrogen mustard as chemotherapy for cancer during World War II meant that the promise of the drug did not become fully apparent until after the war among the nascent community of medical oncologists. Nitrogen mustard became one of many alkylating agents in the oncology arsenal, which work by directly destroying DNA. In the 1950s and 1960s, how to create "durable remissions" with nitrogen mustard and other agents, such as folate antagonists like methotrexate and powerful antibiotics that had antitumor properties like actinomycin-D, was a major goal in pediatric leukemia research. In 1955 the Cancer Chemotherapy National Service Center was established as part of a national program for cancer drug development under the auspices of the NCI and directed by Dr. Kenneth Endicott. A decade later, it was folded into the NCI's chemotherapy program directed by Dr. Gordon Zubrod. Cyclophosphamide, a nitrogen mustard derivative, came to East Africa in the 1950s and 1960s largely through informal connections between British colonial medical officers and staff at the American National Cancer Institute.

Nitrogen mustard is undoubtedly a clunky chemotherapy technology. It is not a targeted therapy that differentiates between the DNA of cancerous cells and the DNA of healthy cells. For a rapidly dividing liquid tumor like Burkitt's lymphoma, which can double in size in a twenty-four- to forty-eight-hour period, the demolition of the DNA of rapidly growing cells is a boon. For slower-growing solid tumors, nitrogen mustard derivatives do not pack the same tumor-destroying punch—they are too indiscriminate in the cells they destroy.

The Katyusha rocket launcher is a Soviet-manufactured multiple-rocket launching system mounted on a heavily armored truck. They are designed to blanket target areas with explosives in a quick and devastating manner. They are not particularly accurate and take a longer time to load than some other forms of artillery. But their mobility and ability to cause mass havoc made them a weapon of choice for the Soviets in World War II. Over ten thousand units were manufactured for the war. After the end of World War II, Soviets continued to manufacture multiple rocket launchers. New generations of multiple rocket-launching systems, modeled after the Katyusha, such as BM-13s and BM-21s, circulated to customers in Libya, Syria, Algeria, India, and elsewhere.[51]

Military sales of Soviet weapons in the 1970s were shaped largely by the politics of supporting oil producers in the Middle East and Africa. In Africa, sales of Soviet arms and equipment were largely concentrated in Libya, the Horn of Africa, and Algeria. In 1973, Egypt ended relations with the Soviets, and Libya became Moscow's top military customer. In 1976, after the Soviets shifted their support from Somalia to Ethiopia, $2 billion worth of weapons were sold to Ethiopia, which "provided a class of sophistication new to the region and far beyond the capabilities of the Ethiopian military establishment to operate or maintain"[52] and consequently led to an extensive training program. Tanzania remained on the margins of these Soviet military purchase packages. Tanzania trained its troops and built its military reserves by drawing upon both Communist and capitalist expertise. Canadians and Chinese both had a hand in training soldiers. Uganda's military might under Amin came largely from its relationship with Libya, which funneled Soviet arms and military support and expertise. Unfortunately, from the records available, it is unclear how many Katyusha-style rocket launchers (whether BM-21s or BM-13s) the Tanzanian army procured in the 1970s and how widely they were used during the war of liberation in 1978 and 1979 in Uganda. Chemotherapy and rocket-launching technologies are both products of secret wartime research and development during both world wars. Both chemotherapy and rocket launchers came to East Africa in the 1960s and 1970s via circuitous routes and on the remote margins of the broader geopolitics and cleavages of the Cold War.[53] The meaning and to an extent the purpose of these relatively old military technologies were refashioned by East Africans on cancer wards and liberation fronts alike.[54]

SUPPLIES AND SENSELESSNESS AT THE MUSEUM

At the time of Dr. M's departure from the UCI in 1993, immediate memories of the collective experience of war in Kampala were fading. Although violence and war in Uganda did not cease with Museveni's government, the geographical locus of unrest markedly shifted to the north. By the early 1990s in Uganda, President Yoweri Museveni and the National Resistance Movement government brought relative peace and stability to Kampala and the surrounding central, western, and eastern regions of the country. North of Lake Kyoga, where the Nile cuts the country in two at Karuma Falls, an ongoing insurgency known as the Lord's Resistance Army fought the National Resistance Army throughout much of northern Uganda. This war would continue for nearly two decades. On the other hand, the ongoing fall out of structural adjustment policies, the underfunding of basic health services, and the procurement politics that shut the UCI out of any sort of reliable drug supply pipeline all contributed to embodied and structural forms of violence in the 1990s and 2000s at the "Museum."

Here, I focus on the story of Dr. Fred Okuku to explore what it meant to work at the UCI in what Kristin Peterson would call a "hollowed-out" or empty space after structural adjustment experiments across much of eastern Africa in the 1980s and 1990s.[55] This was a hollowing that undercut infrastructure, material resources, and sundries. This was a hollowing that stemmed from international decision-making about who should pay for oil booms and busts. Austerity in the 1980s and 1990s instituted draconian fiscal policies and crafted cost-sharing mechanisms that punished the poor in crucial sectors (health, education, sanitation, transportation). Historians and anthropologists alike have directed much of their attention to the immediate material consequences of structural adjustment. In the classic documentary film *Donka: X-ray of an African Hospital*, we see desperate families struggling to pay for medications and procedures to keep their loved ones alive as cash dwindles. This was also the case at UCI. But the fallout of austerity goes beyond burdening impoverished families with the costs of procuring and paying for medical supplies, procedures, tests, and food. It also changes what it means to be a physician. And the impact of austerity also changed the embodied and practical meaning of giving and receiving chemotherapy itself.

Chances are, if you are on a ward round at the UCI and need a translator for a little-known Ugandan language, you will look for Okuku. He grew up near Busia, a vibrant border town and main thoroughfare between Kenya and Uganda. The son of an accountant and homemaker whose family had historic ties to the cattle-selling market and butcheries, Okuku was the first of his family members to pursue a life in medicine and first started working at the UCI as a medical student in the early 2000s. He speaks many of Uganda's forty widely known languages and has a reputation on the wards for smoothing out issues related to end-of-life care or ways forward for dealing with late-stage cancers with a deft, humane, and educational touch.

When he first started at the UCI as a third-year medical student in 2001, he was one of two students on the ward who slept over in the evenings to attend to blood donation and medications.[56] This was a longstanding arrangement at the Institute going back to the 1960s, when bright and energetic medical students were given the opportunity to learn how to do lumbar punctures and blood-type matching. The Institute gave them a roof over their heads and tea in exchange for managing emergencies and being a first line of contact for crises at night.[57] Despite being a "sad place" where if "a patient came with a diagnosis of cancer, there would be no hope for them. Next would be death," Okuku still wanted to work at the UCI, largely because of ongoing mentorship from Orem and Mbidde. "It was a really interesting opportunity to learn." There were no other wards at Mulago where a third-year medical student would be charged with tasks like "getting transfusions done. Clerking for people coming late in the evening because we always had Burkitt's kids coming late, like after 5 p.m. And those kids needed some kind of care." Mbidde, famous for his exacting high standards, taught Okuku how to do a "meticulous examination of the patient," as well as how to manage tumor lysis syndrome through administering adequate fluids. Okuku also learned how to manage pain, prescribe complicated regimens of antibiotics, and even manage some chemotherapy administration.

Okuku continued to work at the UCI for his fourth-year medical school elective and continued to learn. "I started doing [more] procedures. All these procedures we do on kids with Burkitt's like bone marrows. I became very efficient. I taught many post grads. Of course LPs [lumbar punctures] was like daily bread. I did so many lumbar punctures on Burkitt's lymphoma kids. I would do like twenty in a day. I became an expert, really. It was unique to the Institute. Whoever went through there learned so much."

In the 2000s the institutional lore is that staff would receive one shipment of chemotherapy drugs a year, and that supply would run out within a month. They were rarely stocked with morphine. When Okuku was asked to describe what he was doing at the UCI as a medical student and volunteer medical officer, he said, "I'm not sure what kind of care we were providing," but "we weren't doing medicine." I asked him if he was doing palliation: "There was nothing to palliate with. The work went on, but we had serious issues at that point." But at the same time, there were moments of reprieve and patients who did survive and greatly improve. "I personally developed interest in oncology because after working with the patients and seeing some very challenging situations where people died, I was also seeing some success stories." Okuku finished medical school in 2003 and went directly to the UCI as a volunteer medical officer. He was paid "no salary. Nothing." Mulago was still responsible for "all sundries" at the UCI, whose budget was about twenty million Ugandan shillings a year, roughly $7,940. A full chemotherapy cycle of cyclophosphamide, vincristine, and methotrexate (COM) for a Burkitt's lymphoma patient was about $300 at that time.

But the UCI continued to offer a real education, not just in terms of learning new procedures and improvising under circumstances of profound scarcity. Working at the UCI also offered an up-close and often disturbingly intimate look at the reality of poverty facing many of the patients and caretakers who came to this place. It was the only place offering on-cology goods, such as they were, to the public in Uganda. As Okuku put it, "We never saw high clientele come over here for treatment. It was usually this local, rural flock. I guess people who had the money went elsewhere." Destitution and death commingled in unsettling ways. Take the story of Okuku's "worst experience" working at the UCI in the early 2000s:

> FO: We had a situation where there were so many dead, but this was a unique one, where you have a grandmother who brings in a child with HIV and Burkitt's lymphoma. The disease was ad-vanced. There were no drugs at that time [for either BL or HIV]. We knew the child would die. And indeed the child died without receiving any medicines then. And then what happened next was this grandmother didn't have any money to take back the body, like to hire a van or a truck.
>
> So she did what all of us would not imagine. Before the body became stiff she folded the knees of this child and forced the body in to a bag. We had left the child lying on the bed, usually in the area where we do procedures. And I came back and asked, "Eh! Where is the body?" And she showed me the bag. And I said, "What do you mean?" 'The boy's in the bag.' And I said "what? How did you fit him in this short bag this small?" And she said, 'Well, I broke his knees and pushed him in there.'
>
> So in shock I called Angus Robinson [a visiting British hematologist-oncologist who worked at the LTC from 2000 to 2003] to come and experience for himself. We opened the bag because we couldn't believe he [the boy] was in the bag. That was the worst. It traumatized both of us.
>
> We saw that we were working in a place where there was so much poverty that people were forced to do some *extra*ordinary things. Out of this world. To make life easy for them. If it meant hiring a truck, it would have cost lots of money.
>
> MM: But this way she could go on a bus.
>
> FO: She would just go on the bus with a bag. . . . It is still fresh in my mind.[58]

In the 2000s, Okuku and his nursing colleagues worked in a context where death was a common occurrence. With the advent of chemother-apy, syringes, and more reliable morphine stocks since institutional auton-omy in 2009, staff at the UCI still work at a site where caring for late-stage cancers means that many (but certainly not all) patients will die, either on the wards or back in villages and homes. This particular story of the granny and the boy in the bag has become something of an institutional legend, a way to hearken back to the "dark days" of the UCI. In her work on end-of-life care in hospitalizations in the United States, anthropologist Sharon Kaufman writes about the challenges of trying to usher in a "good death" for patients and also for their loved ones. This involves a progression of rituals that medical staff subtly perform for families in order to show they have done everything they can. Meanwhile it is the family's job to "let go" of the patient so the medical staff feel free to "move things along" and usher in a good death for the patient by ending life support or avoiding extreme medical procedures.[59]

At the UCI in the 2000s, and indeed for the three decades the Institute was under the administration of Mulago Hospital, the staff at the UCI were often stripped of their ability to do "everything," be it debulking a late-stage liver tumor with chemotherapy to ease pain or administering antibiotic ointment on Kaposi's sarcoma lesions to prevent fetid infections. They were left to work within a different set of ritual practices that signaled doing everything—a meticulous ward round, a careful diagnostic work-up of cancer stage and histopathological diagnosis (even if the pathology department itself was out of important reagents and that diagnosis languished for six months), writing letters to pharmacists to request cutting the price of cyclophosphamide for this one promising case of early stage Burkitt's lymphoma. For patients and their caretakers, participating in this set of rituals necessitated attending regular chemotherapy treatments and buying coffins and organizing transport when a death on the ward would occur. But as the story of the granny and the boy in the bag shows, the realities of impoverishment often dictated that these rituals of moving things along to a good death were compromised.

As Okuku sees it, money and the ability of a family to purchase the necessary chemotherapy cycles brought the "few success stories" during the early 2000s. Most patients would receive one cycle of chemotherapy and then collect the phone numbers of nursing staff and wait for the call informing them that a new shipment of chemotherapy had arrived.[60] "So then you would have one guy receiving chemo today and then he doesn't come back because he doesn't have money. And he comes back after two months for chemo or another five months. And he gets one injection and goes back again home. So it was senseless. You wouldn't talk about doing any research. Or treatment research to see the outcomes. . . . it was a horrible place."[61] Nonetheless, the staff worked tirelessly and professionally. Mbidde would do a daily "cleanliness round" in which he would walk into the wards and run his finger along the window ledges looking for dirt, and he chided nurses if the toilets smelled bad. Patients were given tea and two meals a day. As "horrible" as it was, the work continued.

CODA: CHEMOTHERAPY AFTER AUSTERITY

Since 2009, the chemotherapy procurement budget for the UCI shifted from less than twenty million Ugandan shillings a year to approximately seven billion Ugandan shillings (about two million US dollars) during my fieldwork in 2012.[62] This has meant far more reliable chemotherapy supplies, although there are still shortages and many more patients. The Institute has grown from twenty to over two hundred employees in a few short years, leading to issues concerning how to transform practice and build institutional cohesion at the "Museum." Redefining the practice of administering chemotherapy has become a major issue. It is no longer a viable option to run a makeshift outpatient unit for patients trickling in with their own drugs in the UCI's reception area. There are now upwards of one hundred outpatients a day coming for their infusions, and this has led to several investments—in additional treatment space, in a chemotherapy reconstitution hood, and in the dedicated training of pharmacists.

During my ethnographic fieldwork on the wards of the UCI, I could hear, see, and smell the violent effects of chemotherapy on the body as drugs destroy DNA, disrupt folic acid reception, and promote cell death. When I talked about saba saba with patients who were treated at the UCI in 2012, some of them remembered the invasion of 1979 but were keen to point out that chemotherapy is no longer saba saba. As they remembered, in the 1980s and 1990s saba saba was related to the violence of administering the drugs through push injections rather than intravenous drips. As one breast cancer survivor put it, "They called it saba saba because they would push it into you. Not like they do today on the wards with the drip." Intravenous drips were seen as more "gentle" and less physically damaging. When I asked nurses who had worked at the UCI in the 1980s and 1990s if they remembered saba saba, they would laugh, clap their hands for emphasis, and say, "Yes, saba saba, the war." These older nurses also confirmed that they had called the drugs saba saba in the past. But even though bodies erupt in the chemotherapy administration room today, chemotherapy is no longer called saba saba among this generation of doctors, nurses, or patients. Younger nurses, most of whom were born in the 1980s, have no visceral, embodied memory of the war, as they had been hired in the late 2000s.[63] For them and for patients, chemotherapy treatments were generally called "the drugs" or *keemo,* the closest Luganda approximation to "chemo" or *empiso mukaaga* (six shots). In patient consultations, this was the terminology Okuku used in sketching out a course of treatment for cancer at the UCI. "You will come back for keemo six times. This is six shots. You must come back for empiso mukaaga even if it makes you sick." He counted it out on his hands as a gesture of clarity and education in consultations with patients and their families. By the end of most afternoons, after the chemo had been administered, the ward was filled with the sounds of retching and the shuffle of parents walking in and out of the ward, with buckets full of sickness to be deposited into the toilets. Whether called saba saba or keemo, cytotoxic drugs are still a source of excruciating violence on the body.

5 ⮀ When Radiotherapy Travels

IN 2012, on any given morning at the radiotherapy bunker at Mulago Hospital, eighty to one hundred cancer patients lined up to be "roasted," as it is known in Luganda, the local language most widely spoken in Kampala and central Uganda. In the early 1990s, the Ugandan government procured a GWGP80 Cobalt-60 machine through a partnership with the International Atomic Energy Agency (IAEA). Manufactured in China and newly refurbished, the GWGP80 was seen as "rugged," "simple," "affordable," and capable of quickly and inexpensively treating cancer patients.[1] While I was researching this book, the machine had a reputation for frequent service disruptions due to breakdowns. In addition, the Cobalt-60 source was severely depleted and should have been replaced in 2005. When I spoke with the Ugandan physician-scientists who trained through IAEA partnerships in radiation oncology and medical physics, they emphasized their moral and medical obligation to continue to run the unit. In order to harness the last of the Cobalt-60's radioactivity, the staff increased the amount of time patients were exposed to the source's gamma rays. But given the weakness of the source, it was unclear to what extent longer exposure times simply harmed and burned rather than healed or alleviated suffering. Nevertheless, women rotting and bleeding from the inside out from cervical cancer, or men with bone cancer, or children with leukemia and central nervous system involvement still spent their time under the "roasting" machine, with the hope that it could provide palliative relief and shrink tumors.[2] Approximately 1,850 patients underwent radiotherapy at the unit per year.[3]

On the one hand, the continued operation of the radiotherapy machine despite its breakdowns and deteriorating source was a remarkable act of creativity in crisis, an extraordinary act of ongoing maintenance and repair. On the other, it was a tragic situation. Patients faced the consequences not only in treatment outcomes but also in terms of how they would spend their last months of life. As Dr. Z, a longtime radiation oncologist at Mulago, said:

> We continue what we do now, which is palliative. The very early cancers we try to treat aggressively. But for anybody who is very advanced, we are very strict and don't give long treatments for that. And it kind of denies them some of the palliative care they can receive and as far as pain control is concerned maybe some of the most distressing symptoms we can control reasonably well with the existing machine. Certainly it's not good, but what can we do where we are working at?[4]

There was a human cost to all of this. Although the work at the unit was mainly to palliate, and the majority of treatments were not aimed at providing cures or even necessarily long-term remissions, that was not always what patients were coming for, whether they were referred from the Uganda Cancer Institute (UCI) or the obstetrics and gynecology ward of Mulago. As Dr. Z put it, this unit was primarily a "lady's unit," and the vast majority of patients who were waiting to get their turn under the weak gamma rays were women with advanced cervical cancer and breast cancer.[5]

Yes, these "lady" patients came to the unit for pain management, but they also came to the unit from remote distances and camped out on the verandahs for months at a time in hopes of renewing biologically and socially reproductive futures. Women with cervical cancer were coming not only to mitigate incessant bleeding but also in the hopes that these beams would restore a sexual life with a partner and the possibility of having a child. And the staff kept these hopes alive, counseling women on how to use their fingers to keep their vaginal walls from collapsing from the treatments and explaining how soon they could return to sexual intercourse.[6] Caring for these hopes of returning to social and biological reproduction, to an ordinary intimate life, was as important as administering chemotherapy and tracking down oral morphine.

Other patients came to the unit after several years of being in remission from cancer. Take the story of Joy.[7] Joy was one of the breast cancer survivors who spent her Friday mornings at the cancer screening clinic educating patients about how to do breast self-exams.[8] She felt a new lump in her remaining breast in 2012, and she was devastated. But she followed up with her oncologist right away, who prescribed a new and punishing regimen of chemotherapy and radiotherapy. While undergoing chemo, Joy tripled her attendance at her Born Again church, in large part to ask God to ensure that the radiotherapy machine would be operational when her name was finally called from the waiting list. "I pray that the machine will be working," she said. The radiotherapy unit's long-term mechanic, Mr. T, was able to scrounge a new electrical component to replace one that had been failing—just in time for Joy to get her treatment with the machine. Her appointment slot was late at night—10 p.m.—because the machine operates twenty hours a day.[9] But after her treatments, Joy did not improve, although her charred skin from the "roasting" and vanished eyebrows remained a reminder of the treatments. She became increasingly ill. She melted away at her home in Ntinda, a suburb of Kampala. Regular hospice attendants managed her pain with oral morphine and kind words until the day of her death. Was it the fact that Joy's cancer was simply too advanced to be treated? Or was it the fact that the radiotherapy machine was operating with a radioactive source that should have been replaced in 2005 and that therefore her radiotherapy treatments were performative rather than efficacious? We will never know.

In this chapter, my aim is not to untangle the ambiguity and uncertainty of diagnosis and therapeutic efficacy in Joy's cancer treatments or those of others coming to Mulago National Referral Hospital for relief from malignancies. It is also not my intention to undermine or call into question the daily efforts of staff and caretakers at the radiotherapy unit to alleviate suffering and to use the tools available for palliation and care. These issues are, of course, tremendously important.[10] On the wards of the radiotherapy unit and at the UCI, uncertainty around the efficacy of treatments, as I discuss elsewhere, is a major topic of concern for medical staff as they try to determine who should be sent home to die and who should undergo a new round of induction therapy.[11] Oncology is an ambivalent constellation of healing technologies under the best of circumstances, where the trinity of practices—poisoning, cutting, and burning—constantly raises concerns about futility, efficacy, and harming.[12]

Here, I am more concerned with untangling the historical, sociotechnical, and political stakes that shaped this reality in 2012. I want to chart the ways in which we can understand why it was possible in the first place for Joy to pray for her time under the weak gamma rays of a radiotherapy machine, which for all intents and purposes was not "working."[13] Every year there were over a thousand patients like Joy who went to the radiotherapy unit in search of treatment, relief, and the possibility to extend life and *live* as they did before. What circumstances led to an ostensibly broken machine being used consistently over twenty hours a day, seven days a week? Why wasn't the machine decommissioned? Why was it so difficult to procure a new radioactive source?

These questions about the material, technological, and political basis of therapeutics and diagnostics were and continue to be part of the core challenges facing oncology care in Uganda. Take the technological challenges of Burkitt's lymphoma treatment, for example, for which treatment outcomes were poorer at the time of my research than they were in Idi Amin's Uganda.[14] Research suggests that this discrepancy may reflect atrophied pathology services in the country. In 2012, on the wards of the UCI, the agreement between clinical diagnosis on the wards and pathological diagnosis for Burkitt's lymphoma was very low. According to a study in 2012 of diagnosis of childhood lymphoma, the agreement between pathological diagnoses made in Uganda and a reference laboratory in the Netherlands was only 36 percent (95 percent CI 28–46). Agreement between Ugandan pathologists and pathologists from the Netherlands on a Burkitt's lymphoma diagnosis occurred only 52 percent of the time. If we were to take the Netherlands diagnoses to be the "right" diagnoses (and to be fair, they most likely were correct, given the limited access to the reagents and laboratory techniques in Uganda), this means that only half the children with Burkitt's lymphoma were being correctly diagnosed.[15] The consequences of this could be devastating. For patients who clinically presented with Burkitt's-like symptoms and received an injection of chemotherapy drugs, this could very well have created drug resistance if it was later decided that the patient actually had a rhabdomyosarcoma.

Untangling why it was so hard to get pathologists to agree on a diagnosis takes us into a thorny briar patch of questions. Why was it so hard to retrofit the pathology laboratory? Why was it such a huge challenge to conduct a biopsy properly and get tissues encased in paraffin with alacrity? Was the responsiveness of Burkitt's lymphoma to a long-established treatment regimen itself changing?[16]

Julie Livingston has argued that improvisation is a fundamental aspect of the practice and provision of biomedicine in Africa. In a context where drugs are constantly in and out of stock, where blood transfusion services are erratic, and where vital reagents for pathology diagnoses are missing, the striking unpredictability of what may or may not be available profoundly shapes medical practice.[17] I agree with Livingston and argue similar issues are in play in oncology services and virtually any biomedical services at Mulago and elsewhere in Uganda. My aim here is to step back and interrogate the technopolitical constellations that make this so.[18]

The history of neoliberal economic reforms that gutted the budgets of African health systems in the 1980s and 1990s is an obvious factor in shaping episodic stock shortages or dilapidated health infrastructures.[19] But scarcity can only partly explain biomedical improvisation. I suggest that one way we can understand this story of the radiotherapy machine is if we contextualize it as a key example of the ramifications of oncology care as a transferred set of technologies.[20] Dr. Z worked in a clinical environment that was the product of a longer history of radiotherapy technology transfer and an example of what it takes to keep technical objects *going* in Uganda. It is but one example of the ways in which transferred technologies are reshaped by a local culture of managing the vagaries of cheap equipment and frequent breakdowns. In Uganda, this logic of care grew at least partially out of experiences of civil war in the 1980s, and it privileges providing *something* to patients, even if it is simply the performance of *doing something*.[21] This desire to give *something* to patients, be it palliation or long-term treatments, was part of what kept the waiting lists long and the machine operating twenty hours a day. Keeping the radiotherapy machine open and operational was shaped also by a local culture of repair and maintenance that is reminiscent of Uganda's automobile repair market. Mechanics, spare parts, and a willingness to keep driving even if the "check engine" light comes on keep vehicles going for the moment; however, repairing roads or potholes is a different story.

In the pages that follow, I show how the technopolitics of eroded infrastructures, an underfunded health-care sector, international partnerships, anticorruption measures around procurement, and (weirdly enough) the global War on Terror and East African military and security concerns shaped the efficacy, practice, and technology of "roasting." I offer a historical overview of radiotherapy services in Uganda and then offer an account of the ways this machine was maintained in a style reminiscent of the ways vehicles are repaired in Kampala. After providing this context, I unpack the broader technopolitical circumstances of procurement and disposal, which made it so challenging to upgrade radiotherapy services. I conclude by discussing some of the implications of technology transfer for the broader arena of oncology services in Uganda.

I draw primarily on accounts from the Ugandan media, reports from the International Atomic Energy Agency (IAEA), academic medical journals on radiotherapy in Africa, and ethnographic research conducted at the radiotherapy unit at Lower Mulago Hospital in 2012. This archival and ethnographic research was further buttressed by interviews with Dr. Z, the pseudonym of one of the longtime radiotherapy oncologists who agreed to be on record about the history of Mulago's radiotherapy services, as well as Dr. Z's mentor, who was one of the individuals responsible for building radiotherapy services at Mulago, and interviews at Lacor Hospital. Luganda translations were discussed and provided by Waalabyeki Magoba. It should also be noted that during the time of conducting this research in 2012, the radiotherapy unit and the UCI were separate bureaucratic entities.

A BRIEF HISTORY OF RADIOTHERAPY SERVICES IN UGANDA: A DEMONSTRATION PROJECT

Radiotherapy technology and expertise came to Uganda through channels of donations, partnerships, and training along two separate geographical and cultural regions in Uganda, rather than being embedded in the UCI's existing experimental infrastructure. In the north, at Lacor Hospital in Gulu, radiotherapy services and a surgical oncology unit opened in the 1970s with the help of an Italian donation. These services were seen as a way to meet the needs of the community in the surrounding area of northern Uganda.[22] At Mulago, radiotherapy services were established in the 1990s independently of the Institute through a partnership with the IAEA.

The radiotherapy unit at Mulago is more commonly referred to as "the bunker," and it was a school of radiography for many years before being converted and reinforced in the early 1990s to house the Cobalt-60 machine. One of the country's first radiation oncologists, Dr. Z worked at the unit from 1994 to 2014. The bunker itself is hot and airless, and when we met, he was wearing a short-sleeve dress shirt to provide some relief from the heat, along with a carefully selected tie. Dr. Z is a busy man and was not afraid to interrupt our interview on a few occasions to follow up on a consultation for a patient.

Mulago's radiotherapy department intimately intertwines with Dr. Z's professional history, the broader history of the hospital's struggles during the Tanzanian war in 1979, its slow restoration in the wake of neoliberal reforms, and an ongoing bush war in the 1980s.[23] Dr. Z first came to Mulago in the late 1970s and became a doctor in 1981, during the worst instability and violence. He recalled:

We were sitting exams. Bombs were going off. A lot of war trauma. And there were no immunizations, so measles was everywhere. Children were dying like anything. We had lost years because things weren't well planned. Programming and prevention and so on. No paper. You would write on some gloves. You would detach the gloves and write clinical notes on the paper. It was really impossible. It was a crazy time. It was a military camp kind of thing. But that's the time we graduated. Very difficult times. Very difficult years. And there was a problem with funding, which has really not improved very much. It's better than it was before, but percentage wise in the national budget, it's a very small percentage.[24]

In the wake of Idi Amin's "disintegrating state"[25] and the uncertainty of war, Dr. Z trained as a radiologist at Mulago but also spent a year and a half studying in Germany. When he returned in the mid-1980s, he was put in charge of operating an X-ray machine, which was used to remove superficial tumors. "I wanted to be a radiologist. I only wanted to become a radiation oncologist after seeing the *need*."[26] In the late 1980s and early 1990s, as Dr. Z was seeing the need for radiation oncology on the wards of Mulago National Hospital, the IAEA started to recognize a growing cancer burden in Africa.[27] Spearheaded in part by emeritus professor of radiotherapy at Cairo University in Egypt, Dr. M. M. Mahfouz, the IAEA presented an agenda for ameliorating the "rather disastrous state of radiation therapy in Africa." Writing in the early 1990s, Mahfouz said: "Only about 35% of the countries in Africa have any facilities for radiation therapy, and in many cases these are grossly ill-equipped and understaffed. There are shortages of radiation oncologists, medical physicists, dosimetrists, radiation technologists, radiotherapy nurses, and other technicians."[28]

A number of factors shaped the absence of radiotherapy services in many African countries. The relative invisibility of cancer as a public health priority, and the tremendous capital and human investments necessary in installing and maintaining radiotherapy services, put radiotherapy facilities at the bottom of the list of health priorities for African governments.[29] As the IAEA noted, "The high cost of developing the basic infrastructure, and buying equipment for establishing a medium-sized radiotherapy center, is probably beyond the means of many African countries. The cost of setting up a unit capable of treating up to 2000 cases per year is about US$2.5 million."[30]

In the early 1990s, the IAEA's leadership decided to address these costs by establishing programs to transfer radiotherapy technology to African countries along with a package of training fellowships and maintenance contracts meant to facilitate the establishment of radiotherapy centers at various national referral hospitals across the continent. This was a demonstration project. For the IAEA, they would show that radiotherapy technologies could be established and used in the developing world safely. African radiotherapy care providers would demonstrate to reluctant ministries of health that if they built radiotherapy bunkers, patients would indeed come from far and wide to the capital in search of relief from their cancer. These investments in radiotherapy equipment and training technologies were meant to establish some of the first but not the only radiotherapy facilities in Africa.

Creating African radiation oncology experts, medical physicists, technicians, and nurses was at the heart of these collaborations, but at least in Uganda, IAEA technocrats and Ministry of Health officials did not create these experts from scratch. Rather, they searched for local talent like Dr. Z, who already had a promising career as a radiologist and was already mentored by the head of the radiology department of Mulago, to send for further training. In Dr. Z's case, he went to train in radiation oncology in Cairo from 1991 to 1993 and returned to Uganda to oversee the operations of Mulago's newly acquired but already used Cobalt-60 machine.

Mulago's secondhand machine was not unique. When the IAEA spearheaded its radiotherapy capacity building in the early 1990s, most of the machines transferred to African countries were refurbished Cobalt-60 units. These machines were cheaper than the ones usually purchased in the Global North and procured as a way to contain costs. As the IAEA noted:

> It becomes obvious, therefore, that the capital outlay has to be reduced to make the units affordable to many countries in Africa. This can be done by encouraging manufacturers of radiotherapy equipment to design cheaper models devoid of costly electronic and mechanical parts, but which will still maintain the same beam quality and optimum radiation safety standards as the more expensive designs. Such a machine will be simple, rugged, and more mechanical than electrical. It is also more likely to withstand damage to electronic parts from fluctuations in electric power supply, and the humid, warm, and dusty climate common in Africa.[31]

In other words, the IAEA was looking for the radiotherapy machine equivalent of the Zimbabwe bush pump—rugged, affordable, simple, and effective. But as the classic piece by Marianne de Laet and Annemarie Mol argues, the Zimbabwe bush pump is a "good" technology not only because it promotes community health and builds the nation but also because "good technologies . . . incorporate the possibility of their own break-down, which have the flexibility to deploy alternative components, and which continue to work to some extent even if some bolt falls out or the user community changes."[32] The Cobalt-60 machine is similarly flexible and open to tinkering; however, what makes a "good" technology can make a bad radiotherapy unit. In the Ugandan case, the machine they received was simply junk. A cast-off unit made and used in China; it was retrofitted for use in Uganda in the name of cutting costs.

There is no equivalent to the word *junk* in Luganda. Things are old (*enkadde*) or very old (*enkadde nnyo*). In English, while colloquially *junk* is defined as useless or worthless stuff (essentially trash), it also refers more generally to material that can be recycled and re-used. Furthermore *to junk* means to discard or scrap a piece of material that is considered useful. Junk, in all of its multiple uses and interpretations here, is an apt way of appraising the quality of the equipment. But I want to be clear here that Ugandan colleagues interviewed for this project did *not* describe the radiotherapy machine in this way. This is my gloss. The closest equivalent to *junk* used by Ugandan colleagues for the unit is "Chinese equipment."[33]

MADE IN CHINA, MAINTAINED IN UGANDA

Over a decade ago, an informant of Dr. Paul Farmer summed up the problem of technology transfer to the developing world in a few sentences. This priest said: "Do you know what 'appropriate' technology means? It means good things for rich people and shit for the poor."[34] Even from the first days of its installation and use, the Cobalt-60 machine operated like "appropriate" technology. It was prone to breakdown and required vigilant care and attention maintenance and small repairs. Within the first several months of being used, a "pilferage of the control panel and TV monitor"[35] late one evening led to the shuttering of the unit for two months while replacement parts were procured from overseas. At other times, issues with Uganda's electricity grid, and "minor" problems such as "cleaning or replacing control switches and fuses or replacing indicator lamps"[36] led to frequent service interruptions of one or two hours at a time.

More dramatic downtimes were caused by the machine's force-back system, which was simply poorly designed. A Cobalt-60 machine's radio-active source is housed in a storage casing of heavy lead and moves into position during treatment where gamma rays irradiate a small surface area on the body. The source is then sucked by a vacuum back into the storage position in the machine after treatment. On one occasion, the motor for the compressor that makes this vacuum possible failed, and the source "had to be hammered back into the safe position," no doubt exposing the mechanic to excess radiation.[37] On another occasion, "the fault was due to a worn-out piston ring" that "could not be obtained locally and an oil seal from a car engine was improvised as a replacement which has been working quite effectively."[38] Today, the improvised oil seal is still in place. The joke at the bunker goes that if Mr. T, the unit's mechanic, is sick for some reason, the machine will be out of commission until he returns.[39]

At the radiotherapy unit, "Chinese equipment" is a polite euphemism for describing the dubious quality of the machine. As Dr. Z says, "This machine I think we have the oldest machine of this type working in the world after seventeen years. It's Chinese equipment. And the thing about Chinese equipment is that they [sic] are not very strong. I think they are an advantage in numbers. You get this, you get a new one. We've had this one for seventeen years. It has many frequent breakdowns."[40] The Cobalt-60 machine is like so many other goods in Uganda. It's a second-hand piece of equipment that in another context would have been junked and dis-posed of, but here it's been given a second chance.[41]

Coping with the quality of "Chinese equipment," which is cheap and easy to come by (but not necessarily robust or high quality), is part of everyday life in Uganda and dovetails more generally with a local culture of repair. One critical way to manage transferred technologies, from auto-mobiles to electronics to medical equipment, is to work with a trusted me-chanic. This mechanic is often charged with finding reliable spare parts as quickly and cheaply as possible, which is a challenge in a parts market where materials are often used, and possibly counterfeit.[42] Maintenance and service guidelines shaped in the metropolitan spaces of conference rooms in Vienna certainly traveled to Uganda. IAEA technocrats knew that the Cobalt-60 machine would be impacted by the dust and the pre-carious power supplies. Mr. T was even sent to China for a couple of months in the 1990s to learn how to keep the refurbished GWGP80 ma-chine operating and well lubricated. The IAEA could not anticipate the ways in which the Cobalt-60 machine would be incorporated into the broader maintenance logic that shapes everyday practices of keeping trans-ferred technologies going in Uganda, where things often break and the necessary spare parts must be radically improvised. Given this innovative culture of repair, is it at all surprising that the maintenance and operations of the radiotherapy unit would be radically different from other forms of repair? Mr. T cares for and maintains the radiotherapy on a day-to-day basis in Uganda much like a *matatu* (a minibus taxi) that must *keep going no matter what.* When I posed this possible analogy between the matatu and the Cobalt-60 machine to Dr. Z, he laughed and said, "Ha ha, exactly. You are moving and moving, and you get out and put in something. But you get to where you need to go eventually."[43]

Ongoing crises around electricity power outages or "load shedding," as well as interruptions in Kampala's water supply are other examples of infrastructural crises where creative repairs keep things going. What is dis-tinctive here is the issue of redundancy and the dilemma of scale. For a radiotherapy unit, a generator cannot be bought at the market, no inverter can be installed, no reserve water tank can be purchased, and there is no child to fetch more water in a jerry can from a burst pipe. If the machine isn't working, you must pray or go to Nairobi or India for care. What are people to do when they cannot maintain, repair, or tinker at a scale be-yond the matatu or a Cobalt-60 unit? Moreover, why is it so hard to repair vital infrastructure such as a road or to buy a new machine?

THE POLITICS AND PRACTICALITIES
OF PROCUREMENT AND DISPOSAL

It seems simple enough to "fix" the problem of an expired Cobalt-60 source. Purchase a new source from a reliable contractor, ship the ma-terial according to international safety standards to the port of Mombasa, move it via truck or train in a hermetically sealed lead box to Kampala, install the source, and dispose of the old radioactive material. After all, this is what was done in years past with great success through the partnership between the Ugandan government and the IAEA at Mulago up until the early 2000s.

The geopolitics of the War on Terror and the fear of "dirty bombs" since the 9/11 World Trade Center terrorist attacks have led to tightened regulations on how radioactive materials may be procured and disposed of. For Mulago staff like Dr. Z, the War on Terror is seen as one of the major obstacles to the timely procurement and mobility of new Cobalt-60. As the current director of Mulago Hospital noted for the record on Ugandan

radio, "The cobalt machine is not an [*sic*] equipment you can buy or-
dinarily. You need International Atomic Energy Association [*sic*] regulations so that actually people don't hijack it and use it for like Shabab or
Al Qaeda."[44] The head of Mulago was not speculating. Since the World
Trade Center attack in 2001, the refusal of airlines to transport radioactive
materials has greatly reduced the mobility of Cobalt-60 and other radioactive sources.[45]

In addition to the challenges of transporting radioactive materials,
new and evolving procurement policies for purchasing materials over
US$1,000, instituted by the Ugandan government to mitigate corruption
and graft, similarly shape and constrain the purchase and movement of
new Cobalt-60. The procurement process involves seven steps of complex
bidding, soliciting tenders, and weighing contracts: all have to be done
according to the cycle of the fiscal year.[46] The manufacture of Cobalt-60
itself is on the decline, as more and more radiotherapy facilities in the
Global North shift their technology to linear acceleration. And there have
been changes in the partnership between the IAEA and the Ugandan government since the early days of the radiotherapy unit. Personal relationships, which were so important in setting up and operating machines in
the first place, shifted and changed as people retired, got promoted, or lost
their energy and willingness to keep one-time technology transfers maintained and viable.

Procurement politics are also shaped by the realities of the challenges
of disposal. What do you do with old sources if a new one comes? On the
disposal side, while the IAEA remains in charge of managing radioactive
waste, the everyday responsibility for safe disposal of radiotherapy sources
often falls on partner governments across the Global South.[47] Despite concerns regarding the mobility and management of radioactive materials like
spent Cobalt-60 sources, countries are still left to deal with these materials
largely on their own and in locally specific ways. Incineration, by far one
of the most common methods of dealing with medical waste at Mulago
Hospital, does not work for disposing of Cobalt-60. In the past, according
to employees, spent sources were taken by the IAEA and dumped out on
"the high seas," usually off the coast of Somalia. Due to the challenges associated with moving these materials to the standards of international regulations, the spent sources remained on Mulago's campus. For much of
the 2000s, depleted Cobalt-60 sources were kept in a small three-by-four-
foot storage facility on Mulago's campus, secured with a padlock and not
kept under particularly close surveillance.[48]

According to US government wires made public by WikiLeaks, in July 2007 a group of thieves broke into the storage area and stole the radioactive materials from the unit, unaware of its value or exactly what it was.[49] Officials from the US National Nuclear Security Administration visited Kampala shortly thereafter to assess the situation and demonstrate a "joint US-Ugandan response to the theft of radiological material from a storage area at Mulago Hospital." (Incidentally, the US ambassador to Uganda responsible for bringing these thefts to the US's attention, Jerry Lanier, went on to work at the State Department as the director of the counterterrorism unit.) On paper, the IAEA is, for all intents and purposes, still responsible for signing off on how radioactive materials are stored in Uganda. As Mulago Hospital spokesman Dan Kimosho said when this story broke in September 2011, "International Atomic Energy Agency clears us for procurement, storage and whatever we do. It's up to them to clear us."[50]

Finally, in addition to the politics of disposal, while the Cobalt-60 source loses its potency, the radiotherapy machine itself continues to break and atrophy, moving from old to extremely old—so old that it is increasingly apparent to staff that the machine should be replaced. And so an ongoing debate has led to a stalemate of sorts. Is it worth buying a new radioactive source and installing it in an old machine that is about to be decommissioned anyway? Would it just be better to wait until the next fiscal year and see if a new machine can actually be procured? In the meantime, is it not just best to house the spent sources on-site rather than spend huge amounts of money to dispose of it properly? In the meantime, the "roasting" continues.[51]

EBOLA: WHAT IT TAKES TO CLOSE A UNIT

So why not just shutter the unit until a new radiotherapy machine is procured or a new Cobalt-60 source is acquired? Dr. Z and many of his colleagues learned how to keep things going and provide care in the midst of civil war. They are used to working creatively in crisis, writing out lab report requests on recycled paper from gloves packaging if need be. In addition, Dr. Z's professional identity is intimately tied to the continued operations of the radiotherapy unit. Dr. Z is an expert, invited to meetings in Geneva and Cape Town. He publishes in international medical journals and has made a better living than most as a senior physician at Mulago. He and his colleagues have a professional stake in keeping the unit open as long as possible.

To shut something like the radiotherapy unit down would probably require a catastrophe. And indeed, catastrophe is what shuttered Uganda's only other radiotherapy unit. Until this point, I have focused mainly on the history of Mulago Hospital's radiotherapy politics and have only discussed Lacor Hospital's radiotherapy unit in passing. In contrast to Mulago's unit, Lacor Hospital's Cobalt-60 machine was procured through the channels of Italian Catholic donors. The secondhand machine was made in Germany by Siemens. It arrived at Lacor Hospital in the mid-1970s via train to Gulu and was assembled on-site with the help of several Italians, including an X-ray technician and mechanic. The machine was installed in a bunker in the middle of the hospital campus and, with a surgical oncology unit, provided cancer care to those living in northern Uganda.[52]

In 2000 the unit closed due to a series of unfortunate circumstances. The Lord's Resistance Army brought havoc to northern Uganda. Lacor Hospital became a war hospital and a space of refuge for nighttime residents fearing kidnappings.[53] The radioactive source needed to be replaced, and it was going to be extremely challenging to move a new Cobalt-60 source in northern Uganda during wartime. The official story of what shuttered the unit, however, was a horrible Ebola outbreak that claimed the lives of over two hundred people, including the hospital's director, Dr. Matthew Lukwiya. His colleague, Dr. Y, who was responsible for running the radiation oncology services at Lacor, suddenly found himself running the hospital. As Dr. Z put it, "He had a weak source and too much administration. He was doing radiology apart from radiotherapy and said, 'Well, radiotherapy. I think it is what? It's closed.'"[54]

Today at Lacor there is no longer a cancer ward. It was converted into a tuberculosis unit. At Lacor Hospital community meetings, people wonder when cancer services will come back to the hospital. While the hospital still sees cancer patients and refers them to Mulago for care, most melt away into their respective northern villages to rot, never to be seen in Kampala. The Cobalt-60 itself is still entombed in its lead chamber, slowly losing its radioactivity as it retreats into its half-life, irradiating all of the old radiotherapy patient records in the process. Ironically, the fallout shelter went nuclear.

With this story, we see what it would take to shut down Mulago's radiotherapy unit, or at least shutter it until a new Cobalt-60 source is procured and installed. Quite frankly, it would probably require something similar to the synergy of the Ebola catastrophe, guerrilla war, and administrative shortfalls that plagued Lacor in the early 2000s. Similar circumstances shuttered Liberia's Cobalt-60 machine in Monrovia during the civil war, as did the full-scale atrophy of Zimbabwe's health services in the early 2000s. Medical staff, as we've seen at Mulago, elsewhere in Uganda, and indeed across Africa, are incredibly adept at acting creatively in times of crisis. But some circumstances are simply too much.

THE HALF-LIFE OF RESEARCH PARTNERSHIPS

The stories of the radiotherapy units, one running on an expired source, the other officially shuttered by an Ebola outbreak and guerrilla war, are just two examples among many of a prominent feature of global health partnerships or international development initiatives. Partnerships often fortuitously bring technological equipment into circumstances in which there is little infrastructural or technological redundancy to begin with. A catastrophe like Ebola can close a hospital ward, or a more gradual shift in the top leadership can lead to the atrophy of a gift that has long outlasted its usefulness.

Radiotherapy bunkers turned radioactive also remind us that there is a fundamental fickleness to biomedical technologies. As Thomas Gieryn suggests, built environments and their material resources shift over time. They can fall into ruin. They can be radically modified. Infrastructures are fluid, consistently being transformed and tinkered with, often through collaboration or political negotiation, even if they are theoretically fixed in mortar and concrete.[55] We can also see that within the context of Uganda, heavy equipment being transferred often consists of donated secondhand machines. Once these are embedded in local maintenance and care logics, these donated machines are difficult to junk or discard. They are more often than not repurposed or used until they break down, and then they are carefully stowed away. In the early 2010s, the UCI was given two mammography vans through international partnerships. The vans themselves often did not have working batteries, and the mammography screening machines did not work. Nevertheless these vans were used in cancer community outreach because they looked impressive and attracted interest when they rolled into towns around Uganda. They also consumed a huge amount of fuel. It seems that the metaphor of the half-life, be it the deterioration of radioactive potency over time, long-standing relationships, or material infrastructure, is apt for describing this process and characterizing the precariousness and long-term ramifications of transferring technologies.

In the end it was neither Ebola nor a civil war that shut down Mulago's radiotherapy unit. It just stopped working in 2016.[56] Ugandan journalists asked how the many cancer patients in need of radiotherapy would find the funds to travel to Kenya, which became the only option for patients from Rwanda to southern Sudan. I do not know why this breakdown was different or why this machine—which was coaxed back to life on so many occasions by Mr. T with duct tape, ingenuity, and care—finally broke. What I do know is that the temporary solution to refer patients to Nairobi for care underscored one of the major consequences of transferring bio-medical technologies on a shoestring. The story of Uganda's "roasting machines" highlights the long-term repercussions of demonstration projects that are shaped to control costs, transfer technology, and build capacity. The Cobalt-60 machine installed in the 1990s at Mulago was never supposed to be the only radiotherapy service in Uganda. It was supposed to be the first among several government-sponsored facilities. Seeking a rugged and simple machine that was affordable, the IAEA transferred a piece of junk that was miraculously maintained by the wits and extraordinary talent of a dedicated group of radiation oncologists, physicists, technicians, and nurses. It is these people, and these people alone, who continue to keep things going long after interest from the IAEA and the Ugandan government has waned, and the half-life of transferred technology has passed.

6 ⌇ "Research Is Our Resource"

IN 2004, Dr. Edward Katongole-Mbidde welcomed Dr. Corey Casper, a new visiting American researcher interested in the possibility of collaboration, to the Uganda Cancer Institute (UCI). Casper, an infectious disease expert, was interested in starting a collaborative project at the Institute focusing on the role of viral infections in the etiology of cancer. Casper knew from data generated by the Kampala Cancer Registry that the Institute saw many patients with Kaposi's sarcoma, cervical cancer, Burkitt's lymphoma, and liver cancer. All are cancers associated with infections and particularly prevalent in patients with HIV/AIDS.[1] The last stop on the visit was the Institute's outpatient facility, a former dental surgery unit. At the time, there was no running water or electricity, but there were plenty of plump, Kampala-sized rats. Behind one of the doors of this shell of a building was a room full of old equipment, freezers, and refrigerators. Someone had painstakingly carved the acronyms of partnerships into these individual pieces of equipment. Some of the freezers dated back to the 1960s, when they were first brought to Kampala by American scientists to store Ugandan cancer patients' tissue samples before they were shipped to the National Cancer Institute (NCI) on dry ice. Other refrigerators stored vials of Adriamycin for liver cancer treatment trials conducted at the Institute in the 1970s. In the midst of unrest in Kampala in the early 1980s, student medical officers kept these freezers and refrigerators running, pouring diesel into generators in between bursts of gunfire exchanged by soldiers and rebels.[2] This room was a mausoleum for research collaborations past.[3]

After opening the door, Mbidde gave his guest a moment to take in the scene and then asked if he would be leaving another abandoned freezer.[4]

Mbidde spoke from four decades of personal experience at the UCI, where partnerships, equipment, drugs, and friendships had come and gone. After years of seeing cycles of international research collaborations, he still welcomed yet another expatriate muzungu (White person) scientist and extended hospitality. Why? The short answer is, I think, that research partnerships, for better or worse, were (and continue to be) an indispensable source of funds, equipment, training, and therapeutics that helped keep things going at the UCI for decades. Casper took the freezer graveyard seriously. As he remembered, "My first thought was, 'What makes you think you could do anything better?' My second thought was, 'What if your legacy in working here was more than just another rusty freezer?'"[5] The result was investment in people and things not seen since the 1960s at the UCI. Since 2004, the Fred Hutchinson Cancer Research Center (FHCRC, or Fred Hutch) in Seattle has spent over $10 million rehabilitating the infrastructure of the UCI and training a new generation of Ugandan oncologists.[6]

Capacity building for cancer research had synergistic effects. While the Fred Hutch helped to expand the number of oncologists in the country from one to eleven in less than a decade, cancer also became a more visible and political problem for the Ugandan government. In the early 2000s, a respected and widely beloved member of parliament, Yefusa Okullo Epak, died of lung cancer, spending many months in and out of care facilities in South Africa and the UCI undergoing palliative chemotherapy. Epak was struck by the profound discrepancies between resources in South Africa and those in Uganda. Receiving chemotherapy in a soft chair with some privacy and strong antiemetics was very different from sitting on a hard wooden bench lined up with other patients in a roofless building. It was Epak's dying wish that his colleagues in the Ugandan government take cancer more seriously and allocate funds and resources accordingly. He worked to pass a bill through parliament that granted the UCI financial and administrative autonomy from Mulago Hospital.[7] The combination of more ministers getting cancer and the visibility of the Fred Hutch partnership politicized oncology in Uganda in the early 2000s. At the same time, Mbidde moved on after nearly forty years at the UCI, and his successor, Dr. Jackson Orem, continued to expand oncology services for the public in Uganda. The Ugandan government made an investment in cancer treatment infrastructure not seen since the 1960s with the construction of a new five-story cancer hospital, which officially opened in 2016.[8]

Just as global health grows and expands as a field of intervention, so too does scholarship interrogating the complexities of health research and care partnerships, especially the question of how to build and sustain both scientific and public health capacity.[9] In the Ugandan context, Johanna Crane writes beautifully about the uneven power dynamics between Ugandan and American scientists engaging in HIV antiretroviral therapy drug resistance research. She highlights struggles for ownership over objects such as patient registries and the structural power dynamics that make true equity in international research partnerships nearly impossible. Writing about toxicology and the challenges of doing science in postcolonial Senegal, Noémi Toussignant highlights the uneven temporalities of scientific capacity, be it "lost," "improvised," "missing," or for "the future." She calls this a "struggle for capacity," in which "rhythms of this struggle have been intermittently set in motion by investments in Senegalese scientific research. . . . More often these rhythms have been stilled and interrupted by stagnating budgets, the end of project funding, the breakdown of equipment, and the wait for an overseas trip."[10]

Capacity can be defined as "the ability or power to do something." A simple example would be the ability to run a polymerase chain reaction (PCR) test today. What I'm more concerned with is the issue of durability—"the ability to withstand wear, pressure, or damage." For example, durability would mean there is an ability to run PCR not only today but also tomorrow and the day after that, which requires a local maintenance contract, not to mention a long-standing pipeline to the necessary reagents ten years after the initial equipment is installed. Framed in this way, capacity is relatively easy to build. Durability is much harder to sustain. We could interpret the freezer room at the UCI in 2004 as the remnants of struggles for capacity akin to the lab Toussignant describes in Senegal. We could, following Wenzel Geissler and others, also frame the freezers as the material manifestations of partnerships that have ended and the detritus of the resources that research partnerships bring.[11] Freezers that were once gifts of goodwill can become symbols of frayed partnerships and relations. We could also see the room as a reminder that each piece of heavy equipment and donated freezer housed in the UCI's freezer graveyard in the early 2000s has an itinerary as complicated and circuitous as Mulago Hospital's radiotherapy machine. Is something like the equipment graveyard the inevitable endpoint of research partnerships, or are there alternatives to abandoned freezers? What if durability, rather than capacity, were the starting point for imagining research collaborations?

Writing about global health partnerships, Iruka Okeke notes:

> In real world partnerships, specifically those built around global health goals, after proposed innovations are tested, community health workers are trained, or an intervention has been piloted, what happens next? A rather too common answer among very different global health partnerships is: little if anything. In sharp contrast to domestic partnerships and even scientific collaborations, one of the uniting characteristics of all but a few very significant global health partnerships is their temporariness. Collaborating biomedical scientists often continue to associate, however informally (and admittedly with fewer administrative and budgetary constraints), but continuity beyond the funded period (or its no-cost extension) is much less common in global health partnerships. Partnerships are for now and not for the distant future.[12]

The remarkable resilience of the UCI over fifty years of creativity, crisis, and cancer in Uganda offers an alternative to the temporariness of global health partnerships Okeke describes.

This chapter examines the ways in which a new generation of Ugandan and American physician-researchers at the UCI and the FHCRC crafted an alternative to the usual temporariness of global health partnerships. By designing and creating new buildings, they sought to make a new and durable experimental infrastructure for cancer care and research in Uganda. I situate these events within a broader set of continuities and changes in the history of research and care at the Institute. I show how older relationships between the UCI and partners in the United States during the early days of Kaposi's sarcoma and HIV research helped to shape the careers and research questions of those like Casper who were interested in the rise of global oncology. I discuss these new investments in people and things with a keen attention to the built environment of the partnership itself. The chapter concludes with an account of the spectacle of the grand opening for the UCI–Fred Hutch Research Center building in 2015. The source materials comprise interviews, ethnographic field-notes from Kampala and Seattle, and medical journal articles. Secondary sources from the anthropology of global health partnerships and threads from the science and technology studies literature on the material politics of buildings and objects provide both an empirical and a theoretical foundation for the chapter.

SLIM DISEASE IN KAMPALA, AIDS IN SAN FRANCISCO

In June 1981, Dr. Alex Coutinho moved into the small living quarters on the UCI's campus to take up residency at the Solid Tumor Center (STC) as part of the Institute's annual prestigious medical training program in oncology for students. During the day, Coutinho and his Sudanese counterpart at the Lymphoma Treatment Center (LTC) were just normal medical students attending classes. But every evening at five o'clock, just as the rest of the students were retiring to have dinner or study for exams, the work picked up for Coutinho. He would walk into the ward of the STC, check in with the nurses, and start the evening ward round. Going from bedside to bedside, he would meet the new patients who had been admitted earlier that day, address the side effects of chemotherapy (particularly kidney failure or dehydration from extreme vomiting), and try to finish up before it got too late or too dark. Then he would return to his quarters, try to ignore the sounds of ongoing gunfire at night, and wait and see if the landline would ring—the signal that there was a patient emergency on the wards of the STC. Or sometimes, there would be a knock on the door, as the landlines were often out of service.[13]

In the aftermath of the war with Tanzania in 1979 and the increasingly violent unrest between the National Resistance Movement's guerrilla army and the Ugandan government's military, the atmosphere in Kampala was decidedly tense and physically insecure.[14] At Mulago Hospital and Makerere Medical School there were shortages of basic supplies and also of teaching staff, making the UCI, headed at the time by Olweny and Mbidde, a decidedly attractive place. As Coutinho remembered, "Hungry students would be looking for someone of caliber to teach them."[15] Ward rounds with Olweny and Mbidde (who had thirty to forty years of experience in oncology between them) made the UCI a hugely desirable place to learn. Despite the flying bullets at night, "the beauty of working there was that you could do proper medicine."[16] Because there were in-house X-ray and laboratory services, they were less dependent on Mulago Hospital, although there were still supply shortages to contend with. "Somehow we were fatalistic. We never complained. We never went to Olweny to say, 'Sorry, we need security guards,' because security guards were also running away."[17]

Despite these insecurities, colleagues at the UCI continued to conduct research and stay connected to the international cancer research community through a combination of reading journals and attending (and sometimes hosting) international conferences. In early 1980, the UCI hosted the second international conference on Kaposi's sarcoma, distilling the key findings conducted at the UCI in the 1970s.[18] Essentially a year later, colleagues agreed that they were seeing more and more cases of Kaposi's sarcoma in women and children on the wards of the STC. "I saw my first HIV patient in the Cancer Institute. I had no idea it was HIV of course. But it was one particular ward round. I remember it clearly. And we were seeing more and more Kaposi's sarcoma in women despite it being historically a male disease. And [Dr. Wilson] Carswell commented I've just been reading a paper that they're seeing a lot of Kaposi's in SF and New York and it's some new disease among gay men. No connection. But I realize now that it was the first HIV case that I saw."[19] At the time of our conversation about his memories of working at the UCI, Coutinho was the director of the Infectious Diseases Institute on Mulago's campus. From his days as a medical student at the UCI to the present, much of his career in medicine was shaped by directing medical services for the care and research of the HIV/AIDS epidemic in Africa: in Uganda but also farther afield in southern and eastern Africa.

In Kampala, UCI staff read about the emerging epidemic in the United States through the international postal system as they saw more and more cases of aggressive Kaposi's sarcoma. The Institute ran a journal club on various topics of interest in oncology. Even in the midst of unrest, current copies of the *New England Journal of Medicine* and the *Lancet* still made it to the Institute for reading and discussion. Sitting around the table, staff at the UCI discussed the papers trickling in on Kaposi's sarcoma in young, White, otherwise healthy males in America. Of course, there was lag time in learning more about how the situation was unfolding in America. As Dr. David Serwadda said, "Remember. No Internet. They [the journals] were coming by post. But they would take a while. [The lag time] was huge. No international calls. You'd have to call the post office and make a booking."[20] As Serwadda, who went on to be a coprincipal investigator in Rakai on numerous HIV-related research studies, recalled:

> Now, on Solid Tumor, we had been dealing with KS for a long time. And so that's why these articles were of interests to us. They talked about aggressive sarcoma among white men. So you know, the KS that we saw at the Cancer Institute was anything but aggressive. It was very mild and usually you would treat it with a cytotoxic drug. I saw a number of people who were cured, really.

Put on their shoes and they went back [home]. But if you saw it in women, it was of the aggressive type that we were seeing in white males in the US.[21]

Colleagues at the UCI were curious about why there were such profound gender and racial differences in the presentation of aggressive Kaposi's sarcoma between the United States and Uganda.

Initial research and publications concerning this new manifestation of Kaposi's sarcoma on the UCI wards continued in a style similar to much of the work at the Institute as it had been practiced since the 1960s.[22] For one, it was highly descriptive and case driven. Serwadda's 1984 publication on Kaposi's sarcoma in Uganda focused on four cases of aggressive Kaposi's sarcoma and included detailed case notes and photographs of two of the four patients, visibly deformed and swelling from the cancer. And in the style of many UCI inquiries, the patients were randomized to different chemotherapy drug regimens. In this case, they either received repeated infusions of a single agent of Adriamycin or a cocktail of actinomycin-D, vincristine, Adriamycin, and imidazole carboxamide. These combinations and single agents followed the treatment regimens for Kaposi's sarcoma established at the Institute first by Vogel and colleagues and then refined by Olweny. And in the spirit of keeping practices within the systems of the Institute, they also made laboratory assays in house, using enzyme-linked immunosorbent assay techniques and HTLV-III antigens derived from local patients.[23]

By 1983, colleagues across East and Central Africa were making similar observations of aggressive Kaposi's sarcoma. For example, in Lusaka, Zambia, the surgeon Dr. Anne Bayley noticed more and more cases of aggressive Kaposi's sarcoma on the wards. Bayley partnered with Olweny, who by then was affiliated with the World Health Organization, to set up Kaposi's sarcoma surveillance and treatment in the country. Between 1983 and 1985 colleagues worked between Kampala and Lusaka to determine if they were in fact seeing the same sort of aggressive Kaposi's sarcoma in both places and if existing drug regimens developed at the UCI in the 1960s and 1970s would help to mitigate aggressive Kaposi's sarcoma. They were also interested in whether patients with either generalized or aggressive Kaposi's sarcoma tested positive for HTLV-III.[24]

Meanwhile, in the early 1980s, Ziegler left the East Coast and the National Cancer Institute for a position at University of California San Francisco (UCSF). The timing of his arrival in the city of sand and fog was auspicious. His colleagues were seeing an explosion of young gay White men in emergency rooms and in hospital beds throughout San Francisco presenting with Kaposi's sarcoma and suppressed immune systems. Ziegler was one of a handful of American physicians who had clinical experience with Kaposi's sarcoma. Much of the working knowledge regarding disease presentation, chemotherapy combination treatment, and staging systems came directly from prior research experiences in Uganda in the 1960s and 1970s. Ziegler also drew upon the experiences of running clinical care systems in underfunded contexts. He and colleagues such as Dr. Paul Volberding spearheaded the initial San Francisco–based Kaposi's sarcoma clinic and later expanded this into what would become the San Francisco AIDS Clinic. In this way, knowledge and practices developed at the UCI made their way far beyond Kampala.[25]

The early work conducted at the Institute on the emergence of the Kaposi's sarcoma epidemic in Uganda in relation to the outbreaks of Kaposi's sarcoma in young adult men in San Francisco and New York proved to be extremely important. Resolving the apparent incommensurability between what would become HIV in San Francisco and HIV in Kampala led to a rich, fiercely productive exchange that relied on knowledge previously generated at the UCI about Kaposi's sarcoma and the patients coming to the STC.[26] But the research agenda that emerged about HIV in Uganda over the next decade—which included the fundamentals of its etiology, the disease's heterosexual patterns of transmission, the time from HIV infection to AIDS, and identifying who was at risk—reflected a set of research priorities that were quite different from the care priorities on the wards where critically ill patients needed immediate comfort and care. The research questions being asked in the 1980s and 1990s (and indeed today) called for blood taking and HIV-positive-persons cohort development.[27]

In contrast to the cancer research at the Institute in the 1960s and 1970s, there were no powerful therapeutics on deck, nothing that would magically make HIV-related issues disappear.[28] Staff at the UCI did not necessarily need chemotherapy clinical trials for Kaposi's sarcoma patients or randomized controlled experiments to see if oral morphine was effective in end-of-life care. Staff knew what was needed from decades of prior experience at the Institute. Saline for rehydration after explosive diarrhea, opiates for crushing pain, antibiotics for opportunistic infections—these were the pressing needs on the wards.[29] At the same time, Ugandan physician-researchers found themselves in a hugely challenging situation where "cutting edge" HIV research did not necessarily map onto their work as clinicians.[30] Ugandan physicians' roles were manifold: they were principal investigators, hosts to international collaborators, cultural brokers, money transfer managers, and ethicists. Above all, they were physicians on the front lines of the protracted social and medical emergency that was the HIV/AIDS epidemic in Uganda in the 1980s and 1990s.

This isn't to say that research collaborations at the Institute were moribund in the 1980s, 1990s, and early 2000s or that Ugandan physicians at the Institute simply worked as gatekeepers. The Institute saw many HIV-positive patients with Kaposi's sarcoma and other AIDS-related malignancies in the 1980s, 1990s, and early 2000s. But these patient populations did not necessarily bring large-scale international investments in the infrastructure of cancer research or care during this period. A collaboration with UCSF physicians did form an active Kaposi's sarcoma study group in the late 1980s and early 1990s.[31] At the UCI, patients with HIV-related Kaposi's sarcoma were (and continue to be) remarkably abundant. Ugandan bodies and communities also provided a wealth of clinical, serological, and epidemiological evidence on the HIV epidemic East Africa. In particular, the community of Rakai in southwestern Uganda was turned into a large-scale population cohort where one could study HIV.[32] Some staff who cut their teeth as medical students at the Institute went on to spearhead the Rakai project and also mobilize some of the largest community-based HIV care operations in the country, such as the AIDS Support Organization.[33] All of this is to say that clinical staff at the UCI, who were operating under a severely constrained budget after being folded into Mulago Hospital, faced the reality that they were now operating under a triple mandate—run a palliative care facility where people were sent to die from Lower Mulago Hospital, try to provide cancer care and treatment support to patients who were able to purchase their own drugs, and serve as a hub for collaborations with international medical researchers.

FROM HIV TO GLOBAL ONCOLOGY

Like many other global health physicians, Casper came to work between Seattle and Kampala largely through experiences with the American HIV-AIDS epidemic.[34] As a medical student on the wards of major teaching hospitals in New York, and then as an infectious diseases resident at UCSF, Casper observed the transformation of AIDS from a death sentence to a pharmaceutically managed chronic illness over the course of the 1990s and early 2000s. He remembered first seeing Kaposi's sarcoma as a medical student in New York. This motivated him to pursue a career in infectious diseases and Kaposi's sarcoma epidemiology and etiology. In the late 1990s and early 2000s, Kaposi's sarcoma cases were declining across the United States, thanks to better patient management and access to long-term antiretroviral therapy. When Casper took a position at the FHCRC in Seattle in the early 2000s, he came with the hopes of building a research cohort of Kaposi's sarcoma patients in the Pacific Northwest. What Casper had not realized was that the year before he arrived, Seattle saw its last Kaposi's sarcoma patient. Casper turned to East Africa under the advice and mentorship of Dr. Merle Sande. Sande was an AIDS physician at UCSF who was instrumental in setting up a major HIV research institute in Uganda. He was also convinced that cancer research in Africa was going to be "the next big thing" after the HIV/AIDS epidemic.[35] With its robust biomedical infrastructure in the form of Makerere Medical School and a cohort of Ugandan physicians who had been instrumental in both publishing on HIV/AIDS in Africa and collaborating with research scientists for long-term cohort studies such as the Rakai project, Uganda seemed an obvious location for setting up a cancer research program.

The UCI had patients—many of whom were suffering from HIV-related malignancies. And thanks to the efforts of Dr. Raphael Owor, Dr. Henry Wabinga, and others, the Kampala Cancer Registry, dating back to 1954, continued to provide population-based data on a variety of cancers, including Kaposi's sarcoma.[36] The registry provided population-based data on cancer incidence and prevalence for Kyadondo County. (Cancer registries in Africa are rare and usually hospital based. And they do not give an accurate count of population-based cancer rates.)[37] Although the registry's work was disrupted throughout much of the late 1970s and 1980s, Wabinga revitalized the registry through ongoing partnerships with the World Health Organization and the International Agency for Research on Cancer in the early 1990s. Wabinga also collaborated extensively with the Uganda Kaposi's Sarcoma Study Group based at the UCI in the 1990s and 2000s on issues of Kaposi's sarcoma epidemiology, HHV-8, and HIV/AIDS infection. Wabinga's work and the collaborative efforts of the Kaposi's Sarcoma Study Group showed that Kaposi's sarcoma was not only a pressing clinical problem in HIV/AIDS care in Uganda but that a study population for long-term Kaposi's sarcoma cohort research was available.

INVESTMENTS IN PEOPLE, INVESTMENTS IN THINGS

When Casper and his colleagues first started working in Uganda in 2004, the term *global oncology* did not exist. *Global oncology*, like *global health*, is a capacious, malleable, and relatively new term to describe what may or may not be a "new" thing. Like global health, global oncology is more of an idea than a discipline. In some circles, global oncology connotes a medical humanitarian agenda for mitigating the vast global inequalities surrounding the prevention, treatment, and palliation of cancers. These inequalities are described as the global cancer divide: "There are glaring disparities between rich and poor in incidence and death from preventable cancers and death from treatable cancers, as well as in the pain, suffering, and stigma associated with the disease. These disparities constitute a cancer divide and demonstrate that increasing access to cancer care and control is also an issue of equity."[38] Numbers tell a stark story about these disparities. According to the World Health Organization, 8.2 million people died from cancer worldwide in 2012; 60 percent of the total new annual cases of cancer occur in Asia, Africa, and Latin America; 30 percent of cancers could be prevented.[39] Julio Frenk, one of the architects of the global oncology movement, argues that "to correct this situation we must address the staggering '5/80 cancer disequilibrium', that is, the fact that low- and middle-income countries account for almost 80 percent of the burden of disease due to cancer yet receive only 5 percent of global resources devoted to deal with this emerging challenge."[40]

Although cancer kills more people every year in the developing world than HIV, tuberculosis, and malaria combined, financial support for addressing the cancer burden outside the United States and Europe remains low. In low- and middle-income countries, it is estimated that there are 4.8 million deaths annually from cancer. It is estimated that there are about 2.1 million deaths from HIV/AIDS annually in the Global South. About 1.1 million deaths from tuberculosis occur in low- and middle-income countries annually. Malaria claims 0.7 million lives annually. Global funding for HIV/AIDS treatment and prevention is $6.2 billion annually. Funding for malaria treatment and prevention receives about $1.3 billion. Tuberculosis prevention and treatment programs receive $903 million annually. Annual global health funding for cancer in low- and middle-income countries is approximately $168 million.[41] In other words, the global funding resources allocated for treating and preventing cancer in low- and middle-income countries annually is much lower than the global funding allocated for treating HIV, tuberculosis, and malaria.

With a high disease burden and many unmet needs in these countries, the research agenda and care priorities for "global oncology" are in the process of being shaped and defined. The FHCRC model for global oncology draws on the language of remediating global inequalities in cancer *and* optimism that certain cancers, particularly Burkitt's lymphoma, are curable, and that "where you live should not determine whether you will survive cancer."[42] To address this burden, the Fred Hutch identified three key areas of intervention over the past decade: improving diagnostic capabilities, optimizing treatment protocols, and also laying the groundwork for better prevention mechanisms for cancers caused by infectious diseases. Vaccines exist for hepatitis B, which is linked to liver cancer, and human papillomavirus (HPV), which is linked to cervical cancer. And as the FHCRC notes, "Infection-related cancers offer an especially promising target for cancer prevention and treatment efforts. Nearly a quarter of the world's cancers are caused by infectious diseases that are preventable or treatable—diseases such as viral hepatitis, Epstein-Barr virus, HIV and HPV. In parts of the developing world, up to 60 percent of all cancers are associated with infectious diseases." The Fred Hutch is already the administrative and scientific home of the HIV Trials Network. It is the institution that laid much of the groundwork on the linkages between HPV and cervical cancer which contributed to HPV vaccine development, and the Hutch is looking for the next big Gardasil-like breakthrough in treating Kaposi's sarcoma and Burkitt's lymphoma. The UCI and FHCRC collaboration endeavors not only to do research that benefits treatment outcomes on the ground but exists largely to do infection-related malignancies research in a setting where access to a large cohort of patients with infection-related cancers is more concentrated than it would be anywhere in the United States.

The UCI–Fred Hutch collaboration was and is serious about building out local oncology capacity and ensuring that every staff member in Seattle works with an "analog" (their words, not mine) in Kampala. These Ugandan physicians are what historian Nancy Rose Hunt would call "middle figures"—in this case mediators between the worlds of oncology research in Seattle and the increasingly visible cancer epidemic in Kampala.[43] They are also seen as the key to the longevity of research efforts in Uganda. "Our goal is to make ourselves redundant," one Seattle-based program operative noted to me. The Ugandan oncologists who see over forty thousand patients a year are brilliant, caring, and cosmopolitan. The vast majority of them also spent a grueling year in Seattle absorbing the ins and outs of how oncology clinics run at the Seattle Cancer Care Alliance while also taking numerous courses in HIV and cancer epidemiology, biology, and biostatistics at the University of Washington. The emphasis of this training program was to create physician-researcher leaders who would then return to the UCI and become publishing scientists.[44]

Roughly eight thousand miles separate Kampala from Seattle. In a pressurized aluminum tube, it takes over twenty-four hours and several international airport connections to travel from Entebbe to Sea-Tac. The dark winters of the chilly Pacific Northwest are a sharp contrast to the equatorial stability of days and nights by Lake Victoria, where rainy seasons and pregnancies coming to full term signal the passing of another year. There is the time difference. As people take their morning coffee and search for an umbrella or all-weather jacket to get out the door in Seattle often by foot or bicycle or bus, Kampala residents are getting into their cars, or onto the backs of motorcycles, or crowding into minibus taxis to face the long jam home to a dinner of steaming soft bananas and sauce. Inside the facilities of the FHRCR and the UCI, the differences are also many. At the Fred Hutch, there is an entire building dedicated to freezer storage. At the UCI, as of September 2013, liquid nitrogen can finally be manufactured on-site to keep the lone container of tissue samples frozen solid. In Uganda, ecstatic prayers on the weekends and church fellowships on the weekdays bring comfort, purpose, and community. In Seattle, email signatures that include holy scriptures are discouraged and may be frowned upon by US government funding agencies. At the Fred Hutch, approximately 90 percent of a physician-research scientist's time is devoted to research. Being on top of the oncology game means being thoroughly engrossed and specialized in a particular kind of cancer.[45] At the UCI, as a colleague noted, most Ugandan practitioners operate at 200 percent on every level. An oncologist is expected to be able to consult with a leukemic child's family, screen for breast cancer, palliate pancreatic cancer, and keep on top of the latest HIV-related malignancy data coming out of sub-Saharan Africa. They are expected to be polymaths, stunningly versatile, and able to seamlessly negotiate back and forth between children and adults, solid tumors and blood cancers.[46]

Dr. Fred Okuku, whom we met in the last chapter as a volunteer medical student at the UCI in the early 2000s, was one of the original promising Ugandan physicians sent to Seattle for training in oncology. People like Okuku, who remember what the UCI was like before institutional autonomy and the collaboration with the Hutch, are relatively rare. For Okuku, the biggest difference between medical practice in Uganda and medical practice in the United States was not necessarily greater access to MRI machines or the latest cancer drugs. What struck Okuku was a "team-based approach to care" and the emphasis placed on spending time with patients and their families. Consider the "family room" approach, which he describes as follows:

> There is a board and the physician is explaining the disease and risk factors and how this all came about. [He discusses] what forms of treatment are available, including survival patterns on different regimens of treatment. That's how detailed! And the guys [patients and family members] come and they have all these data downloaded from the net about different treatments. They are asking very scientific questions and engaging the doctor to the limits. Asking serious questions about side effects. That kind of professionalism wowed me. And I've tried it with patients [here in Uganda] and they love it.[47]

Since returning to the UCI in 2010 as a full-time oncologist, Okuku works to integrate knowledge and practices he assimilated in Seattle into his daily work in Uganda and transfer the technology of the "white board." He also wants to make "contributions to science," as he puts it, by finding time to publish and write grant applications. He balances this with clinical duties. These include getting through eighty to one hundred outpatients every other day as a senior consultant physician. He is responsible for running and overseeing the Solid Tumor Center, which has about twenty beds for forty to sixty inpatients at any given time, many of whom are in late stages of cancer. The National Drug Store Authority in Uganda is an inconsistent drug stocking partner, which means plenty of days when there is no doxorubicin or vincristine on the shelves and no oral morphine on hand. Okuku works to publish his research on Kaposi's sarcoma staging in international medical journals but also tries to find the time to work with the Ministry of Health to improve referral guidelines.

For those who work with and at the UCI, navigating the blurry binary between what constitutes oncology research and what constitutes clinical care is an ongoing dilemma and one that is being constantly negotiated. On one side, there is "research," often more private, of an international project focused on quality control. On the other side, there is "care," often more public, funded by government resources and triaged by necessity. Patients are still financially destitute. And there are far more of them than there used to be. The spaces where Okuku practices research and care at the UCI are also shaped by the historical physical infrastructure of the UCI. Neither the physical structures nor longtime practices such as cleanliness ward rounds are easily changed. What is emerging to cope with the inheritances of the past, promising avenues of infectious disease and cancer research, and mounting pressures on the physical space of the site is a division between "doing a research" and practicing "government medicine." These divisions at the UCI were being spatially inscribed while the UCI–Fred Hutchinson Cancer Center research building and the five-story government-sponsored inpatient facility were being built.

A GRAND OPENING FOR A GRAND BUILDING

On May 21, 2015, the UCI–Fred Hutch Cancer Center officially opened. President Yoweri Museveni attended as the special guest of honor. The opening was a grand spectacle, and here it is helpful to see it through eyes other than my own. As science journalist and Fred Hutch staff writer Mary Engel said:

> People began trickling onto the brick-paved parking lot of the building by 8 a.m. Thursday to go through security set up for the president's arrival. By 9:30, a crowd of around 300 — nurses in their starched white uniforms, colorful belts and dress caps; physician-researchers; university deans, professors and medical students; hospital administrators, government ministers and members of parliament, reporters and others — gathered under a giant white, open-sided party tent. And the dancing began.
> Colorfully costumed dance troupes from around Uganda performed, and their dances were as varied as Uganda's nine indigenous communities and 56 tribes. In one, a courtship dance, men outdid themselves with kicks and jumps to win the hand of a village woman. In another, spear-carrying dancers in long straw-colored wigs imitated the crested crane, Uganda's national symbol. In one dance, men carried big drums on their heads; in another, women with rigid torsos and whirling hips balanced pots on their heads, kneeling to add one at a time until the pots were stacked eight-tall.
> Musicians accompanied the dancers on long wood-framed horns covered in cow hide, xylophones, stringed harps, gourd shakers and drums of every size and shape. Singers joined in. It was impossible not to smile.[48]

There was a collective sigh of relief when President Museveni's convoy arrived. Museveni arrived on the red carpet with a flash of his signature straw hat, flanked by bodyguards in jungle-green army fatigues and sturdy black boots. The booming of welcoming drums commenced, and the blare of trumpets sounded. Then with a deft flick of the wrist, Museveni unveiled the bronze plaque celebrating the commissioning of the building. Wasting no time, the president went on a VIP tour of the building. The rest of the guests sat outside and waited for the next thirty minutes. We were given glasses of juice and made polite conversation, all the while humming to smooth jazz and Toto's "Africa." The usual waiting benches for the X-ray department, which overlook the adult intake space of the new building, were vacant, save a lone special-forces operative diligently scanning the scene.[49]

President Museveni and colleagues finally emerged from the building, pausing for a photo opportunity between the Ugandan and American flags in front of the new center. The guests of honor then entered the tent, which was decorated in the Fred Hutch colors of green, blue, and silver, rather than the Ugandan national colors of red, black, and yellow. This was a departure from past opening ceremonies on the UCI campus, which proudly flew the colors of the Ugandan nation. The trumpets of the national anthem sounded, we prayed, and were seated.

It was Olweny who first took the podium for the hour and a half's worth of speeches from Corey Casper, Larry Corey, the US ambassador, the Ugandan minister of health, and President Museveni himself. "Thanks delayed is thanks denied," noted Olweny as he welcomed the honorable guests to the festivities, especially thanking President Museveni for his presence on this "auspicious occasion." He thanked the Ugandan and US governments and the Fred Hutch for their support and the contractors for completing the building in a timely fashion. "The keyword that's driven the Uganda Cancer Institute since its inception is *collaboration*," noted Olweny. "We do not take the Hutch for granted." He then proceeded to tell the story of the history of collaborative cancer research in Uganda, as he saw it, from the 1960s to the present. What was particularly striking about Olweny's speech was his attention to profound continuities over time. The Institute's original four main objectives—clinical investigation, postgraduate training, active consulting with up-country hospitals, and cancer research—remain the same today. The centrality of collaborative partnership also remains important: "All we need to do is replace the National Cancer Institute with other cancer centers of repute," he noted. This continuity extends also into the centrality of researching the relationships between cancers and viral infections in Africa. As Olweny noted, key cancers of interest, such as Burkitt's lymphoma, Hodgkin's disease, hepatocellular carcinoma, and Kaposi's sarcoma, remain the cornerstones of the research and care agenda at the Institute. But one major point of departure for the UCI is the question of scale. The pursuit of full institutional autonomy on the part of the UCI is being done to ensure that medical and radiation oncology are housed under the same roof. "Cancer care is a very expensive endeavor" and will continue to be in the coming decades, Olweny noted, particularly as the UCI expands its mandate to be East Africa's oncology center of excellence.

There was an unshakable sense that Olweny himself, as well as the UCI, was coming full circle. Here was the first (and for a long time the *only*) Ugandan oncologist who was charged with keeping this research institute alive in the 1970s and whose vision for something more comprehensive was foiled by exile. Olweny's return to Uganda and his new position as the UCI's chairman of the board mark a powerful second chance to see the vision of comprehensive cancer services in the country realized. Olweny's speech was storytelling at its best—Museveni joked, "I have benefitted very much from Olweny's long remarks." Museveni also explicitly thanked Olweny, saying that there is a superstition that the name influences a person. *Olweny*, in some languages spoken in Uganda, means "war." This "Professor Warrior" did a remarkable thing in running a cancer center under Idi Amin. He said, "I would not have done that myself."[50] Olweny's speech also offered some of the necessary context for understanding the history of the UCI for outsiders, both Ugandan and American, who may have been unaware of the Institute's rich history and seen the FHCRC collaboration as something entirely new, rather than an entity built by fifty years of collective action.

At the end of the speeches, everyone rose again for the national anthem. My husband noted to me afterward that Olweny was one of the few with his hand over his heart as the anthem played. Drums again sounded and Museveni's entourage departed. The chair he was sitting on was loaded out to his convoy. Immediately after he departed, they rolled up the red carpet. The nurses dashed to the tea sandwiches and lukewarm eggrolls catered by the Serena Hotel and filled their plates. Patients and caretakers lined up at a catering tent behind the festivities. The air was electric.

The UCI–Fred Hutch Cancer Center is an impressive building. Built in a style of brick and glass reminiscent of the Fred Hutch facilities in Seattle, the facility is, in Casper's words, "audacious and ambitious."[51] It is intended to close the distance between Seattle and Kampala. It is also built on the site of the old LTC. Specifically tailored for examining the linkages between infectious agents and cancers in Uganda, this building is the new experimental infrastructure and the flagship demonstration project for the Fred Hutchinson Cancer Research Center's foray into "global oncology."[52] The Hutch calls this facility a "strategic investment" to help "the UCI grow from a small facility with limited resources—including one oncologist—to a the state-of-the-art UCI–Fred Hutch Cancer Centre, that can treat up to 20,000 patients a year."[53] I wrote the following in my fieldnotes after touring the building in May 2015:

> Walking through the UCI-Fred Hutch Cancer Centre, past the many imported exam tables, the spacious and dare I say inviting chemo bays, the gigantic bathrooms with automatic lights, and the extremely well-equipped histopathology laboratory and PCR station, I am in awe. But then, standing in the adult intake waiting area, I see a group of patients looking in on our building tour from the LTC II, sitting on the benches, waiting for their X-ray films. My heart sinks a little as we eye each other. This beautiful brand-new building cannot possibly see and treat everyone.[54]

"When you are in the building you feel that you are in Seattle," said Dr. K, one of Uganda's new oncologists who has benefitted heavily from the opportunity to train at the Hutch in Seattle.[55] The building is relaxing, air-conditioned, and clean. Walk down the stairs and cross the brick-paved parking area with neat white lines to where the property ends, however, and you are back in a parking lot that is either mud or dust, depending on the rainy season. The most visible divide between the older UCI facilities and the gleaming Fred Hutch collaborative space is a sewage gutter, drawing a literal line in the concrete between the old and the new. It used to take a day in an airplane to close the physical and infrastructural gaps between Seattle and Kampala. Now it takes a five-minute walk and a flight of stairs to exit the bustle of the Institute on top of Mulago Hill and to a space more akin to the US than Uganda.

Months of conversations went into conceptualizing and planning a facility that would meet the basic requirements for conducting clinical drug trials and keep the tools of laboratory research and specimen processing within Uganda. These experiments concerning how patients would encounter the building and experience routine examinations, chemotherapy infusions, and blood draws are written into the building itself and are at their most visible in the spatial separation of children from adults. It sounds obvious, but adult cancer patients find children with Burkitt's lymphoma and other large, distorting tumors to be disturbing. The same goes for pediatric cancer patients, who are turned off by the smells and sights of adults with explosive tumors or cadaverous faces.[56] The building is constructed like a gigantic horseshoe. If you're facing the main steps, you can see an "Adult Patient Clinic" entrance on the left and a "Pediatric Patient Clinic" entrance on the right. There is also a separate "Research Clinic" entrance, which goes up a simple flight of concrete stairs to the second floor, where sunshine yellow tiles and a smiling receptionist greet research subjects for appointments for consent taking, swabbing, and counseling. On the ground floor, there is a small window for the pharmacy tucked into the left-hand corner of the building so patients can just walk to a window and pick up necessary prescriptions. There is also an on-site specimen repository center and generator. The twenty-five-thousand-square-foot center is three stories tall and designed for twenty-thousand patient visits a year.[57]

The UCI–Fred Hutch Cancer Center is so much like America that the building was largely imagined as an interior space. In contrast to the pavilions of Old Mulago (with their large shady outdoor verandahs), the breezy open-air hallways of New Mulago, the large patient-caretaker cooking pavilions of Lacor Hospital, or even the open-air waiting areas of the Infectious Disease Institute, the UCI–Fred Hutch Cancer Center does not utilize outdoor space. The stairs and the entrances to the clinics currently bake in the afternoon sun—in time I imagine they will put up a tent or awning to help mitigate the heat and shelter waiting relatives of patients. In contrast to the Lymphoma Treatment Center and Solid Tumor Center, this is not a residential facility. At its core, this new building is designed for blood taking and chemo administration and research. It is not designed to handle inpatient care. Nor can the twenty thousand slots for patient visits accommodate the number of patients who come through the UCI annually. It would signal a profound continuity if the focus of the research at the new UCI–Fred Hutch Cancer Center remained solely on these two cancers that captured the imaginations of physician-researchers half a century ago: Burkitt's lymphoma and Kaposi's sarcoma.

"RESEARCH IS OUR RESOURCE"

One of the core arguments of this book is that the infrastructure created in order to conduct cancer research and experiments in the 1960s fundamentally shaped the scope and practices of cancer care in Uganda. Cancer care looks, smells, and feels the way it does in Uganda because of the histories of oncology research in this country. Biomedical cancer care is concentrated at the UCI at the top of Mulago Hill in Kampala because oncology's technologies and practices came to the country in the 1960s as part of an internationally supported research enterprise. The concentration of cancer research at the UCI shaped Uganda's singular silo of cancer expertise. The other core argument of the book is that oncology—from treatment technologies to methods for taking a biopsy—largely traveled from metropolitan centers of cancer treatment in the United States and Europe and was then remade by the Ugandan context. The UCI's history shows, over a long arc, how international medical research on human subjects shapes local contexts of care.

Since its founding in 1967, the UCI provided cancer care to patients who fit the criteria for research programs, rather than extending comprehensive oncology services to everyone in need.[58] In the 1960s and 1970s, triage by research agenda influenced who would be given a bed at the UCI. In the 1980s and 1990s, triage on the wards continued even in the absence of robust cancer chemotherapy trials. Patients only received oncology services on the wards if they could produce the funds to pay for their drugs; or if a patient could not afford the cost, in rare cases, the Institute could appeal for drugs and make a strong case that the patient would benefit from treatment.[59] Today, the research focus of the UCI–Fred Hutch Cancer Center alliance is to examine the synergy between infections and cancers. Kaposi's sarcoma and Burkitt's lymphoma are the key targets of inquiry, much as they were in the past during the early days of collaboration between the NCI, Makerere's Department of Surgery, and the British Empire Cancer Campaign. The focus on research operates alongside the contemporary mandate that the Institute provide oncology services as a public good, despite all of the financial, infrastructural, and staff constraints that come with being part of the machinery of Ugandan government health services. The mission to be a center of research excellence in the Great Lakes region of Africa operates alongside the reality that many of the patients seen at the Institute come in the throes of late-stage illness, and while many of them do have Kaposi's sarcoma and Burkitt's lymphoma, a substantial number of other patients do not.[60]

The UCI now technically serves any and all Ugandans seeking oncology relief. Forty beds were never supposed to comprehensively serve the needs of a population catchment of forty million living around the Great Lakes region of Africa but that effectively became the Institute's mandate.[61] The policy shift, that the UCI is a place of hope and treatment for all, has meant that patients who would typically die at home—or would have been told that their cancer is inoperable and then sent directly home after reaching Mulago Hospital—now come to the UCI seeking relief. Patients may be wracked by the rot of advanced breast cancer, such as a beloved matriarch brought to the Institute by a family who can no longer care for her. Or a patient may be a five-year-old child with loose teeth from Burkitt's lymphoma whose parents have exhausted all other treatment options, including long consultations with healers at shrines and courses of herbs.

The partnership between the UCI and the Fred Hutch has, over the past decade, valiantly attempted to address the profound structural inequalities that render Seattle and Kampala incommensurable. Hence the investments in training Ugandans as oncology fellows in Seattle and in building a laboratory facility so research can be done "in-house" on the UCI campus. During my ethnographic fieldwork in 2012, I observed American colleagues setting strategic and practical boundaries at the UCI even as they contributed to new investments in experimental infrastructure. Building patient cohorts, doing HHV-8 shedding studies, and doing some translational research on improving Burkitt's lymphoma outcomes comprised the bulk of activities. Although the offices were located at the UCI, it was clear that many of the late-stage cancer patients who went to the site seeking care would never interact with a research program. This meant that the sort of work that UCI oncologists did for the Fred Hutch on Kaposi's sarcoma staging was often separated from their actual care for Kaposi's patients on the wards of the STC. In other words, these investments in infrastructure and even in staff training hold the possibility of inadvertently cementing inequalities in mortar and concrete on the Institute's campus. The UCI–Fred Hutch Cancer Center's disease-specific research agenda is built into the building's design, and this agenda will mark those whose bodies and cancers will in all likelihood be seen and treated in this space. Closing the "global cancer divide" through infrastructure improvements like the UCI–Fred Hutch Cancer Center has the potential to widen rather than diminish the gaps between "government medicine" and "doing research." Over the next decade, it will be fascinating to see how exactly these differences in research cultures and priorities at the UCI and the UCI–Fred Hutch Cancer Center both re-create and (one hopes) transcend the politics of global cancer inequalities. But that is a different book.

Historians do not like to make predictions, but I'll venture one here. Social, political, epidemiological, economic, and scientific circumstances well beyond the control of the staff and patients at the UCI will, in all likelihood, continue to impact this facility in the next half century. Ugandan citizens will continue to contend with malignancies on the wards and malignant states. Committed Ugandans, these physician-intellectuals, will keep these new investments in cancer services going long after this latest international research partnership with the Fred Hutchinson Cancer Research Center changes or comes to a close. Research is a resource, but it is one fundamentally situated in the temporal shifts of politics, economics, scientific priorities, and personal relationships.

Epilogue
In Memoriam

MOST EVERY Tuesday, somewhere around 1 or 2 p.m., after staff consumed a fast lunch of local food, fish, and groundnut sauce, we piled into the examination and intake room of the Lymphoma Treatment Center (LTC). A wooden table surrounded by hardback chairs dominated the room. A filing cabinet stood in a corner. The social worker, counselor, and I usually assembled on the slightly ragged examination bench with legs dangling. An old sterilizer sat in the corner, donated sometime in the early 1990s by a Christian NGO. Occasionally one of the nursing staff would come in during ward rounds and fire it up, sterilizing piles of cotton gauze that would be used for cleaning up veins after blood draws.

Dr. Joyce Balagadde Kambugu, the head pediatric oncologist at the Uganda Cancer Institute (UCI), would usually rush into the room, apologizing for being late. She would sit down at the seat reserved for her in the middle of the table, surrounded by nursing and laboratory staff, and voluminous piles of pink, manila, blue, and green patient records. Some of the files were so thick they were nearly falling apart. Others were slender, containing only a face sheet and a referral note that had been filled out that very morning. Kambugu would slip a wad of Ugandan shillings to Sister N, the elderly Muganda nurse who had been working on the wards of the UCI since the 1970s. Sister N would come back several minutes later with black *caverras* (plastic bags) of sodas. Coke, Fanta, and Stoney ginger beer would be distributed along with straws to the fifteen or so in attendance, the ward round officially commencing to the sound of bottles being cracked open and the discussion of "very, very sick children."

Quite soon upon returning from a year of training in South Africa, Kambugu, who was running a ward with twenty-four beds and thirty-four to forty more inpatients sleeping outside on the verandah at any given time, decided to initiate comprehensive "sit down" ward rounds in the privacy of the doctor's examination room rather than "standing" ward rounds. Part of this was done to reduce the amount of time spent on one's feet, shuffling from one bed to the next with an entourage in tight quarters. But there was also the question of privacy. "They listen to what you are saying about them," Kambugu says. "They are watching, wondering if you are going to give up on them or if it's game over." "Game over" was the phrase Kambugu invoked time and again for residential cases at the UCI who were for all intents and purposes salvage chemotherapy patients. In a setting that was so public—twenty-four beds jammed on top of one another along with family members and additional kids and relatives coming in to say hello—creating a space for private and frank discussion changed the tenor of the ward round. Given the volume of patients and shortages of space, the long-term goal of admitting a patient—the Luganda phrase *olmuwadde mu'wadde ekitanda* literally means "giving a bed"—was often to discharge that patient as soon as medically and humanely possible. Discharge can come after the side effects of chemotherapy have dissipated, or once the infection from a feeding tube has been abated. Patients who were discharged sometimes come back days later with terrible fevers from immunosuppression, bad headaches, and nausea. Or they might come back two years later with a recurring, newly festering mass. Being discharged and told to come back for follow-up is but one way to leave the UCI. There are other methods—running away, departing in a coffin, or being given a verdict that it is "game over."

On many of these sit-down rounds, we began the day with Baby Winnie. Baby Winnie, an eighteen-month-old who suffered from bladder cancer, was a permanent fixture at the UCI along with her mother for most of 2012. Mama Winnie, a peasant farmer from the central region whose main source of income was selling maize and beans, realized that there was something wrong with her daughter in November 2011 while winnowing beans in her compound. Her child was sitting in a pool of blood. The baby was first taken to elders, who diagnosed the child with a prolapsed uterus, and in "the village style, everyone said they knew the treatment and we started using the local herbs." The child's belly became more and more swollen, and so the child was then taken first to Gombe Hospital, then Nkozi Hospital, and finally Mulago. Mama Winnie recalled:

> When we came to Mulago, the child was so swollen. The swelling was so big and oozing pus and very offensive. We started from the Acute ward where we spent 1 month. We were then sent to ward 2A in New Mulago where she was operated on and a biopsy was done. We spent 2 months in that ward. The biopsy was sent to Wandegeya and the results revealed the child had cancer. After two months, we were sent to the Cancer Institute. When we arrived at the UCI, I found the beds were full. Then I slept outside for two days but since the mosquitoes were so many, I moved in to sleep in the corridors. I stayed there for four days and I was offered a bed in the adult ward. When an adult was admitted, I was requested to leave the bed and waited until I got a bed in the children's ward.[1]

Mama Winnie hung on to her designated bed in the children's ward of the LTC with extreme tenacity throughout 2012, weathering her child's difficult surgery, a feeding tube, and oscillations from chemotherapy cycles, all the while refusing the Institute's attempts to push the family to go home whenever Baby Winnie would stabilize. Away from earning her income from maize and beans, she also became a regular charge of the Uganda Children's Cancer Foundation, which subsidized some of the more expensive tests for Baby Winnie. As Baby Winnie improved over the course of the year, the LTC staff increasingly tried to turn Baby Winnie into an outpatient, to free up the bed, and to have Mama and Baby Winnie come back only for treatment cycles. Mama Winnie refused in stubbornly subtle ways. She would claim that transport money was not available. When transport money was made available, Mama Winnie still refused to leave, preferring to stay on the verandah until the possibility of readmission. The LTC became home.

Next in the stack was Patience and Mama Patience, who lived on the wards of the LTC off and on in 2011 and 2012. Patience suffered from intestinal cancer and was a long-term resident at the UCI for chemotherapy. She was also incontinent from a botched surgery performed for nearly free by a charity hospital located on Entebbe Road. Patience came first to the UCI after several months of searching for a diagnosis. Her story of coming to the UCI captures some of the deep familial conflicts, often about money, regarding how to chart a course of treatment for a patient. These conflicts often emerge over the protracted process of taking biopsies, traveling to referral hospitals, and losing time on the wards. Here is the story relayed by Mama Patience:

> My child fell sick from February 5, 2011. I took her to a clinic but the nurse requested me to go to a main hospital. It started with a swelling from the urethra and would occasionally bleed. I was then referred to Kitovu Hospital, where we were admitted for one week before an operation and a biopsy was taken. We were discharged and told to return after one month for the results. When I went back I did not find him on several occasions. After two weeks, we went back and the growth had grown back, found the doctor who indicated that he had got the results but misplaced them, but they found that the child has cancer. He then asked me to allow him a week to look for them, which I did, and on return he said they were completely lost and we needed to have another biopsy done. This took us another week. There was no transport but the father was still caring and requested the biopsy and brought her to Wandegeya in Kampala.
>
> Meanwhile the child became worse and started oozing pus and had a lot of pain but we kept getting treatment. We then got the results and they said she has cancer and we continued on for two weeks. We were then referred to Mulago but the father decided to take us back home now that the doctor had indicated that there was no hope.
>
> I had cultivated my groundnuts but because I spent a long time in the hospital they were not attended to very well. At this point it was around three months since identifying the problem. I sold my groundnuts for 120,000 [Ugandan shillings, about US$46.50] and by this time my child was bedridden. So with this money, I decided to bring my child to Mulago, where the doctor had advised us to come. So we came in June 2011 and we started from there until now.
>
> I did not inform my husband about my plan as he indicated that he does not have any more money for this case.[2]

Making a cancer diagnosis after the onset of obvious illness can take months or upwards of a year in Uganda. Murky differential diagnoses are one thing, but paperwork is another. At the UCI in 2012, a referral note and a biopsy result must be in hand (or, at the very least, pending) in order for a patient to be admitted to the wards of the UCI. In the 1960s and early 1970s, centralized pathology services at Mulago, which would cooperate with referral hospitals throughout the country and correspond via the post office, ensured that the project of remote diagnosis would take about a week.[3] When the UCI was under serious duress, this referral structure helped to conserve scarce resources from being spent on "hopeless cases," or patients without diagnoses. It was a triage mechanism at the UCI during the 1980s, 1990s, and 2000s, when there were only ten staff members. In 2012, a lost biopsy result could often mean salvage chemotherapy.

By far the largest most complicated file on ward rounds was the file of Baby Angel. For nearly the entirety of 2012, Baby Angel resided in crib number twenty-four, right at the entrance of the pediatric side of the LTC. Her crib was surrounded by a big blue mosquito net, stuffed animals, and a puffy-cheeked doll that mirrored her own cheeks, which were puffed up from steroids. Sponsors and passersby doted on Baby Angel, who had been abandoned by her mother in early 2012. Baby Angel had been left in the care of her father, a peasant farmer from outside of Lira who grew sesame, sorghum, and soya beans. He knew much about the vagaries of rains and planting seasons but less, at least initially, about how to cook or attend to domestic chores. But Tata Angel was a dedicated caretaker. After his wife left for the north, he spent weeks tediously weaning Angel on starchy muffins, tea, and porridge. He would strap Baby Angel to his back and make his way to the market to buy food for cooking at night. Still in contact with his own family members, he would receive weekly shipments of *sim sim* (sesame paste), via bus to be cooked up with sorghum porridge. In the central region, where the diet is based on a starchy banana known as *matooke* and peanut sauce, these packets of sim sim paste offered a taste of home.

Tata Angel was also the "ward chairman" of the LTC. In Uganda, the chairman is a common figure. Chairmen preside over anything requiring meetings or social organization, from boda boda (motorcycle taxi) driver cooperatives to routine UCI general purpose meetings and to National Resistance Movement district government cells. At the LTC, the ward chairman is designated as a point person who welcomes newcomers to the ward, maintains social order and ensures that people and their property are secure, takes grievances to the staff, and oversees hygienic routines like cleaning out the showers and scrubbing the toilets.

In September 2012, Baby Angel was discharged from the LTC permanently. There was no salvage chemotherapy combination left. It was time to go back to their village just outside of Lira. It was "game over." Field-notes from that day capture the heaviness:

> We are sitting in silence. He wears dark-green trousers and
> a pale-colored short-sleeved shirt with a slightly frayed collar. He
> has grooved lines on his forehead and crow's feet around his eyes,
> which are expectant and resigned at the same time. I put my hand
> on his shoulder and he begins: "They have discharged us, me and
> Angel. We are going home. They say that the drugs aren't working
> anymore, that it is time to go home, but I will go home and show
> the family the changes in the body."
> "I am going to the market to buy food. I have food but I do
> not feel like cooking today. I will buy some fish, maybe," said
> Tata Angel as we continued to sit. I listened on. "You see my
> hands—all of this washing. I have been doing so much washing."
> Tata Angel's hands were cracked and chafed at the nail beds. For
> weeks, Baby Angel had suffered from terrible, explosive, bloody
> diarrhea. Her clothes and her bedding needed to be washed
> constantly.
> Tata Angel was tired of cooking, tired of washing, tired of
> being away from home. He packed their possessions from hospice,
> home, and donations into several large cheap plastic zipper bags
> and slept out on the verandah for a night.
> Anxiety among the LTC staff ran high—would he abandon
> the child here on the ward to die or would he take her back to
> Lira? Would he wait around on the verandah after being dis-
> charged to meet his local "sponsors" from the Uganda Children's
> Cancer Foundation who had given money and gifts? "If the spon-
> sors don't have a chance to meet the person they've been sponsor-
> ing then they will feel little incentive to sponsor someone else in
> the future," Dr. R noted. I was headed up to Gulu myself—would
> it make sense to drive them home to their village if it meant that
> Angel would actually safely reach home?
> Tata Angel made the decision to go home via the Gisenyi
> Bus Park on a Saturday morning in September, less than
> 48 hours after being discharged from the LTC. They had two
> motorcycles worth of possessions to take to the bus park. A week
> later, Angel died at home.
> At the LTC, even though her bed was quickly taken over by
> another patient, the crib seemed empty. A few sticker stars were

still plastered onto the wall, but there was no bright blue mosquito net, no chubby cheeked baby splayed out for a nap with her hand resting on a tiny bible, no Tata Angel donning workman's protective gear to clean out the toilets in the afternoon or to partition jackfruit at night.[4]

Only a handful will remember the day in September 2012 that Kirabo's parents found out it was "game over" for their sweet, cherubic little girl. Kirabo had lived off and on at the LTC for months, receiving treatments for her leukemia. Kirabo's mother often wore a blue *gomesi* (a popular floor-length dress style) the color of the noonday Kampala sky, hair wrapped in a flowing white head scarf, usually carrying the new baby on her back. Kirabo's father, who stayed outside of Kampala toward Lugazi, was often at the Institute over the weekend, checking in on his daughter and her progress. Everyone agreed they were a wonderful family. But acute refractory leukemia "in our setting" is not something that can be easily treated. You would need access to bone marrow transplant technologies to even have a fighting chance, and that's just not publicly available in Uganda. On ward rounds that day there was a long discussion about how to slowly and gently break the news to Kirabo's family that it was finally "game over." Kambugu said (and I'm paraphrasing here), "We'll call in hospice to help break the news, send them home with some small juice boxes, some oral morphine, some antibiotics, and what? Anything that can make them more comfortable. It's too bad that we didn't bring in hospice sooner. With them coming in now it just seems like it's game over. It's such a shame. She is the sweetest, most beautiful girl you've ever seen. She doesn't deserve this. Her family doesn't deserve this. But with acute refractory leukemia like this we are out of options without transplantation."[5] Kambugu made a final point to the medical students who were on her service for the next few weeks and were doing master's programs in pediatrics. "Please don't say anything to the family while we are at the bed. We need to be able to break the news."[6] The next day, I saw that the news had been broken. Mama Kirabo was standing next to a hospice vehicle and chatting with them. Kirabo played with some of my arm bracelets and was giggling and wearing her mother's white headscarf like a pirate. She was still cherubic and in high spirits. Even her hair was growing back after the latest round of chemo. And then she was gone.

I remember the departure of Kirabo particularly well only because it was my last day of major ward rounding and I was hoping for some sort of optimistic closure. But for most of the afternoon, a simple wooden coffin sat open and waiting for the deceased on the adult side of the LTC. One of the patient's relatives let out a wail of universal grief when the coffin was finally loaded onto the minibus and driven down the hill. Mama Patience looked slightly exhausted, wearing her faded but formal black suit, walking back and forth between the bathrooms and the ward with a bright-blue bucket to contain the retching. Patience's hair was again shaved close, as she started another intense round of chemo that made her violently retch. Stevie, an adolescent boy being treated for leukemia, was out playing on a seesaw with a friend. "What are you doing, Stevie?"

"We are playing." I could see that.

At the end of the sit-down ward round for the pediatric patients, little Nakkazi from Wobulenzi walked in, sobbing intensely. "Nakkazi, what's *wrong?*" asked Kambugu. In between her eruptions of grief, she said, "I want to go home. I want to go home. I want to go home."[7]

Seeing Kirabo and her family leave with their oral morphine, juice boxes, and instructions for when to go to the hospital for blood, we were all a bit shattered. As I got into my car I asked a colleague, "When on earth will we ever get bone marrow transplant services here in Uganda?" He was hilarious and frank: "Marissa, asking me when we'll get bone marrow transplant services in Uganda is like asking me when I'll be eating chicken every day. There are so many factors—we need infection managers, we need hematologists, we need *everything.* . . . We might as well open a poultry farm. These are things that we might want. But they are just really hard to attain without going slowly by slowly."[8]

During 2012, colleagues shaped systems of care and triage at the LTC through trial, error, the limitations of staffing and resources, and the realities of trying to offer cancer care to patients and families for whom shifting back and forth between the ward and the village was simply too much. As Kambugu worked to build these systems, she did so within a ward space that had been designed largely as a Burkitt's lymphoma research and care facility by Dr. John Ziegler and colleagues in 1967. The old building was nothing special. But it was designed in such a way that the wards had decent cross-ventilation, the verandahs and grassy spaces allowed for play and decompression after ward rounds. There was also a large cooking and washing area in the back. There was a dedicated space for doing bone marrow aspirates and lumbar punctures. In subtle ways, these innovative designs made it easier for staff to do their work and allowed families to camp out at the Institute for weeks or months at a time. The entire time Kambugu and her colleagues worked at the LTC in 2012, they did so with the knowledge that this historical structure was slated for demolition to make way for the new UCI–Fred Hutch Cancer Research Center.

At multiple points in the history of cancer care and research in Uganda, it has been the children—whether deformed by Burkitt's lymphoma or playing with blown-up latex gloves in between chemo cycles—that have given the Institute its international appeal. In October 2011, political dignitaries and international health moguls came to the Institute to celebrate the groundbreaking ceremony for the UCI–Fred Hutch Cancer Research Center that would displace the LTC. And it was the LTC that held the most appeal for the visitors. When I attended the event as a historian-ethnographer, handing out my business cards to American oncologists for follow-up interviews and joking with nurses in Luganda, I remember feeling a sense of horror when I realized that the cancer patients and their family caretakers would not be joining us for the buffet, as they would be expected to at any celebratory Ugandan function such as a wedding or funeral. Instead, patients watched us from the verandah of the LTC. After the ceremony, the visiting oncologists went off for ward rounds to look at exotic cancers. They also saw how oncology is practiced within the LTC, with its outmoded procedures room, children's ward with twenty-five beds, and cribs jammed neatly along walls. "Now I understand why they don't use chemo ports," one of the Americans noted to me after the tour, as patients would be septic in a matter of hours. Another said that it's a shame that survival outcomes for curable cancers remain low, when compared to survival outcomes at the UCI in the 1970s. It was then that I could not help saying, "Well, in the 1970s researchers were paying for transport and buying patients food." The answer was that we should look into building a Ronald McDonald House, as "the kids are just so appealing."[9]

Even after it was slated for demolition, the LTC remained the showpiece of the Institute, used in part to try to marshal further support and donations to furnish the new inpatient cancer hospital. On one such occasion, a prince from a Middle Eastern country announced he was making a visit to the UCI to see the important work being done on noncommunicable diseases in the country. The staff had approximately twenty-four hours to make preparations for his tour of the facilities. Tents needed to be rented. Dancers well versed in "traditional" performances spanning from Kabale to Kitgum were hired to perform hospitality. Box lunches of chicken, samosas, and sodas were ordered. The public relations officer found an imam at the last minute to offer the opening prayer. There was hope that the Middle Eastern country would make a contribution toward

$4 million worth of medical equipment needed to furnish the not-yet-open five-story Ministry of Health–sponsored cancer inpatient facility at the Institute.

That Saturday morning in June 2012, patients and their caretakers were up and out of the LTC before dawn, just as the call to prayer from Mulago National Referral Hospital's mosque started to reverberate up the hill. The floors were scrubbed until they shined. Bleach replaced the smell of vomit and other sicknesses. Beds were made with square hospital corners. Pediatric patients dressed in their best and cleanest outfits. Medical records were stacked neatly on the reception area table, which was cleared of all traces of its usual purpose as a chemotherapy reconstitution lab bench. Overflowing sharps containers were taken down to the incinerator. Rarely used suction machines and blood pressure monitors were wheeled out into prominent view. That morning, the ward sparkled, painted in that unmistakable industrial seafoam green so characteristic of hospitals in East Africa and beyond. The undersea mural of starfish, sea horses, and bobbing fish looked cheerful rather than dreary. All traces of residential life—the cook stoves, cardboard shelters, mats, bedrolls, suitcases, crutches, buckets, and donated stuffed animals clearly loved to death—were erased from the public space of the verandah and the wards and shoved back behind the LTC for the day. Nurses in freshly pressed white government uniforms came to start the morning ward round early, around eight o'clock, ensuring they would finish before the "VIPs" arrived at eleven.

I arrived at the UCI at around 10 a.m. with my camera and notebook to find plenty of police forces standing around in blue security uniforms, but I slipped in easily through the main gate without being searched. There were two tents set up across from one another in the main parking lot, much like they would be at a *kwanjula* (a Baganda introduction ceremony), with ribbons of purple and yellow festively tied to the stakes. The dancers and drummers performed in full force and attracted an audience of patients and caretakers who were watching the scene from the LTC lawn directly outside of the building's main entrance. I walked inside to extend my morning greetings and to check in on a few of the pediatric patients, marveling at how the sparkling walls and tidied supply closets made the space feel less overwhelming, even if there were still a few patients sleeping on the floor.

In particular, I wanted to check on Oliver, an eight-year-old with acute myelogenous leukemia who, upon our first meeting, was a cheerful kid scrawling out his name repeatedly in an exercise booklet and reading from a few donated books to keep up with his schooling while away from his home in Luweero. Tata Oliver, often sporting a Hawaiian shirt, was a maize and beans farmer as well as a blacksmith. He and his wife had seven children, including a new baby. He had put crops and metalwork on hold to care for his favorite son. It was not going well. Months into treatment, the outlook was not good. The treatments had puffed Oliver's face to the point of being barely recognizable. His belly was distended and his arms and legs emaciated. He was only comfortable sleeping in the fetal position and had taken to scratching and biting at his father out of frustration and disorientation. In the United States, Oliver's leukemia would have been a prime candidate for bone marrow transplantation. Here, in Uganda, the oncologists had been working through all lines of salvage therapy. Oliver was very hypertensive, losing weight, and up vomiting morning, noon, and night.

"*Oli otya, mukwano?*" (How are you my friend?) I tried to get a smile.

"He is not fine," said Tata Oliver.

"And how are you doing?" I asked.

"I am not okay," said Tata Oliver. "When he eats, he vomits. When he drinks porridge, he vomits. When he takes water, he vomits. The only thing he can take is tea." Dr. M deftly took Oliver's blood pressure as Tata Oliver continued. "I am not okay. We were told this muzungu is visiting today and that we must put on clean clothes and make the bed. I am happy he is visiting, but"—and here Tata Oliver began to get angrier, louder, and more animated—"I *clean*. I keep my child clean. I make the bed with clean sheets!" he said as he gestured to the perfectly folded corners on the bed. "What is this muzungu bringing me? I have nothing. We have nothing. The doctors said to clean this place. But what are they doing for me? I am not good. I am not fine." I would find out from staff in the next week that in the cleaning frenzy to welcome the prince, someone had thrown out all of Oliver's clothing that had been left to dry on the lawn, leaving them with nothing.

I took my leave to sit down in the tent next to an American colleague who was visiting from Seattle. "What do you think it would take to get a bone marrow transplant unit here?" I asked, filling him in on the scene that had just unfolded.

"It's a strange thing, isn't it?" he said. "There's dancing. And there's dying. I think the only way to make sense of this is to put this into a five-year perspective. If this prince comes, and if the beds are made and clean, perhaps he'll give money. Maybe there will be more second-line drugs. Maybe, someday, the infrastructure for bone marrow transplants."[10]

And so we waited. Then we waited some more. A Ministry of Health vehicle drove up to the gate. An official stepped out and went to talk to the UCI's director. The prince was stuck in traffic across town and would not be coming. He had an afternoon flight to catch out of Entebbe. The imam opened the ceremony with a prayer. We stood for the Ugandan National Anthem. The UCI's director stood with poise and delivered a succinct speech. Kitchen staff distributed warm sodas. The master of ceremonies announced that we were closing the ceremony, and we stood again for the anthem. Patients and staff mingled under the tents and ate the box lunches; among those present was Tata Oliver, who cajoled his son to take another sip of Fanta. I took my leave and told a Ugandan colleague I was very sorry that they had gone to all of this last-minute expense and planning, only to be thwarted by the traffic. "As long as there is money coming," the colleague noted, "it is okay that the prince did not come." To the best of my knowledge, the money never came.[11]

More than a year later, it only took half a day to bulldoze the LTC. It came down easily. The bricks and the plaster and the dreary mural depicting cartoon seahorses swimming in the sea and anthropomorphic starfish crumbled into fine powdery dust. The windows, the doors, and the iron gates were salvaged and piled up behind the Institute's generator. Staff were kindly reminded in internal memos taped on the wall that they were not allowed to re-use these old materials for their own construction needs. Nurses quietly cried and took photographs of their decrepit but beloved LTC. "The heart and soul of the Institute," said Sister A. From their newly improvised temporary space, the Lymphoma Treatment Center II (LTC II), patients and their caretakers watched the building crumble. It was a refurbished tuberculosis outpatient facility with three airless rooms with about seven full-sized beds and a few floor cases apiece, and there was a hallway which had been hastily enclosed to accommodate pediatric cribs. The reception table, which also doubled as a chemotherapy constitution bench in the old LTC, was repurposed outside of the corridors as a place for patients to lean against and store their bedrolls, washing bins, and buckets. This was the temporary fix in 2013. Patients would move into the Ugandan government's newly completed cancer hospital at the top of Mulago Hill as soon as the building was furnished.[12]

When I returned to Uganda the following year in 2014, I was thrilled to be back and fielded inevitable questions like "When are you having a child?" "When are you finishing the book?" "Where are my chocolates?" And I asked my own questions: "Is Oliver still alive?" "How are your chemotherapy supplies these days?" "When did you get married?" "When are you moving up to the new hospital?" "Do you miss the old LTC?" "Tell me what it's like to work in the new LTC?" "How does this new temporary setup shape your day-to-day work?" I filled my notebooks with words. And I share them here with you, not to undermine the efforts to transform the Institute but to offer a fuller historical record of some of the costs of breaking the UCI's original experimental infrastructure.

From the first day I set foot on the wards of the Uganda Cancer Institute in 2010, I was struck by the social intimacy of the place. It seemed to me that the UCI was a lot like a small village, complete with council meetings, weddings, funerals, and a constant procession of increasingly pregnant nurses whose swelling bellies marked the passing of time. Patient families lying out on mats and plaiting one another's hair or preparing a morning meal on tiny cook stoves, the MTN mobile money shacks, the laughter of children, and the rogue goat lunching on the lawn all cemented a sense of village life. Nursing sisters took long and rabble-rousing tea breaks. Mr. K would read the *New Vision* for at least a half hour every morning before he distributed X-ray reports to patients snoozing on benches. Boda bodas would blast into the parking lot, dropping off patients and supplies. Quotidian Kampala pastoral at its best.

Beyond the appearance of village life, there were also complicated kinship networks and intergenerational relations. Some of the older nurses who worked on the wards for three or four decades were much like sisters to one another. The newly trained medical oncology fellows had tended to nighttime emergencies as resident student health officers and were beloved by their surviving patients, many of whom continued to come for follow-up appointments years later and check in as one would do with a relative. Personal histories of staff were often woven into the daily sociality of the Institute, either through intergenerational family ties, personal tragedies, or romance. Mr. S, who was responsible for running orders for blood and platelets back and forth between the UCI and Nakasero Blood Bank had grown up at the Institute. His mother had worked as a cleaner in the X-ray department for years. She had died of colon cancer herself a few years before and had been a patient on the wards.

That summer, scarcely more than a month into fieldwork and energized by this easy analogy, I remarked to a physician colleague that the Institute seemed to resemble a village. He paused for a moment and then looked at me with great seriousness and said, "This isn't a village, Marissa. This is a camp," gesturing to the scene in front of us. It was a revelation. I looked at the bedrolls, the washing basins, and one young patient with debilitating Kaposi's eating away his foot. He had been living on a piece of cardboard outside of the Solid Tumor Center for over three months. It did not take a great leap of imagination to see that my colleague had a point.

I think about this description of the UCI as a camp often as I witness the aftermath of the demolition of the LTC. Forty-five years of carefully planned practices bulldozed for chemotherapy clinical trials that will happen at some point in the future. In the meantime, you have to walk through the toilets to get to the X-ray department or weave through cooking stoves. I expect to see relief tents and multiple hand-washing stations and an army of crisis workers. Where is Doctors without Borders when you need it? Why is there only one water spigot for a hundred-plus people and a cooking area that is a huge accident waiting to happen? This shit stinks—you can literally smell it wafting up from the gutter that separates the LTC II from the construction site while chatting with Mr. K at the X-ray department.

Comments about this tough situation by colleagues spill out over tea and casual conversation. "How do you practice medicine without an examination table?" "I know that the air circulation is poor in that room." "The environment is not good." "We had a flood in February. A flood of patients. They were sleeping and staying on every part of the landing." "There is no space." "We know it's not good that patients are sleeping on the floors." "There have been no pediatric bone marrow needles since October."

Is any of this surprising? This is the sausage-making part of shiny global health initiatives that nobody wants to see or talk about. My Ugandan colleagues aren't happy with it, but *bibaawo*: that's life, what can we do? And my American colleagues who have drawn a strategic line between themselves as researchers and the realities of clinical care at the site are saying, "Well, our new building will be awesome." At the same time, colleagues at the Fred Hutch significantly delayed the construction of the new UCI–Fred Hutch Cancer Center to account for the fact that the LTC patients had nowhere to go and also contributed significant funds to the refurbishment of the temporary LTC II.

Both my colleagues at the UCI and the Fred Hutchinson Cancer Research Center know full well that this temporary ward—hastily made to provide care for lymphoma and leukemia to children and adults while they wait to move into the new building—is far from an ideal situation.[13] They are realistic. They are frustrated. The Institute staff come early to work, and they stay late taking care of patients, running up and down to get chemotherapy drips started and blood transfusions administered. They circumvent the toilets and the cooking stoves as they work. They keep disgust in check in the airless adolescent ward room that smells like bile and wounds. And, in many ways, the Institute sounds and looks much as it did in 2012.

There are silver linings. In the past two years, Kambugu has built a pediatric oncology service that works in "our setting." There are more antibiotics on the wards to prevent infections. There are now standardized treatment protocols for all of the common pediatric cancers. Dr. G, who started on the wards in 2012, has all of the makings of a dedicated pediatric oncologist. Kambugu spends less time in the clinic and more time looking for resources and cultivating partnerships, thanks to Dr. G's dedication and engagement. The six nurses on staff are fully committed to the children. Patients are surviving. Nobody is starving and everyone is getting something warm in their bellies three times a day.

I am keeping my cool and taking notes and trying to gauge the sentiments of my colleagues. I know I'm not in a position to do anything but finish up my work and that the politics of this will speak for itself.[14]

I could easily flip the narrative here and tell an optimistic story of an institution that has defied all odds and miraculously pressured the Ugandan government to take cancer seriously. It has. One could argue that the past decade's investment both from the international community and the national government in oncology goods in Uganda is unprecedented, historical, and miraculous. It is. And these dramatic improvements can be attributed largely to the visionary leadership of Dr. Jackson Orem and his team, who provide care and engage in the political work of making cancer visible. In the years since the LTC was bulldozed, the landscape of cancer care in Uganda transformed dramatically. Referral centers have opened at regional hospitals, new buildings have become equipped and operational, patients have come to the clinic through cancer screening programs, and Ugandan oncology experts have published their research. The temporary LTC II is no more. The LTC is now in its third iteration in the new UCI hospital building, and pediatric patients have a floor of their own. The plans Olweny and colleagues drafted in the early 1980s to rehabilitate the Institute and continue Africanizing oncology are, as I finish this book, coming to full fruition.

And there are surprising moments of survival. In June 2014, while reeling from the changes at the Institute one hot afternoon, I encountered a little boy spinning Ugandan shilling coins like a game of tops on the floor of the verandah space at the new temporary LTC II. He was giggling to himself and wearing shorts and an oversized pinstripe black suit jacket. I only figured out who this cheerful kid was when I made eye contact with Tata Oliver. He sat at the reception bench, and we exploded into smiles, laughter, relief, and joy. "Greet the muzungu!" said Tata Oliver, pulling him away from his coins and up to his feet. We bumped our fists together and had a wonderful laugh. Who knows what will happen next? Dr. G says he has residual disease in his central nervous system. He is one of the last of the leukemia patients I recognize from 2012. Most of the others have "passed."

Notes

PRELUDE

1. Republic of Uganda, *National Population and Housing Census 2014* (Kampala: Uganda Bureau of Statistics, 2014), http://www.ubos.org /onlinefiles/uploads/ubos/NPHC/NPHC%202014%20PROVISIONAL %20RESULTS%20REPORT.pdf.
2. That is, if there is blood available in the country. For more on chronic blood supply shortages in Uganda, see "Major Hospitals Still Lack Blood," *New Vision*, June 5, 2013, http://www.newvision.co.ug/news/643579-major -hospitals-still-lack-blood.html.
3. Fieldnotes, July 2012.

INTRODUCTION

1. Helen Tilley, *Africa as a Living Laboratory* (Chicago: University of Chicago Press, 2011).
2. *Uganda Cancer Institute Annual Report, 1970–1971*, Uganda Cancer Institute Archives.
3. M. S. R. Hutt and D. Burkitt, "Geographical Distribution of Cancer in East Africa: A New Clinicopathological Approach," *British Medical Journal* 2, no. 5464 (September 25, 1965): 719–22.
4. Idi Amin's disastrous effects on Uganda are well known. See David Martin, *General Amin* (London: Faber and Faber, 1974) and A. B. K. Kasozi, Nakanyike Musisi, and James Mukooza Sejjengo, *The Social Origins of Violence in Uganda, 1964–1985* (Montreal: McGill-Queen's University Press, 1994). For a reconsideration of Amin and Ugandan life in the 1970s, see in particular Alicia Decker, *In Idi Amin's Shadow: Women, Gender, and Militarism in Uganda* (Athens: Ohio University Press, 2014); and Derek R. Peterson and Edgar C. Taylor, "Rethinking the State in Idi Amin's Uganda: The Politics of Exhortation," *Journal of Eastern African Studies* 7 (2013): 58–82.
5. While this book is the first full-length monograph on the history of the UCI, others have generated thoughtful accounts of the Institute's history. See, for example, Charles Olweny, "The Uganda Cancer Institute,"

Oncology 37, no. 5 (1980): 367–70; and Harold Varmus, "Medical Research Centers in Mali and Uganda: Overcoming Obstacles to Building Scientific Capacity and Promoting Global Health," *Science and Diplomacy* 3 (2014).

6. Uganda Cancer Institute Staff, interviews by author, 2012.

7. S. D. Desmond-Hellmann and E. Katongole-Mbidde, "Kaposi's Sarcoma: Recent Developments," *AIDS* 5, no. 1 (1991): S135–42.

8. Fieldnotes, May 2015.

9. "Cancer Control in Africa," series, *Lancet Oncology* 14, no. 4 (2013).

10. Fieldnotes, May 2015.

11. Johanna Tayloe Crane, *Scrambling for Africa: AIDS, Expertise, and the Rise of American Global Health Science* (Ithaca, NY: Cornell University Press, 2013).

12. For a sample of knowledge produced at the UCI on cancer, see the selected bibliography of medical and public health research articles in this volume.

13. See Stephen Ellis, "Writing Histories of Contemporary Africa," *Journal of African History* 43, no. 1 (2002): 1–26.

14. Steven Feierman, "Struggles for Control: The Social Roots of Health and Healing in Modern Africa," *African Studies Review* 28, no. 2/3 (1985): 73–147; Steven Feierman and John M. Janzen, eds., *The Social Basis of Health and Healing in Africa* (Berkeley: University of California Press, 1992); Lyn Schumaker, "History of Medicine in Sub-Saharan Africa," in *The Oxford Handbook of the History of Medicine*, ed. Mark Jackson (Oxford: Oxford University Press, 2011), 275–79. Julie Parle and Vanessa Noble, "New Directions and Challenges in Histories of Health, Healing and Medicine in South Africa," *Medical History* 58, no. 2 (April 2014): 147–65, https://doi.org/10.1017/mdh.2014.1; Shula Marks, "What Is Colonial about Colonial Medicine? And What Has Happened to Imperialism and Health?," *Social History of Medicine* 10, no. 2 (August 1, 1997): 205–19; Megan Vaughan, "Healing and Curing: Issues in the Social History and Anthropology of Medicine in Africa," *Social History of Medicine* 7, no. 2 (August 1, 1994): 283–95; and Nancy Rose Hunt, *Suturing New Medical Histories of Africa* (Münster: LIT Verlag, 2013).

15. Hunt, *Suturing New Medical Histories.*

16. Vinh-Kim Nguyen, *The Republic of Therapy: Triage and Sovereignty in West Africa's Time of AIDS* (Durham, NC: Duke University Press, 2010); Didier Fassin, *When Bodies Remember: Experiences and Politics of AIDS in South Africa*, trans. Amy Jacobs and Gabrielle Varro (Berkeley: University of California Press, 2007); Adia Benton, *HIV Exceptionalism: Development through Disease in Sierra Leone* (Minneapolis: University of Minnesota Press, 2015); Shane Doyle, *Before HIV: Sexuality, Fertility and Mortality in East Africa, 1900–1980* (Oxford: Oxford University Press, 2013); Helen Epstein, *The Invisible Cure: Why We Are Losing the Fight*

against *AIDS in Africa* (New York: Farrar, Straus and Giroux, 2007); Paul Farmer, *AIDS and Accusation* (Berkeley: University of California Press, 1992); Mark Hunter, *Love in the Time of AIDS: Inequality, Gender, and Rights in South Africa* (Bloomington: Indiana University Press, 2010); Frederick Klaits, *Death in a Church of Life: Moral Passion during Botswana's Time of AIDS* (Berkeley: University of California Press, 2010); and Susan Reynolds Whyte, ed., *Second Chances: Surviving AIDS in Uganda* (Durham, NC: Duke University Press, 2014).

17. Adia Benton, "The Epidemic Will Be Militarized: Watching Outbreak as the West African Ebola Epidemic Unfolds," *Fieldsights*, October 7, 2014, https://culanth.org/fieldsights/the-epidemic-will-be-militarized-watching-outbreak-as-the-west-african-ebola-epidemic-unfolds; Adia Benton, "Whose Security? Militarization and Securitization during West Africa's Ebola Outbreak," *The Politics of Fear: Médecins sans Frontières and the West African Ebola Epidemic*, ed. Michiel Hofman and Sokhieng Au (New York: Oxford University Press, 2017), 25–50; Paul Farmer, *Fevers, Feuds, and Diamonds: Ebola and the Ravages of History* (New York: Farrar, Straus and Giroux, 2020); and Ibrahim Abdullah and Ismail Rashid, *Understanding West Africa's Ebola Epidemic: Towards a Political Economy* (London: Bloomsbury Academic, 2017).

18. Claire L. Wendland, *A Heart for the Work: Journeys through an African Medical School* (Chicago: University of Chicago Press, 2010); Melissa Graboyes, *The Experiment Must Continue: Medical Research and Ethics in East Africa, 1940–2014* (Athens: Ohio University Press, 2015); Jennifer Tappan, *The Riddle of Malnutrition: The Long Arc of Biomedical and Public Health Interventions in Uganda* (Athens: Ohio University Press, 2017); and Mari K. Webel, *The Politics of Disease Control: Sleeping Sickness in Eastern Africa, 1890–1920* (Athens: Ohio University Press, 2019).

19. Adriana Petryna, *When Experiments Travel: Clinical Trials and the Global Search for Human Subjects* (Princeton, NJ: Princeton University Press, 2009); Cal (Crystal) Biruk, *Cooking Data: Culture and Politics in an African Research World* (Durham, NC: Duke University Press, 2018); Ramah McKay, *Medicine in the Meantime: The Work of Care in Mozambique* (Durham, NC: Duke University Press, 2017); Alice Street, *Biomedicine in an Unstable Place: Infrastructure and Personhood in a Papua New Guinean Hospital* (Durham, NC: Duke University Press, 2014); Crane, *Scrambling for Africa*; Benton, *HIV Exceptionalism*; Elisha P. Renne, *The Politics of Polio in Northern Nigeria* (Bloomington: Indiana University Press, 2010); Whyte, *Second Chances*; João Guilherme Biehl and Adriana Petryna, *When People Come First: Critical Studies in Global Health* (Princeton, NJ: Princeton University Press, 2013); and Simukai Chigudu, *The Political Life of an Epidemic: Cholera, Crisis and Citizenship in Zimbabwe* (Cambridge: Cambridge University Press, 2020).

20. Joseph Ochieng et al., "Evolution of Research Ethics in a Low Resource Setting: A Case for Uganda," *Developing World Bioethics* 20, no. 1 (March 2020): 50–60; Warwick Anderson, "Making Global Health History: The Postcolonial Worldliness of Biomedicine," *Social History of Medicine* 27, no. 2 (May 1, 2014): 372–84.

21. P. Wenzel Geissler and Noémi Tousignant, "Capacity as History and Horizon: Infrastructure, Autonomy and Future in African Health Science and Care," *Canadian Journal of African Studies* (Revue Canadienne Des Études Africaines) 50, no. 3 (September 1, 2016): 349–59; Damien Droney, "Ironies of Laboratory Work during Ghana's Second Age of Optimism," *Cultural Anthropology* 29, no. 2 (2014): 363–84; Julie Livingston, *Improvising Medicine: An African Oncology Ward in an Emerging Cancer Epidemic* (Durham, NC: Duke University Press, 2012), x; Nguyen, *Republic of Therapy*; Biehl and Petryna, *When People Come First*; and Feierman, *When Physicians Meet*.

22. Nancy Rose Hunt, *A Colonial Lexicon: Of Birth Ritual, Medicalization, and Mobility in the Congo* (Durham, NC: Duke University Press, 1999); Paul W. Geissler et al., *Traces of the Future: An Archaeology of Medical Science in Africa* (Chicago: University of Chicago Press, 2016), 106–73.

23. Hunt, *Colonial Lexicon*; Stoler, "Imperial Debris"; Paul W. Geissler et al., *Traces of the Future*; and Droney, "Ironies of Laboratory Work," 363–84.

24. Frederick Cooper, *Africa since 1940: The Past of the Present*, New Approaches to African History (New York: Cambridge University Press, 2002), 91–131.

25. Nolwazi Mkhwanazi, "Medical Anthropology in Africa: The Trouble with a Single Story," *Medical Anthropology* 35, no. 2 (March 3, 2016): 199.

26. My own attempts to wrestle with this challenge include Marissa Mika, "Cytotoxic: Notes on Chemotherapy at the Lymphoma Treatment Center, Uganda Cancer Institute, Kampala," *BioSocieties* 14, no. 4 (December 1, 2019): 573–82; Marissa Mika, "The Half-Life of Radiotherapy and Other Transferred Technologies," *Technology and Culture* 61, no. 2 (2020): S135–57; and Marissa Mika, "Fifty Years of Creativity, Crisis, and Cancer in Uganda," *Canadian Journal of African Studies* (Revue Canadienne Des Études Africaines) 50, no. 3 (September 1, 2016): 395–413.

27. This argument is informed by theories of technology transfer as a tool of empire, incoming technologies such as the gun, and writing on the rugged, simple, affordable technofix such as the Zimbabwean bush pump. See Daniel R. Headrick, *The Tools of Empire: Technology and European Imperialism in the Nineteenth Century* (New York: Oxford University Press, 1981); Clapperton Chakanetsa Mavhunga, *Transient Workspaces: Technologies of Everyday Innovation in Zimbabwe* (Cambridge, MA: MIT Press, 2014); and Marianne de Laet and Annemarie Mol, "The Zimbabwe Bush Pump: Mechanics of a Fluid Technology," *Social Studies of Science* 30, no. 2 (April 2000): 225–63.

28. Petryna, *When Experiments Travel*; Peter Redfield, *Life in Crisis: The Ethical Journey of Doctors without Borders* (Berkeley: University of California Press, 2013).

29. Olweny, "Uganda Cancer Institute," 367–370; and Alfred Jatho et al., "Capacity Building for Cancer Prevention and Early Detection in the Ugandan Primary Healthcare Facilities: Working toward Reducing the Unmet Needs of Cancer Control Services," *Cancer Medicine* 10, no. 2 (January 2021): https://doi.org/10.1002/cam4.3659.

30. John Ziegler, interview by author, June 2012.

31. Vickie Mujuzi, interview by author, March 2012; Tom Tomusange, interview by author, March 2012; John Ziegler, interview by author, June 2012.

32. Vickie Mujuzi, interview by author, March 2012; Tom Tomusange, interview by author, March 2012; John Ziegler, interview by author, June 2012.

33. Margaret Lock and Vinh-Kim Nguyen, *An Anthropology of Biomedicine* (Malden, MA: Wiley-Blackwell, 2010), 23.

34. S. Løchlann Jain, *Malignant: How Cancer Becomes Us* (Berkeley: University of California Press, 2013), 68.

35. *Uganda Cancer Institute Annual Reports, 1967–1977*, Uganda Cancer Institute Archives.

36. David Arnold, *Colonizing the Body: State Medicine and Epidemic Disease in Nineteenth-Century India* (Berkeley: University of California Press, 1993).

37. Susan Leigh Star, "The Ethnography of Infrastructure," *American Behavioral Scientist* 43, no. 3 (November 1, 1999): 377–91.

38. Paul Edwards, "Infrastructure and Modernity: Force, Time and Social Organization in the History of Sociotechnical Systems," in *Modernity and Technology*, ed. Thomas J. Misa, Philip Brey, and Andrew Feenberg (Cambridge, MA: MIT Press, 2003), 185–226; Brian Larkin, "The Politics and Poetics of Infrastructure," *Annual Review of Anthropology* 42, no. 1 (2013): 327–43; Wiebe E. Bijker, Thomas Parke Hughes, and Trevor Pinch, *The Social Construction of Technological Systems: New Directions in the Sociology and History of Technology* (Cambridge, MA: MIT Press, 2012); David Edgerton, "Innovation, Technology, or History: What Is the Historiography of Technology About?," *Technology and Culture* 51, no. 3 (August 15, 2010): 680–97; and David Edgerton, *The Shock of the Old: Technology and Global History since 1900* (Oxford: Oxford University Press, 2006).

39. Edwards, "Infrastructure and Modernity," 188.

40. Edwards, 188.

41. Nikhil Anand, Akhil Gupta, and Hannah Appel, *The Promise of Infrastructure* (Durham, NC: Duke University Press, 2018); Antina von Schnitzler, *Democracy's Infrastructure: Techno-politics and Protest after Apartheid* (Princeton, NJ: Princeton University Press, 2016); Nikhil Anand, *Hydraulic City: Water and the Infrastructures of Citizenship in Mumbai* (Durham,

NC: Duke University Press, 2017); Filip De Boeck, "'Poverty' and the Politics of Syncopation: Urban Examples from Kinshasa (DR Congo)," *Current Anthropology* 56, no. 11 (October 1, 2015): S146–58; Brenda Chalfin, *Neoliberal Frontiers: An Ethnography of Sovereignty in West Africa* (Chicago: University of Chicago Press, 2010); Gabrielle Hecht, "Interscalar Vehicles for an African Anthropocene: On Waste, Temporality, and Violence," *Cultural Anthropology* 33 no. 1 (2018): 109–41.

42. Brian Larkin, *Signal and Noise: Media, Infrastructure, and Urban Culture in Nigeria* (Durham, NC: Duke University Press, 2008); Headrick, *Tools of Empire*; Robyn D'Avignon, "Spirited Geobodies: Producing Subterranean Property in Nineteenth-Century Bambuk, West Africa," *Technology and Culture* 61, no. 2 (2020): S20–48, https://doi.org/10.1353/tech.2020.0069.

43. Steven Feierman, "A Century of Ironies in East Africa," in Philip D. Curtin et al., *African History* (London: Longman, 1995), 352–76; Randall M. Packard, *White Plague, Black Labor: Tuberculosis and the Political Economy of Health and Disease in South Africa* (Berkeley: University of California Press, 1989); Jennifer Ann Dawe, "History of Cotton Growing in East and Central Africa: British Demand, African Supply" (PhD diss., University of Edinburgh, 1993).

44. For more on the history of the repercussions of medical experiment and research in sub-Saharan Africa, see Crane, *Scrambling for Africa*; Epstein, *Invisible Cure*; Feierman and Janzen, *Social Basis of Health and Healing in Africa*; Duana Fullwiley, *The Encultured Gene: Sickle Cell Health Politics and Biological Difference in West Africa* (Princeton, NJ: Princeton University Press, 2011); Wenzel P. Geissler and Catherine Molyneux, eds., *Evidence, Ethos and Experiment: The Anthropology and History of Medical Research in Africa* (New York: Berghahn, 2011); P. W. Geissler et al., "He Is Now Like a Brother, I Can Even Give Him Some Blood'—Relational Ethics and Material Exchanges in a Malaria Vaccine 'Trial Community' in the Gambia," *Social Science and Medicine* 67, no. 5 (2008): 696–707; P. W. Geissler and R. Pool, "Editorial: Popular Concerns about Medical Research Projects in Sub-Saharan Africa—a Critical Voice in Debates about Medical Research Ethics," *Tropical Medicine and International Health* 11, no. 7 (2006): 975–82; Maryinez Lyons, *The Colonial Disease: A Social History of Sleeping Sickness in Northern Zaire, 1900–1940* (New York: Cambridge University Press, 1992); Vinh-Kim Nguyen, "Government-by-Exception: Enrolment and Experimentality in Mass HIV Treatment Programmes in Africa," *Society and Health* 7 (2009): 196–217; Vinh-Kim Nguyen, *The Republic of Therapy: Triage and Sovereignty in West Africa's Time of AIDS* (Durham, NC: Duke University Press, 2010); Packard, *White Plague, Black Labor*; Richard Rottenburg, "Social

and Public Experiments and New Figurations of Science and Politics in Postcolonial Africa," *Postcolonial Studies* 12, no. 4 (2009): 423–40; Megan Vaughan, *Curing Their Ills: Colonial Power and African Illness* (Cambridge, UK: Polity, 1991); and Luise White, *Speaking with Vampires: Rumor and History in Colonial Africa* (Berkeley: University of California Press, 2000).

45. John Iliffe, *East African Doctors: A History of the Modern Profession* (Kampala: Fountain, 2002); Vaughan, *Curing Their Ills*; Doyle, *Before HIV*; Jennifer Tappan, "The True Fiasco: The Treatment and Prevention of Sever Acute Malnutrition in Uganda 1950–1974," in *Global Health in Africa: Historical Perspectives on Culture, Epidemiology, and Disease Control*, ed. Tamara Giles Vernick and James Webb Jr. (Athens: Ohio University Press, 2013), 92–113; and Diane Zeller, "The Establishment of Western Medicine in Buganda" (PhD diss., Columbia University, 1971).

46. James Ferguson, *Global Shadows: Africa in the Neoliberal World Order* (Durham, NC: Duke University Press, 2006).

47. Farmer, *Fevers, Feuds, and Diamonds*.

48. Siddhartha Mukherjee, *The Emperor of All Maladies: A Biography of Cancer* (New York: Scribner, 2010), 204.

49. See, for example, D. M. Parkin et al., eds., *Cancer in Africa: Epidemiology and Prevention* (Lyon: International Agency for Research on Cancer, 2003).

50. Livingston, *Improvising Medicine*; Darja Djordjevic, "Pluripotent Trajectories: Public Oncology in Rwanda," *BioSocieties* 14, no. 4 (2019): 553–70, https://doi.org/10.1057/s41292-019-00160-w; and see Benson Mulemi's extensive corpus on living with cancer in Kenya, including *Coping with Cancer and Adversity: Hospital Ethnography in Kenya* (Leiden: African Studies Center, 2010).

51. Megan Vaughan, Kafui Adjaye-Gbewonyo, and Marissa Mika, eds., *Epidemiological Change and Chronic Disease in Sub-Saharan Africa: Social and Historical Perspectives* (London: UCL Press, 2021); Julie Livingston, "Pregnant Children and Half-Dead Adults: Modern Living and the Quickening Life Cycle in Botswana," *Bulletin of the History of Medicine* 77, no. 1 (March 20, 2003): 133–62; Emily Mendenhall and Shane A. Norris, "When HIV Is Ordinary and Diabetes New: Remaking Suffering in a South African Township," *Global Public Health* 10, no. 4 (2015): 449–62.

52. Emily Mendenhall, "Syndemics: A New Path for Global Health Research," *Lancet* 389, no. 10072 (2017): 889–91; Florence K. Baingana and Eduard R. Bos, "Changing Patterns of Disease and Mortality in Sub-Saharan Africa: An Overview," in *Disease and Mortality in Sub-Saharan Africa*, ed. Dean T. Jamison et al., 2nd ed. (Washington, DC: World

Bank, 2006), http://www.ncbi.nlm.nih.gov/books/NBK2281/; Vaughan, Adjaye-Gbewonyo, and Mika, *Epidemiological Change*.

53. Vaughan, Adjaye-Gbewonyo, and Mika, *Epidemiological Change*.

54. Satish Gopal and Patrick J. Loehrer Sr., "Global Oncology," *JAMA* 322, no. 5 (August 6, 2019): 397–98; Rachel M. Abudu et al., "Landscape of Global Oncology Research and Training at National Cancer Institute–Designated Cancer Centers: Results of the 2018 to 2019 Global Oncology Survey," *Journal of Global Oncology* 5 (November 22, 2019): 1–8; Jackson Orem and Henry Wabinga, "The Roles of National Cancer Research Institutions in Evolving a Comprehensive Cancer Control Program in a Developing Country: Experience from Uganda," *Oncology* 77, no. 5 (2009): 272–80.

55. Livingston, *Improvising Medicine*, 43–56. Daniel H. Low et al., "Engagement in HIV Care and Access to Cancer Treatment among Patients with HIV-Associated Malignancies in Uganda," *Journal of Global Oncology* 5 (February 2019): 1–8.

56. Manoj P. Menon et al., "Association between HIV Infection and Cancer Stage at Presentation at the Uganda Cancer Institute," *Journal of Global Oncology* 4 (September 2018): 1–9; Anna E. Coghill et al., "Contribution of HIV Infection to Mortality among Cancer Patients in Uganda," *AIDS* 27, no. 18 (November 28, 2013): 2933–42.

57. Phiona Bukirwa et al., "Trends in the Incidence of Cancer in Kampala, Uganda, 1991 to 2015," *International Journal of Cancer* 148, no. 9 (May 1, 2021): 2129–38. https://doi.org/10.1002/ijc.33373.

58. Livingston, *Improvising Medicine*, x.

59. On the contradictions of Museveni's Uganda, see Aili Mari Tripp, *Museveni's Uganda: Paradoxes of Power in a Hybrid Regime* (Boulder, CO: Rienner, 2010); Hölger Bernt Hansen and Michael Twaddle, eds., *Uganda Now: Between Decay and Development* (London: J. Currey, 1988); J. Oloka-Onyango, "'New-Breed' Leadership, Conflict, and Reconstruction in the Great Lakes Region of Africa: A Sociopolitical Biography of Uganda's Yoweri Kaguta Museveni," *Africa Today* 50 (2004): 29–52; Stefan Lindemann, "Just Another Change of Guard? Broad-Based Politics and Civil War in Museveni's Uganda," *African Affairs* 110 (2011): 387–416; Sverker Finnstrom, "Wars of the Past and War in the Present: The Lord's Resistance Movement/ Army in Uganda," *Africa* 76 (2006): 200–220; and Ben Jones, *Beyond the State in Rural Uganda* (Edinburgh: Edinburgh University Press, 2009).

60. Derek Peterson, "Uganda's History from the Margins," *History in Africa* 40, no. 1 (November 2013): S23–25; Andrew Rice, *The Teeth May Smile but the Heart Does Not Forget: Murder and Memory in Uganda* (New York: Picador, 2010); Sverker Finnstrom, *Living with Bad Surroundings: War, History, and Everyday Moments in Northern Uganda* (Durham, NC: Duke University Press 2008); and Michel-Rolph Trouillot, *Silencing the Past: Power and the Production of History* (Boston: Beacon, 1995).

61. For more on the topography of African archives since decolonization, see Ellis, "Writing Histories of Contemporary Africa"; and Jean Allman, "Phantoms of the Archive: Kwame Nkrumah, a Nazi Pilot Named Hanna, and the Contingencies of Postcolonial History-Writing," *American Historical Review* 118 (2013): 104–29.

62. See Veena Das, *Critical Events: An Anthropological Perspective on Contemporary India* (Oxford: Oxford University Press, 1997) and the way historian Lynn Thomas invokes critical events as a way to engage with African history in *Politics of the Womb: Women, Reproduction, and the State in Kenya* (Berkeley: University of California Press, 2003), 6–9. I am referring to the period of Uganda's history since 1962 as the postindependence period. This is how colleagues and the popular press in Uganda write, speak, and describe the time after the end of British Protectorate rule on October 9, 1962. Describing this period as "postcolonial," while appropriate in an academic intellectual setting, does not ring true with the vernacular Ugandan English description of Uganda's recent past. For more on celebrations of Ugandan independence, see James Magara, *Uganda Jubilee Handbook 2012: Commemorate. Celebrate. Contemplate* (Kampala: New Life, 2012).

63. On Obote's presidency, see the following: A. G. G. Gingyera-Pinycwa, *Apolo Milton Obote and His Times* (New York: NOK, 1978); Godfrey Nsubuga, *The Person of Dr. Milton Obote: A Classic Personality Study* (Kampala: Nissi, 2012); Omongole R. Anguria, ed., *Apollo Milton Obote: What Others Say* (Kampala: Fountain, 2006); and Kenneth Ingham, *Obote: A Political Biography* (New York: Routledge, 2014).

64. R. H. Morrow et al., "Survival of Burkitt's Lymphoma Patients in Mulago Hospital, Uganda," *British Medical Journal* 4 (1967): 323–27; Richard Morrow, interview by author, November 2012; Aloysius Kisuule, interview by author, March 2012; John Ziegler, interviews by author, June 2012, February 2013; Patient Records, Uganda Cancer Institute Archives

65. Avrum Bluming, interview by author, February 2015.

66. John Ziegler, interview by author, June 2012

67. As Iliffe argues, Uganda in the 1970s was a "disintegrating state," and this could be seen quite clearly at Mulago, where "its [Mulago's] piped water supply broke down in 1974 for a decade. The mortuary's refrigeration system was out of action from 1975 and sewerage ceased to function at about the same period. . . . At that time [1978] not one of the hospital's twelve X-ray units was functioning. . . . Yet they kept the hospital functioning." See Iliffe, *East African Doctors*, 147.

68. David Serwadda, interview by author, July 2012.

69. Sjaak van der Geest and Kaja Finkler, "Hospital Ethnography: Introduction," *Social Science and Medicine* 59, no. 10 (November 2004): 1995–2001.

70. John Ziegler, personal correspondence with author, May 2012.

71. See, for example, Denise Grady, "Uganda's Neglected Epidemic of Breast Cancer," *New York Times*, October 21, 2013, https://www.nytimes.com/2013/10/29/health/the-epidemic-uganda-is-neglecting.html.

72. Susan Reverby and David Rosner, "Beyond the Great Doctors," in *Health Care in America: Essays in Social History*, ed. Susan Reverby and David Rosner (Philadelphia: Temple University Press, 1979), 3–16; Susan Reverby and David Rosner, "Beyond the Great Doctors Revisited," in *Locating Medical History*, ed. Frank Huisman and John Harley Warner (Baltimore: Johns Hopkins University Press, 2004), 167–93; Leslie Butt, "The Suffering Stranger: Medical Anthropology and International Morality," *Medical Anthropology* 21, no. 1 (January 1, 2002): 1–24.

73. Nolwazi Mkhwanazi, "Medical Anthropology in Africa: The Trouble with a Single Story," *Medical Anthropology* 35, no. 2 (March 3, 2016): 199.

74. Steven Feierman, *Peasant Intellectuals: Anthropology and History in Tanzania* (Madison: University of Wisconsin Press, 1990); and Stacey Langwick, *Bodies, Politics, and African Healing: The Matter of Maladies in Tanzania* (Bloomington: Indiana University Press, 2011).

75. Feierman, "Struggles for Control"; Sunita Puri, *That Good Night: Life and Medicine in the Eleventh Hour* (New York: Viking, 2019); and Jain, *Malignant*.

CHAPTER 1: THE AFRICAN LYMPHOMA

1. This account is drawn from the following materials: Denis Burkitt, Mss. Afr.s. 1872/20, Burkitt Memories, Denis Parsons Burkitt Papers, Rhodes House; Anthony Epstein and M. A. Eastwood, "Denis Parsons Burkitt, 28 February 1911–23 March 1993," *Biographical Memoirs of Fellows of the Royal Society* 14 (1995): 89–102; Jon A. Story and David Kritchevsky, "Denis Parsons Burkitt," *Journal of Nutrition* 124 (1994): 1551–54; Venita Jay, "Extraordinary Epidemiological Quest of Dr. Burkitt," *Pediatric and Developmental Pathology* 1 (1998): 562–64; Cliff L. Nelson and Norman J. Temple, "Tribute to Denis Burkitt," *Journal of Medical Biography* 2, no. 3 (August 1994): 180–83; and Bernard Glemser, *Mr. Burkitt and Africa* (Cleveland: World Publishing, 1970).

2. J. N. P. Davies to Canon R. Moore, September 21, 1982, Mss. Afr.s. 1872, J. N. P. Davies Papers, Rhodes House.

3. J. N. P. Davies, "Answers to Aide Memoire," Mss. Afr.s. 1872, Rhodes House.

4. J. N. P. Davies to Canon R. Moore, September 21, 1982, J. N. P. Davies Papers.

5. J. N. P. Davies to Canon R. Moore, September 21, 1982, J. N. P. Davies Papers.

6. J. N. P. Davies to Canon R. Moore, September 21, 1982, J. N. P. Davies Papers.

7. See in particular the papers of J. N. P. Davies et al., Mss. Afr.s. 1872, Rhodes House; Denis Burkitt Papers, Trinity College, Dublin; Sir Albert Ruskin Cook, *Uganda Memories, 1897–1940* (Kampala: Uganda Society, 1945).

8. Victoria Walusansa, Fred Okuku, and Jackson Orem, "Burkitt Lymphoma in Uganda, the Legacy of Denis Burkitt and an Update on the Disease Status," *British Journal of Haematology* 156, no. 6 (March 2012): 757–60; Owen Smith, "Denis Parsons Burkitt CMG, MD, DSc, FRS, FRCS, FTCD (1911–93) Irish by Birth, Trinity by the Grace of God," *British Journal of Haematology* 156, no. 6 (March 2012): 770–76; and John Ziegler, "Into and Out of Africa—Taking Over from Denis Burkitt," *British Journal of Haematology* 156, no. 6 (March 2012): 766–69.

9. Fieldnotes, May 2012.

10. For alternative approaches to writing about colonial medical ethics in East Africa, see Jennifer Tappan, "Blood Work and 'Rumors' of Blood: Nutritional Research and Insurrection in Buganda, 1935–1970," *International Journal of African Historical Studies* 47, no. 3 (September 2014): 473–94; Melissa Graboyes, *The Experiment Must Continue: Medical Research and Ethics in East Africa, 1940–2014* (Athens: Ohio University Press, 2015); and Luise White, *Speaking with Vampires: Rumor and History in Colonial Africa* (Berkeley: University of California Press, 2000).

11. The following account is derived from Davies, "Answers to Aide Memoire."

12. John Iliffe, *East African Doctors: A History of the Modern Profession* (Kampala: Fountain, 2002), 60–91; and Anna Crozier, *Practicing Colonial Medicine: The Colonial Medical Service in British East Africa* (London: I. B. Taurus, 2007).

13. Davies, "Answers to Aide Memoire."

14. Davies.

15. Davies.

16. Davies.

17. Denis Burkitt, "Answers to Aide Memoire," Mss. Afr.s. 1872, Rhodes House.

18. Denis Wright, interview by author, November 2012.

19. Burkitt, "Answers to Aide Memoire."

20. Burkitt.

21. J. N. P. Davies, Barbara Wilson, John Knowelden, "Cancer in Kampala: A Survey in an Underdeveloped Country," *British Medical Journal* 2 (1958): 439–43.

22. Shane Doyle, *Before HIV: Sexuality, Fertility and Mortality in East Africa, 1900–1980* (Oxford: Oxford University Press, 2013), 299.

23. Iliffe, *East African Doctors*, 141–42.

24. Davies, "Answers to Aide Memoire."

25. Davies.

26. Davies.

27. Davies.

28. Davies.

29. Davies.

30. Davies; Iliffe, *East African Doctors*, 140–44; Denis P. Burkitt, "Some Diseases Characteristic of Modern Western Civilization: A Possible Common Causative Factor," *Clinical Radiology* 24, no. 3 (January 1, 1973): 271–80.

31. Davies et al., "Cancer in Kampala," 439–43; J. N. P. Davies and B. A. Wilson, "Cancer in Kampala, 1952–1953," *East African Medical Journal* 31 (1954): 395–416.

32. Davies, "Answers to Aide Memoire."

33. Davies et al., "Cancer in Kampala," 440.

34. Davies et al., 440.

35. Davies et al., 440.

36. J. N. P. Davies et al., "Cancer in an African Community, 1897–1956: An Analysis of the Records of Mengo Hospital, Kampala, Uganda: Part I," *British Medical Journal* 1, no. 5378 (1964): 260.

37. See, for example, Denis Burkitt, "The Discovery of Burkitt's Lymphoma," *Cancer* 51, no. 10 (1983): 1777–86; Epstein and Eastwood, "Denis Parsons Burkitt"; Story and Kritchevsky, "Denis Parsons Burkitt," 1551–54; Jay, "Extraordinary Epidemiological Quest of Dr. Burkitt," 562–64; and Nelson and Temple, "Tribute to Denis Burkitt," 180–83.

38. J. N. P. Davies to Canon R. Moore, September 21, 1982, J. N. P. Davies Papers.

39. Glemser, *Mr. Burkitt and Africa*.

40. Epstein and Eastwood, "Denis Parsons Burkitt."

41. Burkitt, "Answers to Aide Memoire."

42. Mary Louise Pratt, *Imperial Eyes: Travel Writing and Transculturation* (London: Routledge, 2003).

43. Denis Burkitt, "A Sarcoma Involving the Jaws in African Children," *British Journal of Surgery* 46, no. 197 (1958): 218–23.

44. Burkitt, "A Sarcoma Involving the Jaws in African Children," 218–23.

45. Burkitt, "Answers to Aide Memoire."

46. Burkitt, "A Sarcoma Involving the Jaws in African Children."

47. Denis Burkitt, "A 'Tumour Safari' in East and Central Africa," *British Journal of Cancer* 16 (1962): 379–86.

48. A. J. Haddow, "An Improved Map for the Study of Burkitt's Lymphoma Syndrome in Africa," *East African Medical Journal* 40 (1963): 429–32.

49. Burkitt, "Answers to Aide Memoire."

50. Burkitt, "A 'Tumour Safari'"; Denis Burkitt, "Determining the Climatic Limitations of a Children's Cancer Common in Africa," *British Medical*

Journal 2, no. 5311 (October 20, 1962): 1019–23. https://doi.org/10.1136/bmj
.2.5311.1019.

51. Burkitt, "Answers to Aide Memoire."
52. Julia R. Cummiskey, "'An Ecological Experiment on the Grand Scale':
    Creating an Experimental Field in Bwamba, Uganda, 1942–1950," *Isis* 111,
    no. 1 (March 1, 2020): 3–21.
53. Burkitt, "Answers to Aide Memoire."
54. Burkitt.
55. Burkitt.
56. Burkitt.
57. Burkitt, "A 'Tumour Safari.'"
58. Burkitt.
59. Ian Magrath, "Denis Burkitt and the African Lymphoma," *Ecancermedi-
    calscience* 3 (2009): 159, https://doi.org/10.3332/ecancer.2009.159.
60. Magrath, 159.
61. Burkitt, "Answers to Aide Memoire."
62. Joseph Burchenal, "Burkitt's Tumor as a Stalking Horse for Leukemia,"
    JAMA 222, no. 9 (1972): 1165.
63. Gretchen Krueger, *Hope and Suffering: Children, Cancer, and the Par-
    adox of Experimental Medicine* (Baltimore: Johns Hopkins University
    Press, 2008).
64. Siddhartha Mukherjee, *The Emperor of All Maladies: A Biography of
    Cancer* (New York: Scribner, 2010), 143–44.
65. For more on the history of treating pediatric leukemia, see Krueger, *Hope
    and Suffering*, 82–162; and John Laszlo, *The Cure of Childhood Leukemia:
    Into the Age of Miracles* (New Brunswick, NJ: Rutgers University Press,
    1996).
66. Burchenal, "Burkitt's Tumor as a Stalking Horse for Leukemia," 1165.
67. Burchenal, 1165.
68. Burkitt, "Answers to Aide Memoire."
69. Denis Burkitt, M. S. R. Hutt, and D. H. Wright, "The African Lym-
    phoma: Preliminary Observations on Responses to Therapy," *Cancer* 18
    (April 1965): 399–410.
70. Glemser, *Mr. Burkitt and Africa*, 133. Initially, Burkitt also treated some
    patients with nitrogen mustard. See Burkitt, "Sarcoma Involving the Jaws
    in African Children."
71. Burkitt.
72. Denis Burkitt, "The Reasons for Going to Africa," in *Pioneers in Pediatric
    Oncology*, ed. Grant Taylor (Houston: University of Texas MD Anderson
    Cancer Center, 1990), 43.
73. John L. Ziegler and Daniel G. Miller, "Lymphosarcoma Resembling the
    Burkitt Tumor in a Connecticut Girl," *JAMA* 198, no. 10 (1966): 1071.
74. Burkitt, "Sarcoma Involving Jaws in African Children," 218–23; Denis
    Burkitt and G. T. O'Conor, "Malignant Lymphoma in African Children:

I. A Clinical Syndrome," *Cancer* 14 (April 1961): 258–69; Burkitt, Wright, and Hutt, "African Lymphoma: Preliminary Observations on Responses to Therapy," 339–410.

75. Ziegler and Miller, "Lymphosarcoma Resembling the Burkitt Tumor," 1071.
76. John Ziegler, interview by author, June 2012.
77. John Ziegler, interview by author, June 2012.
78. For the proceedings of this conference, see Peter Clifford, Allen Linsell, and Geoffrey Timms, eds., *Cancer in Africa: A Selection of Papers Given at the East African Medical Research Council Scientific Conference in Nairobi in January 1967* (Evanston, IL: Northwestern University Press, 1968).
79. John Ziegler, interview by author, 2013.
80. John Ziegler, interview by author, 2013. Others who worked at the UCI in the 1960s and 1970s echoed Ziegler's sentiments. See, for example, interviews with Robert Comis, Avrum Bluming, Richard Morrow, Denis Wright, Tom Tomusange, Alosyius Kisuule, Nsalabwa, and Charles Olweny. See also memoirs by Chuck Vogel and Avrum Bluming; fieldnotes from a conversation with Keith McAdam, April 2012; and fieldnotes from Uganda Cancer Institute Symposium, August 2014. See also Calvin M. Kunin, M.D. Professor and Chairman, University of Virginia to Gordon Zubrod, National Cancer Institute, April 28, 1969, John Ziegler Personal Papers.
81. Iliffe, *East African Doctors*; John Ziegler, interview by author, June 2012; Richard Morrow, interview by author, November 2012; *Uganda Cancer Institute Annual Report, 1970* (Kampala: Uganda Cancer Institute, 1970); Kenneth Endicott, Director of the National Cancer Institute, to Joseph Palmer, American Ambassador, Lagos, Nigeria, July 30, NCI Files AR 6307–00319, National Institutes of Health Archives.

CHAPTER 2: A HOSPITAL BUILT FROM SCRATCH

1. John Ziegler, interview by author, June 2012.
2. For more on Kampala and its environs in the 1950s, see Aidan W. Southall and Peter C. W. Gutkind, *Townsmen in the Making: Kampala and Its Suburbs* (Kampala: East African Institute of Social Research, 1957).
3. John Ziegler, interview by author, June 2012. See also: John L. Ziegler, "Early Studies of Burkitt's Tumor in Africa," *American Journal of Pediatric Hematology/Oncology* 8, no. 1 (1986): 63–65.
4. Ian McAdam, "Welcoming Speech for the LTC Opening, 1967," John Ziegler Papers. See also *Uganda Cancer Institute Annual Report* (Kampala: Uganda Cancer Institute, 1970), John Ziegler Papers.
5. Paul Farmer, *Fevers, Feuds, and Diamonds: Ebola and the Ravages of History* (New York: Farrar, Straus and Giroux, 2020).
6. John Ziegler, interview by author, June 2012.
7. John Ziegler, interview by author, June 2012.

8. John Ziegler, interview by author, June 2012.
9. John Ziegler, interview by author, June 2012.
10. John Ziegler, interview by author, June 2012.
11. John Ziegler, interview by author, June 2012.
12. Aloysius Kisuule, interview by author, February 2012; Tom Tomusange, interview by author, May 2012; Charles Olweny, interview by author, May 2012; and Richard Morrow, interview by author, November 2012. See also Bus Travel Vouchers, Uganda Cancer Institute Archives.
13. John Ziegler, interview by author, June 2012.
14. John Iliffe, *East African Doctors: A History of the Modern Profession* (Kampala: Fountain, 2002); J. N. P. Davies, Barbara Wilson, and John Knowelden, "Cancer in Kampala: A Survey in an Underdeveloped Country," *British Medical Journal* 2 (1958): 439–43; J. N. P. Davies and B. A. Wilson, "Cancer in Kampala, 1952–1953," *East African Medical Journal* 31 (1954): 395–416; Sir Albert Ruskin Cook, *Uganda Memories, 1897–1940* (Kampala: Uganda Society, 1945); Megan Vaughan, *Curing Their Ills: Colonial Power and African Illness* (Cambridge, UK: Polity, 1991); and Diane Zeller, "The Establishment of Western Medicine in Buganda" (PhD diss., Columbia University, 1971).
15. See, for example, interviews by author with John Ziegler, Robert Comis, Avrum Bluming, Richard Morrow.
16. Richard Morrow, interview by author, November 2012.
17. Iliffe, *East African Doctors.*
18. John Ziegler, interview by author, June 2012; NCI Oral History collection with Joseph Burchenal, Gordon Zubrod; and Gretchen Krueger, *Hope and Suffering: Children, Cancer, and the Paradox of Experimental Medicine* (Baltimore: Johns Hopkins University Press, 2008).
19. John Ziegler, interview by author, June 2012; Charles Vogel, memoirs unpublished and in the author's possession.
20. Ian McAdam, "Welcoming Speech for the LTC Opening, 1967," John Ziegler Papers.
21. Archival collections consulted in the US include the National Institute of Health Office of History, Bethesda; the National Institute of Health Oral Histories repository; American Philosophical Society Archives, Philadelphia; John Ziegler's Personal Papers, San Francisco (now in the UCI's possession). Collections consulted in the UK and Ireland include Rhodes House Archives, Oxford University; Wellcome Collection Archives, London; Trinity College Archives, Dublin; National Archives, Kew. Collections consulted in Uganda include the Uganda Cancer Institute Archives, Kampala; and Albert Cook Library, Kampala.
22. *Uganda Cancer Institute Annual Reports, 1967–1977*, Uganda Cancer Institute Archives.
23. Denis Burkitt, "Answers to Aide Memoire," Mss. Afr.s. 1872, Rhodes House Archives, Oxford University.

24. Burkitt, "Answers to Aide Memoire."
25. Burkitt.
26. For more on the politics of manners in central Uganda, see Carol Summers, "Radical Rudeness: Ugandan Social Critiques in the 1940s," *Journal of Social History* 39 (2006): 741–70. Also see Holly Elizabeth Hanson, *Landed Obligation: The Practice of Power in Buganda* (Portsmouth, NH: Heinemann, 2003).
27. S. K. Kyalwazi, "Carcinoma of the Penis: A Review of 153 Patients Admitted to Mulago Hospital, Kampala, Uganda," *East African Medical Journal* 43 (1966): 415–25; S. K. Kyalwazi, "Chemotherapy of Kaposi's Sarcoma: Experience with Trenimon," *East African Medical Journal* 45 (1966): 17–26; S. K. Kyalwazi, "Kaposi's Sarcoma: Clinical Features, Experience in Uganda," *Antibiotic Chemotherapy* 29 (1971): 59–69.
28. Fieldnotes from conversation with Keith McAdam, April 2012. See also L. A. Reynolds and E. M. Tansye, eds., *British Contributions to Medical Research and Education in Africa after the Second World War*, Wellcome Witnesses to Twentieth Century Medicine 10 (London: Wellcome Trust Centre for the History of Medicine at UCL, 2001), 36–37.
29. David Carter, "Sir Ian William James McAdam," *British Medical Journal* 318 (1999): 1216.
30. Fieldnotes, April 2012.
31. For an example of this abundance of clinical material, see A. C. Templeton, *Tumors in a Tropical Country: A Survey of Uganda 1964–1968* (New York: Springer-Verlag, 1973). Also see J. N. P. Davies, "The Pattern of African Cancer in Uganda," *East African Medical Journal* 38 (1961): 486–91.
32. Ian McAdam, "Lymphoma Treatment Center Opening Speech, August 1967," John Ziegler Personal Papers.
33. McAdam, "Lymphoma Treatment Center Opening Speech, August 1967."
34. Photograph of Uganda Minister of Health John Lwamafa hanging the commemorative plaque at the Lymphoma Treatment Center Honoring Denis Burkitt, August 1967, John Ziegler Personal Papers.
35. Photograph of Sebastian Kyalwazi, Denis Burkitt, and others at the grand opening of the Lymphoma Treatment Center, August 1967, John Ziegler Personal Papers.
36. For more on Obote, see A. G. G. Gingyera-Pinycwa, *Apolo Milton Obote and His Times* (New York: NOK, 1978); Godfrey Nsubuga, *The Person of Dr. Milton Obote: A Classic Personality Study* (Kampala: Nissi, 2012); Omongole R. Anguria, ed., *Apollo Milton Obote: What Others Say* (Kampala: Fountain, 2006); Kenneth Ingham, *Obote: A Political Biography* (London: Routledge, 2014).
37. Richard Morrow, interview by author, November 2012.
38. Denis P. Burkitt and Dennis Howard Wright, eds., *Burkitt's Lymphoma* (Edinburgh: Livingstone, 1971).

39. Vickie Mujuzi, interview by author, February 2012; Tom Tomusange, interview by author, May 2012; Aloysius Kisuule, interview by author, February 2012.

40. Photograph of Mulago Hospital, 1960s or 1970s, John Ziegler Personal Papers.

41. Steven Feierman's forthcoming book is a history of care from below in East and Central Africa. For a recent discussion of this work in progress, see "Colonial Medicine and the Political Economy of Care" (presentation given during workshop, History and Sociology of Science Department, University of Pennsylvania, March 2021); Julie Livingston, *Debility and the Moral Imagination in Botswana*, African Systems of Thought (Bloomington: Indiana University Press, 2005).

42. John Ziegler, interview by author, June 2012.

43. John Ziegler, interview by author, June 2012; Joseph Burchenal, interview, NCI Oral Histories, National Cancer Institute Archives; Gordon Zubrod, interview, NCI Oral Histories, National Cancer Institute Archives; Krueger, *Hope and Suffering*.

44. On the importance of food and medical care, see Ramah McKay, *Medicine in the Meantime: The Work of Care in Mozambique* (Durham, NC: Duke University Press, 2017), 88–141; Susan Reynolds Whyte, ed., *Second Chances: Surviving AIDS in Uganda* (Durham, NC: Duke University Press, 2014), 191–214.

45. Vickie Mujuzi, interview by author, February 2012.

46. John M. Janzen and William Arkinstall, *The Quest for Therapy in Lower Zaire*, Comparative Studies of Health Systems and Medical Care (Berkeley: University of California Press, 1978); Julie Livingston, *Improvising Medicine: An African Oncology Ward in an Emerging Cancer Epidemic* (Durham, NC: Duke University Press, 2012).

47. John Ziegler, interviews by author, June 2012, November 2013; Avrum Bluming, interview by author, March 2015; Robert Comis, interview by author, September 2013; Charles Vogel, unpublished memoirs in author's possession; photographs of the Uganda Cancer Institute from the 1960s, John Ziegler Personal Papers.

48. John Ziegler, interview by author, June 2012.

49. Marissa Mika, "Fifty Years of Creativity, Crisis, and Cancer in Uganda," *Canadian Journal of African Studies* (Revue Canadienne Des Études Africaines) 50, no. 3 (September 1, 2016): 395–413.

50. Richard Morrow, interview by author, November 2012.

51. Richard Morrow, interview by author, November 2012.

52. Aloysius Kisuule, interview by author, February 2012.

53. Richard Morrow, interview by author, November 2012.

54. Aloysius Kisuule, interview by author, February 2012.

55. Aloysius Kisuule, interview by author, February 2012.

56. Over the past fifty years this face sheet has been largely unchanged at the Institute.

57. Aloysius Kisuule, interview by author, February 2012.
58. Aloysius Kisuule, interview by author, February 2012.
59. Aloysius Kisuule, interview by author, February 2012.
60. R. H. Morrow, M. C. Pike, and A. Kisuule, "Survival of Burkitt's Lymphoma Patients in Mulago Hospital, Uganda," *British Medical Journal* 4 (1967): 323–27.
61. Aloysius Kisuule, interview by author, February 2012.
62. Fieldnotes, October 2012.
63. Charles Olweny, interview by author, May 2012.
64. Fieldnotes, May 2012.
65. Avrum Bluming, interview by author, March 2015.
66. Avrum Bluming, interview by author, March 2015.
67. Robert Comis, interview by author, September 2013.
68. Vogel, memoirs.
69. *Uganda National Cancer Institute Annual Reports*, John Ziegler Personal Papers.
70. *Uganda National Cancer Institute Annual Reports*.
71. Jacob Dlamini, *Native Nostalgia* (Auckland Park, South Africa: Jacana, 2017).

CHAPTER 3: AFRICANIZING ONCOLOGY IN IDI AMIN'S UGANDA

1. On the history of cancer chemotherapy research, see Peter Keating and Alberto Cambrosio, *Cancer on Trial: Oncology as a New Style of Practice* (Chicago: University of Chicago Press, 2012); Siddhartha Mukherjee, *The Emperor of All Maladies: A Biography of Cancer* (New York: Scribner, 2010).
2. Denis P. Burkitt and Dennis Howard Wright, eds., *Burkitt's Lymphoma* (Edinburgh: Livingstone, 1971); "Special Issue: Burkitt's Lymphoma," *British Journal of Haematology* 156 (2012): 689–783.
3. National Institute of Health Archives, "Progress in Cancer Chemotherapy," *Medical World News*, November 17, 1972, 52.
4. Z. Lalani, *Uganda Asian Expulsion: 90 Days and Beyond through the Eyes of the International Press* (Bloomington: Indiana University Press, 1997); and Mahmood Mamdani, *From Citizen to Refugee: Uganda Asians Come to Britain* (Cape Town: Pambazuka, 2011).
5. For more on violence in Idi Amin's Uganda, see A. B. K. Kasozi, Nakanyike Musisi, and James Mukooza Sejjengo, *The Social Origins of Violence in Uganda, 1964–1985* (Montreal: McGill-Queen's University Press, 1994).
6. Charles L. M. Olweny et al., "Long-Term Experience with Burkitt's Lymphoma in Uganda," *International Journal of Cancer* 26, no. 3 (1980): 261–66.
7. Charles L. M. Olweny et al.
8. John Iliffe, *East African Doctors: A History of the Modern Profession* (Kampala: Fountain, 2002), 136.

9. Iliffe, 147.
10. Charles Olweny et al., "Epstein-Barr Virus Genome Studies in Burkitt's and Non-Burkitt's Lymphomas in Uganda," *Journal of the National Cancer Institute* 58, no. 5 (May 1977): 1191–96; Charles Olweny et al., "Childhood Kaposi's Sarcoma: Clinical Features and Therapy," *British Journal of Cancer* 33, no. 5 (May 1976): 555–60; Charles Olweny et al., "Further Experience in Treating Patients with Hepatocellular Carcinoma in Uganda," *Cancer* 46, no. 12 (December 15, 1980): 2717–22; Charles Olweny et al., "Treatment of Burkitt's Lymphoma: Randomized Clinical Trial of Single-Agent versus Combination Chemotherapy," *International Journal of Cancer* 17, no. 4 (April 15, 1976): 436–40.
11. Vickie Mujuzi, interview by author, March 2012. See Charles Olweny to the Chief Engineer, Uganda Electricity Board, November 10, 1975, Uganda Cancer Institute Archives.
12. Charles Olweny, *A Rolling Stone: An Autobiography of Charles L. M. Olweny* (Kampala: Uganda Martyrs University Research Directorate, 2014).
13. Warwick Anderson, *The Collectors of Lost Souls: Turning Kuru Scientists into Whitemen* (Baltimore: Johns Hopkins University Press, 2008); P. Wenzel Geissler and Catherine Molyneaux, eds., *Evidence, Ethos, and Experiment: The Anthropology and History of Medical Research in Africa* (New York: Berghahn, 2011); and Adriana Petryna, *When Experiments Travel: Clinical Trials and the Global Search for Human Subjects* (Princeton, NJ: Princeton University Press, 2009).
14. Aloysius Kisuule, interview by author, February 2012.
15. Iliffe, *East African Doctors*, 136–68.
16. Steven J. Jackson, "Rethinking Repair," in *Media Technologies: Essays on Communication, Materiality, and Society*, ed. Tarleton Gillespie, Pablo J. Boczkowski, and Kirsten A. Foot (Cambridge, MA: MIT Press, 2014), 221–39.
17. Andrea Stultiens, *The Photographer: Deo Kyakulagira* (Edam, The Netherlands: YDoc, 2012).
18. Olweny, *A Rolling Stone*, 51.
19. See Mark Leopold, *Inside West Nile: Violence, History and Representation on an African Frontier*, World Anthropology (Oxford: J. Currey, 2005); A. B. K. Kasozi, Nakanyike Musisi, and James Mukooza Sejjengo, *The Social Origins of Violence in Uganda, 1964–1985* (Montreal: McGill-Queen's University Press, 1994); and David Martin, *General Amin* (London: Faber and Faber, 1974).
20. See Godfrey Asiimwe, *The Impact of Post-colonial Policy Shifts in Coffee Marketing at the Local Level in Uganda: A Case Study of Mukono District, 1962–1998* (London: Shaker, 2002).
21. "Uganda Cancer Institute 5 Year Plan," John L. Ziegler Personal Papers.
22. "Uganda Cancer Institute 5 Year Plan."
23. Charles Olweny, interview by author, May 2012.

24. John Ziegler, interview by author, November 2013.
25. Charles Olweny et al., "Adult Hodgkin's Disease in Uganda," *Cancer* 27, no. 6 (June 1971): 1295–1301.
26. Charles Olweny, interview by author, May 2012.
27. Edgar C. Taylor, "Asians and Africans in Ugandan Urban Life, 1959–1972" (PhD diss., University of Michigan, 2016); Michael Twaddle, *Expulsion of a Minority: Essays on Ugandan Asians* (London: Athlone Press for the Institute of Commonwealth Studies, 1975); Mamdani, *From Citizen to Refugee*; Mahmood Mamdani, "The Ugandan Asian Expulsion: Twenty Years After," *Journal of Refugee Studies* 6, no. 3 (January 1, 1993): 265–73; Anneeth Kaur Hundle, "Exceptions to the Expulsion: Violence, Security and Community among Ugandan Asians, 1972–79," *Journal of Eastern African Studies* 7, no. 1 (February 1, 2013): 164–82.
28. Timothy M. Shaw, "Uganda under Amin: The Costs of Confronting Dependence," *Africa Today* 20, no. 2 (1973): 32–45; Michael J. Schultheis, "The Ugandan Economy and General Amin, 1971–1974," *Studies in Comparative International Development* 10, no. 3 (September 1, 1975): 3–34.
29. Shaw, "Uganda under Amin."
30. See Janet MacGaffey, *The Real Economy of Zaire: The Contribution of Smuggling and Other Unofficial Activities to National Wealth* (London: J. Currey, 1991).
31. Charles Vogel to John Ziegler, October 16, 1972, John Ziegler Personal Papers.
32. Charles Vogel to John Ziegler, October 16, 1972, John Ziegler Personal Papers.
33. Charles Vogel to John Ziegler, October 16, 1972, John Ziegler Personal Papers.
34. Charles Vogel to John Ziegler, October 16, 1972, John Ziegler Personal Papers.
35. Charles Vogel to John Ziegler, October 16, 1972, John Ziegler Personal Papers.
36. Fieldnotes, April 2012.
37. Charles Olweny, interview by author, May 2012; Olweny, *A Rolling Stone*.
38. Charles Olweny, interview by author, May 2012; Olweny, *A Rolling Stone*, 100.
39. Iliffe, *East African Doctors*, 136–68.
40. Charles Olweny, interview by author, May 2012.
41. Raphael Owor, interview by author, June 2012.
42. Nsalwabwa, interview by the author, February 2012.
43. Charles Olweny, interview by author, May 2012.
44. Burkitt and Wright, *Burkitt's Lymphoma*.
45. *Proposal Contract for the Uganda Cancer Institute*, 1975/1976, Uganda Cancer Institute Archives.

46. See Public Health Service contracts from the National Cancer Institute, Uganda Cancer Institute Archives; Charles Olweny, interview by author, May 2012; John Ziegler, interview by author, June 2012; Olweny, *A Rolling Stone*; *Proposal Contract for the Uganda Cancer Institute, 1975/1976*, Uganda Cancer Institute Archives.

47. Olweny et al., "Long-Term Experience with Burkitt's Lymphoma in Uganda."

48. Olweny et al., 263.

49. Charles Olweny, interview by author, May 2012.

50. *Proposal Contract for the Uganda Cancer Institute, 1975/1976*, Uganda Cancer Institute Archives.

51. Aloysius Kisuule, interview by author, February 2012.

52. *Report on Trip to Northern Region By Gerald and Emmanuel 13.10.72 to 22.10.72 Inclusive*, Uganda Cancer Institute Archives.

53. "Follow up Teso-Lango Trip by E. B. Tomusange. 1.6.71–16.6.71," Uganda Cancer Institute Archives.

54. "Follow up Teso-Lango Trip."

55. "Follow up Teso-Lango Trip."

56. "Follow up Teso-Lango Trip."

57. "Follow up Teso-Lango Trip."

58. "Follow up Teso-Lango Trip."

59. "Follow up Teso-Lango Trip."

60. "Follow up Teso-Lango Trip."

61. Luise White, *Speaking with Vampires: Rumor and History in Colonial Africa* (Berkeley: University of California Press, 2000); Wenzel Geissler et al., "'He Is Now Like a Brother, I Can Even Give Him Some Blood'—Relational Ethics and Material Exchanges in a Malaria Vaccine 'Trial Community' in the Gambia," *Social Science and Medicine* 67, no. 5 (2008): 696–707; Melissa Graboyes, *The Experiment Must Continue: Medical Research and Ethics in East Africa, 1940–2014* (Athens: Ohio University Press, 2015); Jennifer Tappan, *The Riddle of Malnutrition: The Long Arc of Biomedical and Public Health Interventions in Uganda* (Athens: Ohio University Press, 2017).

62. Anderson, *Collectors of Lost Souls*.

63. Southall and Gutkind, *Townsmen in the Making*.

64. "Follow up Teso-Lango Trip."

65. John M. Janzen and William Arkinstall, *The Quest for Therapy in Lower Zaire*, Comparative Studies of Health Systems and Medical Care (Berkeley: University of California Press, 1978).

66. On maintenance, see David Edgerton, *The Shock of the Old: Technology and Global History since 1900* (Oxford: Oxford University Press, 2006), 75–102.

67. Andrea Stultiens and Marissa Mika, *Staying Alive: Documenting the Uganda Cancer Institute* (Stockholm: Paradox, 2017); photographs of fieldwork from the 1970s, John Ziegler Personal Papers.

68. John Ziegler, interview by author, November 2013; fieldnotes, May 2012.
69. Fieldnotes, May 2012.
70. Fieldnotes, May 2012.
71. "Report Trip to Bukedi, Bugishu, Sebei, Teso, Lango and Acholi by Geral Angala Beginning 22.7.74 to 4.8.74," Uganda Cancer Institute Archives.
72. "Report Trip to Bukedi."
73. "Report Trip to Bukedi."
74. "Report Trip to Bukedi."
75. "Report Trip to Bukedi."
76. Professor Charles Olweny to General Manager, Food and Beverages LTD, April 20, 1976, Uganda Cancer Institute Archives.
77. Professor Charles Olweny to General Manager, Food and Beverages LTD, April 20, 1976, Uganda Cancer Institute Archives.
78. John Ziegler, interview by author, June 2012; Tom Tomusange, interview by author, May 2012; Aloysius Kisuule, interview by author, February 2012; Charles Olweny, interview by author, May 2012; Vickie Mujuzi, interview by author, March 2012.
79. Correspondence with drug companies in the 1970s, Uganda Cancer Institute Archives.
80. Charles Olweny, interview by author, May 2012.
81. Charles Olweny, interview by author, May 2012.
82. Charles Olweny, interview by author, May 2012.
83. Charles Olweny, interview by author, May 2012.
84. Fieldnotes, February 2012, March 2012, May 2012.
85. Olweny, A Rolling Stone.
86. Iliffe, East African Doctors; Cole P. Dodge and Paul D. Wiebe, Crisis in Uganda: The Breakdown of Health Services (New York: Pergamon, 1985), 1–14.
87. Charles Olweny, interview by author, May 2012.
88. Professor Charles Olweny to Chief Engineer, Uganda Electricity Board, November 10, 1975, Uganda Cancer Institute Archives.
89. Derek Peterson and Edgar Taylor, "Rethinking the State in Idi Amin's Uganda: The Politics of Exhortation," Journal of Eastern African Studies 7 (2013): 58–82.
90. John Ziegler, interview by author, June 2012.
91. Charles Olweny, interview by author, May 2012.
92. Charles Olweny, interview by author, May 2012.
93. Proposal contract for the Uganda Cancer Institute, 1974–1975, Uganda Cancer Institute Archives.
94. "Shipping Instructions for the Unit of Biological Carcinogenesis," Uganda Cancer Institute Archives.
95. "Shipping Instructions for the Unit of Biological Carcinogenesis."
96. Vicky Mujuzi, interview by author, February 2012.
97. Technician of Professor G. Klein to Professor Olweny, date unknown, Uganda Cancer Institute Archives.

98. W. Serumaga to All Members of Staff, Medical School, Head of Medical Illustration Department, August 26, 1976, Uganda Cancer Institute Archives.
99. Nsalabwa, interview by author, February 2012.
100. Fieldnotes, March 2012.
101. Fieldnotes, July 2012.
102. Nsalabwa, interview by author, February 2012.
103. Nsalabwa, interview by author, February 2012.
104. Nsalabwa, interview by author, February 2012.
105. Nsalabwa, interview by author, February 2012.
106. Charles Olweny, interview by author, May 2012. Amin's status at the UCI during this period is also institutional lore at the site. See fieldnotes about the memories of Amin and his relationship with the Institute, 2012.
107. Iliffe, *East African Doctors*; and Hölger Bernt Hansen, "Uganda in the 1970s: A Decade of Paradoxes and Ambiguities," *Journal of Eastern African Studies* 7, no. 1 (2003): 83–103.
108. John Ziegler, interview by author, November 2012.
109. Tom Tomusange to the Engineer in Charge, October 17, 1977, Uganda Cancer Institute Archives.
110. Charles Olweny, interview by author, May 2012.

CHAPTER 4: ROCKET LAUNCHERS AND TOXIC DRUGS

1. Tony Avirgan and Martha Honey, *War in Uganda: The Legacy of Idi Amin* (Westport, CT: Lawrence Hill, 1982).
2. Peter Nayenga, "The Overthrowing of Idi Amin: An Analysis of the War," *Africa Today* 31 (1984): 69–91.
3. John Iliffe, *East African Doctors: A History of the Modern Profession* (Kampala: Fountain, 2002), 149.
4. *Lancet* editor to John Ziegler, September 12, 1979, Uganda Cancer Institute Archive.
5. David Serwadda, interview by author, June 2012; Alex Coutinho, interview by author, April 2012.
6. Patient Files, Uganda Cancer Institute.
7. Henry Lubega, "Dr. Olweny Went on Leave but Never Returned to Office," *Daily Monitor*, October 6, 2013, http://www.monitor.co.ug/Magazines/PeoplePower/Dr-Olweny-went-on-leave-but-never-returned-to-office/-/689844/2019912/-/6x35nw/-/index.html.
8. David Serwadda, interview by author, April 2012; Alex Coutinho, interview by author, April 2012; and fieldnotes from conversation with Edward Mbidde, August 2014.
9. MK, interview by author, March 2012; Fred Okuku, interview by author, March 2012; SB, interview by author, August 2012. These accounts are corroborated by patient records from the 1980s, 1990s, and 2000s.
10. MK, interview by author, March 2012; Fred Okuku, interview by author, March 2012; SB, interview by author, August 2012.

11. S. D. Desmond-Hellmann and E. Katongole-Mbidde, "Kaposi's Sarcoma: Recent Developments," *AIDS* 5, no. 1 (1991): S135–42; S. D. Desmond-Hellmann et al., "The Value of a Clinical Definition for Epidemic KS in Predicting HIV Seropositivity in Africa," *Journal of Acquired Immune Deficiency Syndrome* 4, no. 7 (1991): 647–51.

12. S. Chuck et al., "Frequent Presence of a Novel Herpesvirus Genome in Lesions of Human Immunodeficiency Virus-Negative Kaposi's Sarcoma," *Journal of Infectious Diseases* 173, no. 1 (January 1996): 248–51.

13. M. Pfaller et al., "Molecular Epidemiology and Antifungal Susceptibility of *Cryptococcus neoformans* Isolates from Ugandan AIDS Patients," *Mycology* 32 (1988): 191–99.

14. Fred Okuku, interview by author, March 2012; and NM, interview by author, March 2012.

15. *Uganda Cancer Institute Annual Reports 1967–1978*, Uganda Cancer Institute Archives; Charles Olweny, "The Uganda Cancer Institute," *Oncology* 37, no. 5 (1980): 367–70.

16. John Ziegler, interview by author, June 2012; and Robert Comis, interview by author, September 2013.

17. John Ziegler, interview by author, June 2012; Charles Olweny, interview by author, May 2012.

18. Cole P. Dodge and Paul D. Wiebe, eds., *Crisis in Uganda: The Breakdown of Health Services* (New York: Pergamon, 1985), 1–14; Hölger Bernt Hansen and Michael Twaddle, eds., *Uganda Now: Between Decay and Development* (London: J. Currey, 1988); Hölger Bernt Hansen and Michael Twaddle, eds., *Changing Uganda: The Dilemmas of Structural Adjustment and Revolutionary Change* (London: J. Currey, 1991). For general accounts of the HIV/AIDS epidemic in Uganda, see Johanna Tayloe Crane, *Scrambling for Africa: AIDS, Expertise, and the Rise of American Global Health Science* (Ithaca, NY: Cornell University Press, 2013); Helen Epstein, *The Invisible Cure: Why We Are Losing the Fight against AIDS in Africa* (New York: Farrar, Straus, and Giroux, 2007); John Iliffe, *The African AIDS Epidemic: A History* (Athens: Ohio University Press, 2005); Noerine Kaleeba, *We Miss You All: AIDS in the Family* (Kampala: AIDS Support Organization, 1991).

19. Susan Sontag, *Illness as Metaphor and AIDS and Its Metaphors* (New York: Picador, 2001); Audre Lorde, *The Cancer Journals* (New York: Penguin, 2020); S. Løchlann Jain, *Malignant: How Cancer Becomes Us* (Berkeley: University of California Press, 2013).

20. *Summary Proposal for the Rehabilitation of Makerere Medical School Mulago Hospital Complex in Kampala, Uganda*, Uganda Cancer Institute Archives.

21. *Summary Proposal*.

22. *Summary Proposal*.

23. *Summary Proposal*.

24. *Summary Proposal.*
25. "Public Voucher for Purchases and Services Other Than Personal: Uganda Cancer Institute Voucher for chemotherapy purchase, January 4, 1980," Uganda Cancer Institute Archives, photographed June 22, 2012, timestamp 13.25.44.
26. *Report on Visit to USA and UK by CLM Olweny, October 29, 1979,* Uganda Cancer Institute Archives.
27. *Report on Visit to USA and UK.*
28. Hansen and Twaddle, *Uganda Now.*
29. Charles Olweny, interview by author, May 2012.
30. Fieldnotes, May 2012.
31. Fieldnotes, August 2014.
32. Fieldnotes, August 2014.
33. Fieldnotes, August 2014.
34. Fieldnotes, August 2014.
35. Fieldnotes, August 2014.
36. Steven Feierman, "When Physicians Meet: Local Medical Knowledge and Global Public Goods," in *Evidence, Ethos, and Experiment: The Anthropology and History of Medical Research in Africa,* ed. P. Wenzel Geissler and Catherine Molyneux (New York: Berghahn, 2011), 193.
37. John Ziegler, interview by Gretchen A. Case, August 4, 1998, 32, National Cancer Institute Oral History Project.
38. For a thoughtful account of the embodied memories of violence in South Africa in the context of the HIV epidemic, see Didier Fassin, *When Bodies Remember: Experiences and Politics of AIDS in South Africa,* trans. Amy Jacobs and Gabrielle Varro (Berkeley: University of California Press, 2007).
39. Dr. M, interview by author, June 2012.
40. Steven Zaloga and James Grandsen, *Soviet Tanks and Combat Vehicles of World War Two* (London: Arms and Armour, 1984), 153.
41. Dr. M, interview by author, June 2012.
42. This account is derived from conversations with nurses and staff who worked on the wards during this period and is corroborated by patient records from the 1980s and the 1990s.
43. Dr. M, interview by author, June 2012.
44. Dr. M, interview by author, June 2012.
45. Dr. M, interview by author, June 2012.
46. MK, interview by author, March 2012.
47. Fieldnotes, 2012.
48. George C. Bond and Joan Vincent, "Living on the Edge: Changing Social Structures in the Context of AIDS," in Hansen and Twaddle, *Changing Uganda,* 113–29.
49. Rose Papac, "Origins of Cancer Therapy," *Yale Journal of Biology and Medicine* 74 (2001): 391–98; and Siddhartha Mukherjee, *The Emperor of All Maladies: A Biography of Cancer* (New York: Scribner, 2010).

50. Papac, "Origins of Cancer Therapy," 391–98.
51. A. B. Tokaty, "Soviet Rocket Technology," *Technology and Culture* 4, no. 4 (1963): 515–28. On the circulation of Soviet arms and assistance during the Cold War, see Orah Cooper and Carol Fogarty, "Soviet Economic and Military Aid to the Less Developed Countries, 1954–78," *Soviet and Eastern European Foreign Trade* 2, nos. 1–3 (1985): 54–73.
52. Cooper and Fogarty, "Soviet Economic and Military Aid," 54–73.
53. Elizabeth Schmidt, *Foreign Intervention in Africa* (Cambridge: Cambridge University Press, 2013).
54. David Edgerton, *The Shock of the Old: Technology and Global History since 1900* (Oxford: Oxford University Press, 2006), xi.
55. Kristin Peterson, "AIDS Policies for Markets and Warriors: Dispossession, Capital, and Pharmaceuticals in Nigeria," in *Medicine, Mobility, and Power in Global Africa: Transnational Health and Healing*, ed. Hansjorg Dilger, Abdoulaye Kane, and Stacey Langwick (Bloomington: Indiana University Press, 2012), 138–62.
56. Fieldnotes, November 2011; Fred Okuku, interview by author, March 2012.
57. Many internationally recognized Ugandan physician-researchers initially started their careers as third-year medical student residents at the UCI, including Professor David Serwadda, now the head of the School of Public Health and one of the first physicians to publish on the SLIM syndrome that would eventually be identified as AIDS in the early 1980s, and Dr. Alex Coutinho, head of the Infectious Diseases Institute. Dr. Robert Comis, an American breast cancer specialist who now heads up ECOG, was one of the first medical students to do this rotation in 1970.
58. Fred Okuku, interview by author, March 2012.
59. Sharon Kaufman, *And a Time to Die: How American Hospitals Shape the End of Life* (Chicago: University of Chicago Press, 2005).
60. Claims about how many chemotherapy shipments the UCI actually received per year in the early 2000s vary across and within accounts. Some say once a year. Some say quarterly. Some say every month.
61. Fred Okuku, interview by author, March 2012.
62. Fieldnotes, June 2012.
63. Fieldnotes, July 2012.

CHAPTER 5: WHEN RADIOTHERAPY TRAVELS

1. F. A. Durosinmi-Etti, M. Nofal, and M. M. Mahfouz, "Radiotherapy in Africa: Current Needs and Prospects," *IAEA Bulletin* 33, no. 4 (December 1991): 25.
2. Sasha Garrey, "Uganda's Lone Radiotherapy Machine," *Pulitzer Center Crisis Reporting*, September 4, 2014, http://pulitzercenter.org/reporting/africa-uganda-cervical-cancer-radiotherapy-cobalt.
3. These estimates are drawn from Joseph Kigula Mugambe and P. Wegoye, "Pattern and Experience with Cancers Treated with the Chinese

GWGP80 Cobalt Unit at Mulago Hospital, Kampala," *East African Medical Journal* 77 (2000): 523–26, and were verified by the head of the radiotherapy department at Mulago Hospital in 2012.

4. Dr. Z, interview by author, June 2012.

5. A range of solid tumors, most commonly head and neck cancers, are also treated at the unit, as are some patients with lymphoma and leukemia of the central nervous system.

6. Fieldnotes from conversations with nurses at the radiotherapy unit, June 2012.

7. "Joy" is a pseudonym. Some identifying features of illness progression and where they are from have been altered to preserve patient privacy.

8. Breast cancer activism is practiced by a small but growing community in Kampala, Uganda, and spearheaded by the inspirational and courageous women at the Uganda Women's Cancer Support Organization. They do weekly breast cancer education sessions at the Friday Screening Clinic at the UCI, headed by Dr. N.

9. Garrey, "Uganda's Lone Radiotherapy Machine."

10. As we know, therapeutic efficacy has long occupied the interests of historians and anthropologists of medicine and is particularly salient in the history and anthropology of cancer. On issues of therapeutic efficacy in the history of medicine in general, see Allan Brandt, *No Magic Bullet: A Social History of Venereal Disease in the United States since 1880* (Oxford: Oxford University Press, 1987); Jeremy Greene, *Prescribing by Numbers: Drugs and the Definition of Disease* (Baltimore: Johns Hopkins University Press, 2007); Charles E. Rosenberg, "The Therapeutic Revolution: Medicine, Meaning and Social Change in Nineteenth-Century America," *Perspectives in Biology and Medicine* 20, no. 4 (1977): 485–506; John Harley Warner, *The Therapeutic Perspective: Medical Practice, Knowledge, and Identity in America* (Princeton, NJ: Princeton University Press, 2014). On cancer and therapeutic efficacy, see Robert Aronowitz, *Unnatural History: Breast Cancer and American Society* (New York: Cambridge University Press, 2007); Allan M. Brandt, *The Cigarette Century: The Rise, Fall, and Deadly Persistence of the Product That Defined America* (New York: Basic Books, 2009); S. Løchlann Jain, *Malignant: How Cancer Becomes Us* (Berkeley: University of California Press, 2013); Julie Livingston, *Improvising Medicine: An African Oncology Ward in an Emerging Cancer Epidemic* (Durham, NC: Duke University Press, 2012); Ilana Löwy, *Preventive Strikes: Women, Precancer, and Prophylactic Surgery* (Baltimore: Johns Hopkins University Press, 2010); and Siddhartha Mukherjee, *The Emperor of All Maladies: A Biography of Cancer* (New York: Scribner, 2010).

11. See my discussion of "game over" in the epilogue.

12. Of course, I am not the first nor unfortunately the last person to make this point. On healing and harming in oncology, see Aronowitz, *Unnatural*

History; Jain, *Malignant*; Livingston, *Improvising Medicine*; Lowy, *Preventive Strikes*; and Mukherjee, *Emperor of All Maladies*. For a general discussion of this tension in African healing, see Steven Feierman, *Peasant Intellectuals: Anthropology and History in Tanzania* (Madison: University of Wisconsin Press, 1990).

13. Even with a weak Cobalt-60 source, you can still treat patients, but treatment must be for longer and longer periods, which means that patients must lie still for a long time and will also experience more severe burns. If the source is as old as the machine at Mulago, then it is also possible that treatment efficacy is reduced because of the ability of tumors to repair themselves. All of this is to say that while radiotherapists at Mulago are doing their best and following the general logic of Cobalt-60 decay, the source is so old that it is nearly impossible to gauge whether or not the treatments offered have much efficacy. See Dr. Charles Simone, personal communication, October 3, 2014.

14. Charles Olweny et al., "Long-Term Experience with Burkitt's Lymphoma in Uganda," *International Journal of Cancer* 26, no. 3 (1980): 261–66.

15. Jackson Orem et al., "Agreement between Diagnoses of Childhood Lymphoma Assigned in Uganda and by an International Reference Laboratory," *Clinical Epidemiology* 4 (2012): 339–47.

16. For more on the issue of laboratories and capacity in Africa, see Iruka Okeke, *Divining without Seeds: The Case for Strengthening Laboratory Medicine in Africa* (Ithaca, NY: Cornell University Press, 2011).

17. Livingston, *Improvising Medicine*, 6–7.

18. On technopolitics, see Gabrielle Hecht, *The Radiance of France* (Cambridge, MA: MIT Press, 2009); Warwick Anderson, "Introduction: Postcolonial Technoscience," *Social Studies of Science* 32, nos. 5–6 (2002): 643–58; Timothy Mitchell, *Rule of Experts: Egypt, Techno-politics, Modernity* (Berkeley: University of California Press, 2002). On the history of technology transfer in Africa, see Daniel R. Headrick, *The Tools of Empire: Technology and European Imperialism in the Nineteenth Century* (New York: Oxford University Press, 1981). On the repurposing of transferred technologies and their use in everyday life, see David Arnold, *Everyday Technology: Machines and the Making of India's Modernity* (Chicago: University of Chicago Press, 2013); and David Edgerton, *The Shock of the Old: Technology and Global History since 1900* (Oxford: Oxford University Press, 2006).

19. On the ramifications of structural adjustment policies on the health sector in Africa, see Meredeth Turshen, *Privatizing Health Services in Africa* (New Brunswick, NJ: Rutgers University Press, 1999). For a discussion of structural adjustment in Uganda specifically, see C. P. Dodge, "Uganda — Rehabilitation, or Redefinition of Health Services?," *Social Science and Medicine* 22, no. 7 (1986): 755–61; Hölger Bernt Hansen and Michael Twaddle, eds., *Changing Uganda: The Dilemmas of Structural*

Adjustment and Revolutionary Change, Eastern African Studies (London: J. Currey, 1991). See also Kristin Peterson, *Speculative Markets: Drug Circuits and Derivative Life in Nigeria* (Durham, NC: Duke University Press, 2014).

20. See Wiebe E. Bijker, Thomas P. Hughes, and Trevor Pinch, eds., *The Social Construction of Technological Systems: New Directions in the Sociology and History of Technology* (Cambridge, MA: MIT Press, 2012). I first heard of this conceptualization from Steve Feierman in his comparative medicine course for which I was a teaching assistant in 2009 at the University of Pennsylvania. I have found this to be a helpful way of framing the fragmentations and limitations of biomedicine in sub-Saharan Africa since this initial suggestion.

21. Uganda's postcolonial history of violence is bleak. While Idi Amin's tenure from 1972 to 1979 was economically, politically, and socially devastating, the Tanzanian War of Liberation (or the Tanzanian Invasion War, depending on who you talk to) of 1979–81 was also catastrophic. On the history of violence in Uganda, see A. B. K. Kasozi, Nakanyike Musisi, and James Mukooza Sejjengo, *The Social Origins of Violence in Uganda, 1964–1985* (Montreal: McGill-Queen's University Press, 1994). For an account of the Tanzanian War of Liberation, see Tony Avirgan and Martha Honey, *War in Uganda: The Legacy of Idi Amin* (Westport, CT: Lawrence Hill, 1982). For an account of the toll of the war on Mulago Hospital, see John Iliffe, *East African Doctors: A History of the Modern Profession* (Kampala: Fountain, 2002), 136–68.

22. Dr. Y, interview by author, September 2012.

23. See Avirgan and Honey, *War in Uganda*; and Kasozi et al., *Social Origins of Violence in Uganda 1964–1985*.

24. Dr. Z, interview by author, June 2012.

25. Iliffe, *East African Doctors*, 136.

26. Dr. Z, interview by author, June 2012. Emphasis on the *need* is from Dr. Z.

27. On the status of radiotherapy services in Africa and the developing world, see May Abdel-Wahab et al., "Status of Radiotherapy Resources in Africa: An International Atomic Energy Agency Analysis," *Lancet Oncology* 14 (2013): e168–75; Brandon J. Fisher et al., "Radiation Oncology in Africa: Improving Access to Cancer Care on the African Continent," *International Journal of Radiation Oncology Biology Physics* 89, no. 3 (July 2014): 458–61; G. P. Hanson et al., "An Overview of the Situation in Radiotherapy with Emphasis on the Developing Countries," *International Journal of Radiation Oncology Biology Physics* 19, no. 5 (November 1990): 1256–61; and C. V. Levin et al., "Radiation Therapy in Africa: Distribution and Equipment," *Radiotherapy and Oncology* 52, no. 1 (July 1999): 79–84. On radiotherapy in Uganda, see J. B. Kigula-Mugambe and F. A. Durosinmi, "Radiotherapy in Cancer Management at Mulago Hospital, Kampala, Uganda," *East African Medical Journal* 73 (1996): 611–13.

28. Durosinmi-Etti, Nofal, and Mahfouz, "Radiotherapy in Africa," 24.
29. Keep in mind that during the 1980s and the 1990s, African health systems were undergoing a challenging set of neoliberal economic reforms that would make it impossible for countries to reasonably purchase radiotherapy technologies or to tackle cancer as a serious public health problem. For more on this issue, see Turshen, *Privatizing Health Services in Africa*.
30. Durosinmi-Etti, Nofal, and Mahfouz, "Radiotherapy in Africa," 25.
31. Durosinmi-Etti, Nofal, and Mahfouz, 26.
32. Marianne de Laet and Annemarie Mol, "The Zimbabwe Bush Pump: Mechanics of a Fluid Technology," *Social Studies of Science* 30, no. 2 (April 2000): 252.
33. For more on joking about the quality of broken things in postcolonial Africa, see Damien Droney, "Ironies of Laboratory Work during Ghana's Second Age of Optimism," *Cultural Anthropology* 29, no. 2 (2014): 363–84.
34. Paul Farmer, *Infections and Inequalities: The Modern Plagues* (Berkeley: University of California Press, 1999), 21.
35. Kigula Mugambe and Wegoye, "Pattern and Experience with Cancers."
36. Kigula Mugambe and Wegoye.
37. Kigula Mugambe and Wegoye.
38. Kigula Mugambe and Wegoye.
39. Akrich would cite this improvised oil seal as a prime example of "mechanisms of reciprocal adjustment between the technical object and its environment." For more on the plasticity of technological objects and how they travel, see Madeleine Akrich, "The De-scription of Technical Objects," in *Shaping Technology/Building Society: Studies in Sociotechnical Change*, ed. Wiebe E. Bijker and John Law (Cambridge, MA: MIT Press, 1992), 205–24.
40. Dr. Z, interview by author, June 2012.
41. For more on the quality of "Chinese" manufactured goods in Africa, see Jane I. Guyer, *Marginal Gains: Monetary Transactions in Atlantic Africa* (Chicago: University of Chicago Press, 2004), 83–96.
42. On everyday corruption in Uganda, see Godfrey Asiimwe, "Of Extensive and Elusive Corruption in Uganda: Neo-patronage, Power, and Narrow Interests," *African Studies Review* 56, no. 2 (2013): 129–44. In addition, some of the most evocative writing about these issues comes from scholars of Nigeria. See Brian Larkin, *Signal and Noise: Media, Infrastructure and Urban Culture in Nigeria* (Durham, NC: Duke University Press, 2008); and Daniel Jordan Smith, *A Culture of Corruption: Everyday Deception and Popular Discontent in Nigeria* (Princeton, NJ: Princeton University Press, 2008).
43. Dr. Z, interview by author, June 2012.
44. The current executive director of Mulago Hospital, as quoted in Olive Nakatudde, "PAC Grills Mulago Officials Over the Delayed Purchase

of a Cobalt Machine," Uganda Radio Network, February 3, 2014, https://
ugandaradionetwork.com/story/pac-grills-mulago-officials-over-the
-delayed-purchase-of-a-cobalt-machine.

45. International Civil Aviation Agency, *Refusing Radioactive Material Shipments for Transfer by Air*, Information Paper no. 20, February 2013, https://www.icao.int/safety/DangerousGoods/Working%20Group%20of%20the%20Whole/IP08%20Att.pdf#search=Refusing%20Radioactive%20Material%20Shipments%20for%20Transfer%20by%20Air. For a discussion of the politics of nuclearity in Africa, see Gabrielle Hecht, *Being Nuclear: Africans and the Global Uranium Trade* (Cambridge, MA: MIT Press, 2012).

46. Maria Kiwanuka, *The Public Procurement and Disposal of Public Assets (Contracts) Regulations 2014*, Statutory Instruments Supplement no. 3 (Entebbe, Uganda: UPPC, 2014), https://www.ppda.go.ug/download/regulations/regulations/central_government_regulations/2014/PPDA-Regs-2014.pdf. This analysis is also based on multiple conversations with staff at the UCI about the challenges they face in the procurement process.

47. International Atomic Energy Agency, *Disposal of Radioactive Waste*, IAEA Safety Standards (Vienna: IAEA, 2011).

48. R. Kasasira, "WikiLeaks: America Feared Theft of Nuclear Material from Mulago," *Daily Monitor*, September 10, 2011, https://www.monitor.co.ug/uganda/news/national/wikileaks-america-feared-theft-of-nuclear-material-from-mulago-1499818.

49. The situation in Uganda is not unique. Recall the recent theft of radioactive waste in Mexico. Randall C. Archibold and Paulina Villegas, "6 Arrested in Theft of Truck with Radioactive Waste," *New York Times*, December 6, 2013.

50. Kasasira, "WikiLeaks."

51. See Javier Auyero, *Patients of the State: The Politics of Waiting in Argentina* (Durham, NC: Duke University Press, 2012); and Akhil Gupta, *Red Tape: Bureaucracy, Structural Violence, and Poverty in India* (Durham, NC: Duke University Press, 2012). On "slow violence," see Rob Nixon, *Slow Violence and the Environmentalism of the Poor* (Cambridge, MA: Harvard University Press, 2011).

52. Fieldnotes, September 2012; Dr. Y, interview by author, September 2012. For more on the history of Lacor Hospital itself, see Piero Corti and Lucille Teasdale, *To Make a Dream Come True: Letters from Lacor Hospital Uganda* (Bergamo, Italy: Corponove Editrice, 2009).

53. See Tim Allen and Koen Vlassentoot, eds., *The Lord's Resistance Army: Myth and Reality* (London: Zed, 2010); Adam Branch, *Displacing Human Rights: War and Intervention in Northern Uganda* (Oxford: Oxford University Press, 2011); and Sverker Finnstrom, *Living with Bad Surroundings: War, History, and Everyday Moments in Northern Uganda* (Durham, NC: Duke University Press, 2008).

54. Dr. Z, interview by author, June 2012.
55. Thomas F. Gieryn, "What Buildings Do," *Theory and Society* 31 (2002): 35–74.
56. Since the completion of the research for this book, radiotherapy access has been restored and expanded in Uganda. See Omar Yusuf, "From Emergency to Expansion: With IAEA Support, Uganda Recovers and Improves Its Radiotherapy Services," *IAEA News*, January 28, 2020, https://www.iaea.org/newscenter/news/from-emergency-to-expansion -with-iaea-support-uganda-recovers-and-improves-its-radiotherapy -services.

CHAPTER 6: "RESEARCH IS OUR RESOURCE"

1. Jackson Orem and Henry Wabinga, "The Roles of National Cancer Research Institutions in Evolving a Comprehensive Cancer Control Program in a Developing Country: Experience from Uganda," *Oncology* 77, no. 5 (2009): 272–80; Corey Casper, "The Increasing Burden of HIV-Associated Malignancies in Resource-Limited Regions," *Annual Review of Medicine* 62 (2011): 157–70.
2. This description of the inventory of the freezer graveyard is drawn from fieldnotes from discussions with Corey Casper in 2012 and interviews. See Vicki Mujuzi, interview by author, March 2012; and Alex Coutinho, interview by author, April 2012.
3. Ann Laura Stoler, ed., *Imperial Debris: On Ruins and Ruination* (Durham, NC: Duke University Press, 2013).
4. This anecdote is drawn from fieldnotes and several conversations with Corey Casper in 2012 and 2013.
5. Mary Engel, "Building a Legacy of Hope," Fred Hutchinson Cancer Research Center, February 3, 2015, http://www.fredhutch.org/en/news /center-news/2015/02/hutch-uganda-world-cancer-day.html.
6. Jackson Orem, interview by author, July 2012. See also Engel, "Building a Legacy of Hope."
7. Joyce Namutebi and John Odkyek, "Oyam South MP Okullo Epak Dead," *New Vision*, April 25, 2007; Charles Mwanguhya, "Uganda: Faire Thee Well Dr. Okullo Epak," *Daily Monitor* May 2, 2007, http:// allafrica.com/list/aans/post/full/day/20070502.html. Fieldnoted discussion with Corey Casper, June 2012; Fred Okuku, interview by author, March 2012.
8. UCI, Ministry of Health Website, https://www.health.go.ug/projects /ongoing-projects/uganda-cancer-institute/.
9. P. Wenzel Geissler and Noémi Tousignant, "Capacity as History and Horizon: Infrastructure, Autonomy and Future in African Health Science and Care," *Canadian Journal of African Studies* (Revue Canadienne Des Études Africaines) 50, no. 3 (September 1, 2016): 349–59, https://doi .org/10.1080/00083968.2016.1267653.

10. Noémi Tousignant, *Edges of Exposure: Toxicology and the Problem of Capacity in Postcolonial Senegal* (Durham, NC: Duke University Press, 2018), 4–21.

11. Paul W. Geissler et al., *Traces of the Future: An Archaeology of Medical Science in Africa* (Chicago: University of Chicago Press, 2016).

12. Iruka Okeke, "Partnerships for Now?," *Medicine Anthropology Theory* 5, no. 2 (May 15, 2018): https://doi.org/10.17157/mat.5.2.531.

13. Alex Coutinho, interview by author, April 2012.

14. A. B. K. Kasozi, Nakanyike Musisi, and James Mukooza Sejjengo, *The Social Origins of Violence in Uganda, 1964–1985* (Montreal: McGill-Queen's University Press, 1994).

15. Alex Coutinho, interview by author, April 2012.

16. Alex Coutinho, interview by author, April 2012.

17. Alex Coutinho, interview by author, April 2012.

18. C. L. Olweny et al., *Kaposi's Sarcoma: 2nd Symposium, Kampala, January 8–11, 1980* (Basel: Karger, 1981).

19. Alex Coutinho, interview by author, April 2012.

20. David Serwadda, interview by author, June 2012.

21. David Serwadda, interview by the author, June 2012.

22. Olweny et al., *Kaposi's Sarcoma*.

23. David Serwadda et al., "Slim Disease: A New Disease in Uganda and Its Association with HTLV-III Infection," *Lancet* 2 (1985): 849–52.

24. Ann Bayley to Charles Olweny, WHO Tropical Diseases Research Centre Box 71769 Ndola, November 26, 1982, Ann Bayley Papers, PP/Bay/F/3, Wellcome Library.

25. John Ziegler, interview by author, June 2012; Paul Volberding, interview by author, April 2012. See A. Moss, "AIDS in the 'Gay' Areas of San Francisco," *Lancet* 1 (1983): 923–24. Also see the AIDS Oral Histories series, accessed August 24, 2015, https://www.library.ucsf.edu/collections/archives/manuscripts/aids/oh.

26. John Ziegler, interview by author, June 2012; Paul Volberding, interview by author, April 2012.

27. Johanna Tayloe Crane, *Scrambling for Africa: AIDS, Expertise, and the Rise of American Global Health Science* (Ithaca, NY: Cornell University Press, 2013); Helen Epstein, *The Invisible Cure: Why We Are Losing the Fight against AIDS in Africa* (New York: Farrar, Straus and Giroux, 2007).

28. Didier Fassin, *When Bodies Remember: Experiences and Politics of AIDS in South Africa*, trans. Amy Jacobs and Gabrielle Varro (Berkeley: University of California Press, 2007); Crane, *Scrambling for Africa*.

29. Elly T. Katabira et al., *HIV Infection. Diagnostic and Treatment Strategies for Health Care Workers* (Kampala: STD/AIDS Control Programme, Ministry of Health, 2000).

30. Crane, *Scrambling for Africa*.

31. S. D. Desmond-Hellmann and E. Katongole-Mbidde, "Kaposi's Sarcoma: Recent Developments," *AIDS* 5, no. 1 (1991): S135–42; S. D. Desmond-Hellmann et al., "The Value of a Clinical Definition for Epidemic KS in Predicting HIV Seropositivity in Africa," *Journal of Acquired Immune Deficiency Syndromes* 4, no. 7 (1991): 647–51.

32. Julia R. Cummiskey, "Early AIDS Research in Rakai: Ugandan Experiences and Expertise in the Creation of the African AIDS Paradigm," *International Journal of African Historical Studies* 53, no. 1 (2020): 1–26.

33. Noerine Kaleeba, *We Miss You All: AIDS in the Family* (Kampala: AIDS Support Organization, 1991); Jan Kuhanen, "The Historiography of HIV and AIDS in Uganda," *History in Africa* 35, no. 1 (January 14, 2009): 301–25; Peter Kitonsa Ssebbanja, *United Against AIDS: The Story of TASO* (Oxford: Strategies for Hope Trust, 2007).

34. Fieldnotes, June 2012, May 2013; and Engel, "Building a Legacy of Hope."

35. Conversation with Corey Casper, fieldnotes 2012.

36. J. N. P. Davies, Barbara Wilson, and John Knowelden, "Cancer in Kampala: A Survey in an Underdeveloped Country," *British Medical Journal* 2 (1958): 439–43.

37. Jackson Orem and Henry Wabinga, "The Roles of National Cancer Research Institutions in Evolving a Comprehensive Cancer Control Program in a Developing Country: Experience from Uganda," *Oncology* 77, no. 5 (2009): 272–80.

38. Felicia Knaul, Julio Frenk, and Lawrence Shulman, "Closing the Cancer Divide: A Blueprint to Expand Access in Low and Middle Income Countries," SSRN Scholarly Paper, Rochester, New York, Social Science Research Network, 2011, https://papers.ssrn.com/abstract=2055430.

39. World Health Organization Global Cancer Burden, http://www.who.int/cancer/en/.

40. Global Oncology and Global Health, http://www.hsph.harvard.edu/news/press-releases/global-health-cancer/.

41. *Fred Hutch Global Oncology Brochure* (Seattle: Fred Hutchinson Cancer Research Center, 2015).

42. *Fred Hutch Global Oncology Brochure.*

43. Nancy Rose Hunt, *A Colonial Lexicon of Birth Ritual, Medicalization, and Mobility in the Congo* (Durham, NC: Duke University Press, 1999), 2.

44. Fieldnotes, February 2014.

45. Fieldnotes, September 2013.

46. Fieldnotes, September 2013.

47. Fred Okuku, interview by author, March 2012.

48. Mary Engel, "Singing, Dancing, Dignitaries Mark Opening of UCI-Fred Hutch Cancer Centre," *Fred Hutch News Service*, May 21, 2015, http://www.fredhutch.org/en/news/center-news/2015/05/uci-fred-hutch-cancer-centre-opens.html.

49. Fieldnotes, May 2015.

50. Fieldnotes, May 2015.
51. Mary Engel, "An 'Audacious and Ambitious Building' Seattle Celebrates the Opening of the new Uganda-Fred Hutch Cancer Center," *Fred Hutch News Service*, June 4, 2015, http://www.fredhutch.org/en/news/center -news/2015/06/an-audacious-ambitious-building.html.
52. See *Fred Hutch Global Oncology Brochure*; and Shulman et al., "Bringing Cancer Care to the Poor: Experiences from Rwanda," *Nature Reviews Cancer* 14 (2014): 815–21.
53. *Fred Hutch Global Oncology Brochure*.
54. Fieldnotes, May 2015.
55. Fieldnotes, May 2015.
56. Fieldnotes, May 2015.
57. Fieldnotes, May 2015, June 2012, October 2013.
58. On the problem of triage in global health, see Vinh-Kim Nguyen, *The Republic of Therapy: Triage and Sovereignty in West Africa's Time of AIDS* (Durham, NC: Duke University Press, 2010), 89–110; Peter Redfield, *Life in Crisis: The Ethical Journey of Doctors Without Borders* (Berkeley: University of California Press, 2013), 155–78; João Guilherme Biehl, *Will to Live: AIDS Therapies and the Politics of Survival* (Princeton, NJ: Princeton University Press, 2007), 53–105. On health access, triage, and its relationship to pharmaceutical research, see Adriana Petryna, *When Experiments Travel: Clinical Trials and the Global Search for Human Subjects* (Princeton, NJ: Princeton University Press, 2009), 89–138. On triage and the cancer ward, see Julie Livingston, *Improvising Medicine: An African Oncology Ward in an Emerging Cancer Epidemic* (Durham, NC: Duke University Press, 2012), 152–58.
59. "Letter Requesting Chemotherapy," Charles Olweny Notes, Uganda Cancer Institute Archives.
60. According to data from the Kampala Cancer Registry, the number of Kaposi's sarcoma cancer cases reported between 1991 and 2010 for Kyadondo County was 6,003. The total number of prostate cancer cases was 1,158 while breast cancer cases totaled 1,572. Age standard rates per 100,000 for Kaposi's sarcoma in men from 1991 to 1995 was 39.7. For 2006–10, it was 29.3. In other words, Kaposi's sarcoma age standard rates have declined since the height of the HIV/AIDS epidemic. Prostate cancer age standard rates have increased. From 1991 to 1995, the age standard rate for prostate cancer was 25.7. In 2006–10, the age standard rate was 58.0. Breast cancer age standard rates in women have similarly increased over time. From 1991 to 1995, the age standard rate for breast cancer (in women) was 18.0. From 2006 to 2010, it was 31.2. This is not to say that "HIV related malignancies" are suddenly no longer a problem. The implication here is that there is a need for better cancer screening programs. And there is still much to do in ensuring that patients who come to the UCI with advanced cancers and who would not benefit from aggressive treatment still receive

care. See Wabinga et al., "Trends in the Incidence of Cancer in Kampala, Uganda 1991–2010," *International Journal of Cancer* 135 (2014): 432–39.

61. "Comprehensive Plan for Cancer Hospital in the Early 1980s," Charles Olweny Notes, Uganda Cancer Institute Archives.

IN MEMORIAM

1. Mama Winnie, interview conducted and translated by Irene Nassozi, June 2012.
2. Mama Patience, interview conducted and translated by Irene Nassozi, June 2012.
3. Raphael Owor, interview by author, June 2012.
4. Fieldnotes, September 2012.
5. Fieldnotes, September 2012.
6. Fieldnotes, September 2012.
7. Fieldnotes, September 2012.
8. Fieldnotes, September 2012.
9. Fieldnotes, October 2011.
10. Fieldnotes, June 2012.
11. Fieldnotes, June 2012.
12. Fieldnotes, July 2014.
13. Fieldnotes, July 2014.
14. Fieldnotes, June, July, and August 2014.

Bibliography

ARCHIVES

American Philosophical Society, Philadelphia, PA, United States
British National Archives, Kew, UK
National Cancer Institute Archives, Bethesda, MD, United States
National Institutes of Health Archives, Bethesda, MD, United States
Sir Albert Cook Library, Kampala, Uganda
Rhodes House, Oxford, UK
Trinity Library, Dublin, Ireland
Uganda Cancer Institute Archives, Kampala, Uganda
Uganda National Archives, Entebbe, Uganda
Wellcome Library, London, UK

PERSONAL PAPERS, PHOTOGRAPHS, AND MEMOIRS
IN AUTHOR'S POSSESSION

Avrum Bluming, unpublished memoir, Encino, CA, United States.
Paul Carbone, Columbus, OH, United States, courtesy of David Carbone.
Photographs from John Ziegler's collection.
Charles Vogel, unpublished memoir, Florida, United States.
John Ziegler, correspondence, *Uganda Cancer Institute Annual Reports*, photography collection, San Francisco, CA, United States.

PUBLISHED BIOMEDICAL AND PUBLIC HEALTH WORKS

This section lists publications that are indebted to the Uganda Cancer Institute's contributions to biomedical and public health research on cancer and oncology.

Abdel-Wahab, May, Jean-Marc Bourque, Yaroslav Pynda, Joanna Iżewska, Debbie Van der Merwe, Eduardo Zubizarreta, Eduardo Rosenblatt. "Status of Radiotherapy Resources in Africa: An International Atomic Energy Agency Analysis." *Lancet Oncology* 14 (2013): e168–75.
Abimbola, Seye, and Madhukar Pai. "Will Global Health Survive Its Decolonisation?" *Lancet* 396, no. 10263 (November 21, 2020): 1627–28.

Abudu, Rachel M., Mishka K. Cira, Doug H. M. Pyle, and Kalina Duncan. "Landscape of Global Oncology Research and Training at National Cancer Institute–Designated Cancer Centers: Results of the 2018 to 2019 Global Oncology Survey." *Journal of Global Oncology* 5 (November 22, 2019): 1–8.

Adesina, Adekunle, David Chumba, Ann M. Nelson, Jackson Orem, Drucilla J. Roberts, Henry Wabinga, Michael Wilson, and Timothy R. Rebbeck. "Improvement of Pathology in Sub-Saharan Africa." *Lancet Oncology* 14, no. 4 (April 2013): e152–57.

Baik, Sonya, Mike Mbaziira, Makeda Williams, Martin D. Ogwang, Tobias Kinyera, Benjamin Emmanuel, John L. Ziegler, Steven J. Reynolds, and Sam M. Mbulaiteye. "A Case-Control Study of Burkitt Lymphoma in East Africa: Are Local Health Facilities an Appropriate Source of Representative Controls?" *Infectious Agents and Cancer* 7, no. 1 (March 13, 2012): 5.

Baingana, Florence K., and Eduard R. Bos. "Changing Patterns of Disease and Mortality in Sub-Saharan Africa: An Overview." In *Disease and Mortality in Sub-Saharan Africa*, edited by Dean T. Jamison, Richard G. Feachem, Malegapuru W. Makgoba, Eduard R. Bos, Florence K. Baingana, Karen J. Hofman, and Khama O. Rogo. 2nd ed. Washington, DC: World Bank, 2006. http://www.ncbi.nlm.nih.gov/books/NBK2281/.

Banura, Cecily, Florence M. Mirembe, Jackson Orem, Anthony K. Mbonye, Simon Kasasa, and Edward K. Mbidde. "Prevalence, Incidence and Risk Factors for Anogenital Warts in Sub Saharan Africa: A Systematic Review and Meta Analysis." *Infectious Agents and Cancer* 8, no. 1 (July 10, 2013): 27.

Bateganya, Moses H., Jeffrey Stanaway, Paula E. Brentlinger, Amalia S. Magaret, Anna Wald, Jackson Orem, and Corey Casper. "Predictors of Survival after a Diagnosis of Non-Hodgkin Lymphoma in a Resource-Limited Setting: A Retrospective Study on the Impact of HIV Infection and Its Treatment." *Journal of Acquired Immune Deficiency Syndromes* 56, no. 4 (April 2011): 312–19.

Bornkamm, Georg W. "Epstein-Barr Virus and the Pathogenesis of Burkitt's Lymphoma: More Questions than Answers." *International Journal of Cancer* 124, no. 8 (April 15, 2009): 1745–55.

Brown, Theodore M., Marcos Cueto, and Elizabeth Fee. "The World Health Organization and the Transition from 'International' to 'Global' Public Health." *American Journal of Public Health* 96 (2006): 62–72.

Buckle, Geoffrey C., Jennifer Pfau Collins, Peter Odada Sumba, Beccy Nakalema, Dorine Omenah, Kristine Stiffler, Corey Casper, Juliana A. Otieno, Jackson Orem, and Ann M. Moormann. "Factors Influencing Time to Diagnosis and Initiation of Treatment of Endemic Burkitt Lymphoma among Children in Uganda and Western Kenya: A Cross-Sectional Survey." *Infectious Agents and Cancer* 8, no. 1 (September 30, 2013): 36.

Bukhman, Gene, John Ziegler, and Eldryd Parry. "Endomyocardial Fibrosis: Still a Mystery after 60 Years." *PLoS Neglected Tropical Diseases* 2, no. 2 (February 27, 2008): e97.

Bukirwa, Phiona, Henry Wabinga, Sarah Nambooze, Phoebe Mary Amulen, Walburga Yvonne Joko, Biying Liu, and Donald Maxwell Parkin. "Trends in the Incidence of Cancer in Kampala, Uganda, 1991 to 2015." *International Journal of Cancer* 148, no. 9 (May 1, 2021): 2129–38. https://doi.org /10.1002/ijc.33373.

Burchenal, Joseph. "Burkitt's Tumor as a Stalking Horse for Leukemia." *JAMA* 222, no. 9 (1972): 1165.

Burkitt, Denis P. "The Beginnings of the Burkitt's Lymphoma Story." *IARC Scientific Publications*, no. 60 (1985): 11–15.

———. "A Children's Cancer Dependent on Climatic Factors." *Nature* 194 (April 21, 1962): 232–34.

———. "Determining the Climatic Limitations of a Children's Cancer Common in Africa." *British Medical Journal* 2, no. 5311 (October 20, 1962): 1019–23. https://doi.org/10.1136/bmj.2.5311.1019.

———. "The Discovery of Burkitt's Lymphoma." *Cancer* 51, no. 10 (1983): 1777–86.

———. "Distribution of Cancer in Africa." *Proceedings of the Royal Society of Medicine* 66, no. 4 (April 1973): 312–14.

———. "The Reasons for Going to Africa." In *Pioneers in Pediatric Oncology*, edited by Grant Taylor. Houston: University of Texas MD Anderson Cancer Center, 1990.

———. "A Sarcoma Involving the Jaws in African Children." *British Journal of Surgery* 46, no. 197 (November 1958): 218–23.

———. "Some Diseases Characteristic of Modern Western Civilization: A Possible Common Causative Factor." *Clinical Radiology* 24, no. 3 (January 1, 1973): 271–80.

———. "A Study of Cancer Patterns in Africa." *Scientific Basis of Medicine Annual Reviews* (1969): 82–94.

———. "A 'Tumour Safari' in East and Central Africa." *British Journal of Cancer* 16 (September 1962): 379–86.

Burkitt, Denis P., M. S. Hutt, and G. Slavin. "Clinico-Pathological Studies of Cancer Distribution in Africa." *British Journal of Cancer* 22, no. 1 (March 1968): 1–6.

Burkitt, Denis P., M. S. Hutt, and D. H. Wright. "The African Lymphoma: Preliminary Observations on Response to Therapy." *Cancer* 18 (April 1965): 399–410.

Burkitt, Denis P., and S. K. Kyalwazi. "Spontaneous Remission of African Lymphoma." *British Journal of Cancer* 21, no. 1 (March 1967): 14–16.

Burkitt, Denis, and G. T. O'Conor. "Malignant Lymphoma in African Children: I. A Clinical Syndrome." *Cancer* 14 (April 1961): 258–69.

Burkitt, Denis P., J. P. Stanfield, and J. C. Church. "A Medical Research Safari: Fruits and Frustrations." *Central African Journal of Medicine* 16, no. 9 (September 1970): 197–201.

Burkitt, Denis P., E. H. Williams, and L. Eshleman. "The Contribution of the Voluntary Agency Hospital to Cancer Epidemiology." *British Journal of Cancer* 23, no. 2 (June 1969): 269–74.

Burkitt, Denis P., and Dennis Howard Wright, eds. *Burkitt's Lymphoma.* Edinburgh: Livingstone, 1971.

———. "A Lymphoma Syndrome in Tropical Africa with a Note on Histology, Cytology, and Histochemistry." *International Review of Experimental Pathology* 2 (1963): 67–138.

Büyüm, Ali Murad, Cordelia Kenney, Andrea Koris, Laura Mkumba, and Yadurshini Raveendran. "Decolonising Global Health: If Not Now, When?" *BMJ Global Health* 5, no. 8 (August 1, 2020): e003394. https://doi .org/10.1136/bmjgh-2020-003394.

Byamugisha, Josaphat, Ian G. Munabi, Aloysius G. Mubuuke, Amos D. Mwaka, Mike Kagawa, Isaac Okullo, Nixon Niyonzima et al. "A Health Care Professionals Training Needs Assessment for Oncology in Uganda." *Human Resources for Health* 18, no. 1 (September 1, 2020): 62.

Cady, Blake. "Denis Parsons Burkitt, an Overlooked Surgical Oncologist." *Annals of Surgical Oncology* 25, no. 5 (May 2018): 1112–15. https://doi.org/10 .1245/s10434-018-6386-9.

"Cancer Control in Africa." Series, *Lancet Oncology* 14, no. 4 (2013).

Carpenter, Lucy M., Robert Newton, Delphine Casabonne, John Ziegler, Sam Mbulaiteye, Edward Mbidde, Henry Wabinga, Harold Jaffe, and Valerie Beral. "Antibodies against Malaria and Epstein-Barr Virus in Childhood Burkitt Lymphoma: A Case-Control Study in Uganda." *International Journal of Cancer* 122, no. 6 (March 15, 2008): 1319–23.

Carter, David. "Sir Ian William James McAdam." *British Medical Journal* 318 (1999): 1216.

Casper, Corey. "The Increasing Burden of HIV-Associated Malignancies in Resource-Limited Regions." *Annual Review of Medicine* 62 (2011): 157–70.

Chabner, B. A., G. P. Canellos, C. L. Olweny, and V. T. DeVita. "Late Recurrence of Testicular Tumor." *New England Journal of Medicine* 287, no. 8 (August 24, 1972): 413.

Chang, Y., J. Ziegler, H. Wabinga, E. Katangole-Mbidde, C. Boshoff, T. Schulz, D. Whitby et al. "Kaposi's Sarcoma-Associated Herpesvirus and Kaposi's Sarcoma in Africa. Uganda Kaposi's Sarcoma Study Group." *Archives of Internal Medicine* 156, no. 2 (January 22, 1996): 202–4.

Chêne, Arnaud, Daria Donati, Jackson Orem, E. R. Mbidde, Fred Kironde, Mats Wahlgren, and Maria Teresa Bejarano. "Endemic Burkitt's Lymphoma as a Polymicrobial Disease: New Insights on the Interaction between Plasmodium Falciparum and Epstein-Barr Virus." *Seminars in Cancer Biology* 19, no. 6 (December 2009): 411–20.

Chêne, Arnaud, Daria Donati, André Ortlieb Guerreiro-Cacais, Victor Levitsky, Qijun Chen, Kerstin I. Falk, Jackson Orem, Fred Kironde, Mats Wahlgren, and Maria Teresa Bejarano. "A Molecular Link between

Malaria and Epstein-Barr Virus Reactivation." *PLoS Pathogens* 3, no. 6 (June 2007): e80.

Chikanza, I. C., A. S. Latif, P. Neill, P. Mason, and C. L. Olweny. "Unusual Complications of Typhoid Fever." *Central African Journal of Medicine* 32, no. 2 (February 1986): 31–34.

Chuck, S., R. M. Grant, E. Katongole-Mbidde, M. Conant, and D. Ganem. "Frequent Presence of a Novel Herpesvirus Genome in Lesions of Human Immunodeficiency Virus-Negative Kaposi's Sarcoma." *Journal of Infectious Diseases* 173, no. 1 (January 1996): 248–51.

Clifford, Peter, Allen Linsell, and Geoffrey Timms, eds. *Cancer in Africa: A Selection of Papers Given at the East African Medical Research Council Scientific Conference in Nairobi in January 1967.* Evanston, IL: Northwestern University Press, 1968.

Coghill, Anna E., Polly A. Newcomb, Margaret M. Madeleine, Barbra A. Richardson, Innocent Mutyaba, Fred Okuku, Warren Phipps, Henry Wabinga, Jackson Orem, and Corey Casper. "Contribution of HIV Infection to Mortality among Cancer Patients in Uganda." *AIDS* 27, no. 18 (November 28, 2013): 2933–42.

Coghill, Anna E., Jeannette M. Schenk, Zeina Mahkoul, Jackson Orem, Warren Phipps, and Corey Casper. "Omega-3 Decreases IL-6 Levels in HIV and Human Herpesvirus-8 Coinfected Patients in Uganda." *AIDS* 32, no. 4 (February 20, 2018): 505–12.

Cook, P. J., and D. P. Burkitt. "Cancer in Africa." *British Medical Bulletin* 27, no. 1 (January 1971): 14–20.

Cook-Mozaffari, P., R. Newton, V. Beral, and D. P. Burkitt. "The Geographical Distribution of Kaposi's Sarcoma and of Lymphomas in Africa before the AIDS Epidemic." *British Journal of Cancer* 78, no. 11 (December 1998): 1521–28.

Coutinho, Alex, Uchechi Roxo, Henry Epino, Alex Muganzi, Emily Dorward, and Billy Pick. "The Expanding Role of Civil Society in the Global HIV/AIDS Response: What Has the President's Emergency Program for AIDS Relief's Role Been?" *Journal of Acquired Immune Deficiency Syndromes* 60, no. 3 (August 15, 2012): S152–57.

Davies, J. N. P. "The Pattern of African Cancer in Uganda." *East African Medical Journal* 38 (1961): 486–91.

Davies, J. N. P., Sally Elmes, M. S. R. Hutt, L. A. R. Mtimavalye, R. Owor, and Lorna Shaper. "Cancer in an African Community, 1897–1956: An Analysis of the Records of Mengo Hospital, Kampala, Uganda: Part I." *British Medical Journal* 1, no. 5378 (1964): 259–64.

Davies, J. N. P., and B. A. Wilson. "Cancer in Kampala, 1952–1953." *East African Medical Journal* 31 (1954): 395–416.

Davies, J. N. P., Barbara Wilson, and John Knowelden. "Cancer in Kampala: A Survey in an Underdeveloped Country." *British Medical Journal* 2 (1958): 439–43.

Ddungu, Henry, Elizabeth M. Krantz, Isaac Kajja, Sandra Naluzze, Han-ifah Nabbanja, Flavia Nalubwama, Warren Phipps, Jackson Orem, Noah Kiwanuka, and Anna Wald. "How Low Can You Go: What Is the Safe Threshold for Platelet Transfusions in Patients with Hemato-logic Malignancy in Sub-Saharan Africa." *PloS One* 14, no. 2 (2019): e0211648.

Ddungu, Henry, Elizabeth M. Krantz, Isaac Kajja, Sandra Naluzze, Hani-fah Nabbanja, Flavia Nalubwama, Warren Phipps, Jackson Orem, Anna Wald, and Noah Kiwanuka. "Transfusion Challenges in Patients with Hematological Malignancies in Sub-Saharan Africa: A Prospective Ob-servational Study from the Uganda Cancer Institute." *Scientific Reports* 10, no. 1 (February 18, 2020): 2825.

Ddungu, Henry, Elizabeth M. Krantz, Warren Phipps, Sandra Naluzze, Jackson Orem, Noah Kiwanuka, Anna Wald, and Isaac Kajja. "Survey to Assess Knowledge and Reported Practices Regarding Blood Transfusion among Cancer Physicians in Uganda." *Journal of Global Oncology* 4 (Oc-tober 2018): 1–12.

De Boer, Christopher, Nixon Niyonzima, Jackson Orem, John Bartlett, and S. Yousuf Zafar. "Prognosis and Delay of Diagnosis among Kaposi's Sar-coma Patients in Uganda: A Cross-Sectional Study." *Infectious Agents and Cancer* 9 (2014): 17.

Denburg, Avram E., Nazeefah Laher, Innocent Mutyaba, Suzanne McGol-drick, Joyce Kambugu, Erica Sessle, Jackson Orem, and Corey Casper. "The Cost Effectiveness of Treating Burkitt Lymphoma in Uganda." *Cancer* 125, no. 11 (June 1, 2019): 1918–28.

Desmond-Hellmann, S. D., and E. Katongole-Mbidde. "Kaposi's Sarcoma: Recent Developments." *AIDS* 5, no. 1 (1991): S135–42.

Desmond-Hellmann, S. D., E. K. Mbidde, A. Kizito, N. S. Hellmann, and J. L. Ziegler. "The Value of a Clinical Definition for Epidemic KS in Predicting HIV Seropositivity in Africa." *Journal of Acquired Immune De-ficiency Syndromes* 4, no. 7 (1991): 647–51.

Downing, Julia, Henry Ddungu, Fatia Kiyange, Mwazi Batuli, James Kafeero, Harriet Kebirungi, Rose Kiwanuka et al. "United against Cancer: Preven-tion to End-of-Life Care-Highlights from the Uganda Cancer Institute-Palliative Care Association of Uganda Joint International Conference on Cancer and Palliative Care and the 7th Palliative Care Conference, 24–25 August 2017, Kampala, Uganda." *Ecancermedicalscience* 11 (2017): 790. https://doi.org/10.3332/ecancer.2017.790.

Durosinmi-Etti, F. A., M. Nofal, and M. M. Mahfouz. "Radiotherapy in Af-rica: Current Needs and Prospects." *IAEA Bulletin* 33, no. 4 (December 1991): 24–28.

Epstein, Anthony, and M. A. Eastwood. "Denis Parsons Burkitt, 28 February 1911–23 March 1993." *Biographical Memoirs of Fellows of the Royal Society* 14 (1995): 89–102.

Epstein, M. A. "Historical Background; Burkitt's Lymphoma and Epstein-Barr Virus." *IARC Scientific Publications* 60 (1985): 17–27.

Esau, Daniel. "Denis Burkitt: A Legacy of Global Health." *Journal of Medical Biography* 27, no. 1 (February 2019): 4–8.

Fisher, Brandon J., Larry C. Daugherty, John P. Einck, Gita Suneja, Mira M. Shah, Luqman K. Dad, Robert W. Mutter, J. Ben Wilkinson, Arno J. Mundt. "Radiation Oncology in Africa: Improving Access to Cancer Care on the African Continent." *International Journal of Radiation Oncology Biology Physics* 89, no. 3 (July 2014): 458–61.

Foster, W. D. "Doctor Albert Cook and the Early Days of the Church Missionary Society's Medical Mission to Uganda." *Medical History* 12, no. 4 (October 1968): 325–43.

Gagliardi, Alessia, Vanessa L. Porter, Zusheng Zong, Reanne Bowlby, Emma Titmuss, Constance Namirembe, Nicholas B. Griner et al. "Analysis of Ugandan Cervical Carcinomas Identifies Human Papillomavirus Clade-Specific Epigenome and Transcriptome Landscapes." *Nature Genetics* 52, no. 8 (August 2020): 800–810.

Gantt, Soren, Abel Kakuru, Anna Wald, Victoria Walusansa, Lawrence Corey, Corey Casper, and Jackson Orem. "Clinical Presentation and Outcome of Epidemic Kaposi Sarcoma in Ugandan Children." *Pediatric Blood and Cancer* 54, no. 5 (May 2010): 670–74.

Gantt, Soren, Jackson Orem, Elizabeth M. Krantz, Rhoda Ashley Morrow, Stacy Selke, Meei-Li Huang, Joshua T. Schiffer et al. "Prospective Characterization of the Risk Factors for Transmission and Symptoms of Primary Human Herpesvirus Infections among Ugandan Infants." *Journal of Infectious Diseases* 214, no. 1 (July 1, 2016): 36–44.

Gao, S. J., L. Kingsley, M. Li, W. Zheng, C. Parravicini, J. Ziegler, R. Newton et al. "KSHV Antibodies among Americans, Italians and Ugandans with and without Kaposi's Sarcoma." *Nature Medicine* 2, no. 8 (August 1996): 925–28.

Gopal, Satish, and Patrick J. Loehrer Sr. "Global Oncology." *JAMA* 322, no. 5 (August 6, 2019): 397–98.

Gunvén, P., G. Klein, J. L. Ziegler, I. T. Magrath, C. L. Olweny, W. Henle, G. Henle, A. Svedmyr, and A. Demissie. "Epstein-Barr Virus-Associated and Other Antiviral Antibodies during Intense BCG Administration to Patients with Burkitt's Lymphoma in Remission." *Journal of the National Cancer Institute* 60, no. 1 (January 1978): 31–37.

Haddow, A. J. "An Improved Map for the Study of Burkitt's Lymphoma Syndrome in Africa." *East African Medical Journal* 40 (1963): 429–32.

Hamilton, P. J., M. S. Hutt, N. E. Wilks, C. Olweny, R. L. Ndawula, and L. Mwanje. "Idiopathic Splenomegaly in Uganda. 1. Pathological Aspects." *East African Medical Journal* 42 (May 1965): 191–95.

———. "Idiopathic Splenomegaly in Uganda. 2. Geographical Aspects." *East African Medical Journal* 42 (May 1965): 196–202.

Hanson, G.P., J. Stjernswärd, M. Nofal, and F. Durosinmi-Etti. "An Overview of the Situation in Radiotherapy with Emphasis on the Developing Countries." *International Journal of Radiation Oncology Biology Physics* 19, no. 5 (November 1990): 1256–61.

Harford, Joe B. "Viral Infections and Human Cancers: The Legacy of Denis Burkitt." *British Journal of Haematology* 156, no. 6 (March 2012): 709–18.

Hosseinipour, Mina C., Minhee Kang, Susan E. Krown, Aggrey Bukuru, Triin Umbleja, Jeffrey N. Martin, Jackson Orem et al. "As-Needed vs. Immediate Etoposide Chemotherapy in Combination with Antiretroviral Therapy for Mild-to-Moderate AIDS-Associated Kaposi Sarcoma in Resource-Limited Settings: A5264/AMC-067 Randomized Clinical Trial." *Clinical Infectious Diseases: An Official Publication of the Infectious Diseases Society of America* 67, no. 2 (July 2, 2018): 251–60.

Hume, Heather A., Henry Ddungu, Racheal Angom, Hannington Baluku, Henry Kajumbula, Dorothy Kyeyune-Byabazaire, Jackson Orem, Sandra Ramirez-Arcos, and Aaron A. R. Tobian. "Platelet Transfusion Therapy in Sub-Saharan Africa: Bacterial Contamination, Recipient Characteristics, and Acute Transfusion Reactions." *Transfusion* 56, no. 8 (August 2016): 1951–59.

Hutt, M. S. R., and D. Burkitt. "Geographical Distribution of Cancer in East Africa: A New Clinicopathological Approach." *British Medical Journal* 2, no. 5464 (September 25, 1965): 719–22.

Jatho, Alfred, Noleb M. Mugisha, James Kafeero, George Holoya, Fred Okuku, Nixon Niyonzima, and Jackson Orem. "Capacity Building for Cancer Prevention and Early Detection in the Ugandan Primary Healthcare Facilities: Working toward Reducing the Unmet Needs of Cancer Control Services." *Cancer Medicine* 10, no. 2 (January 2021): 745–56. https://doi.org/10.1002/cam4.3659.

Jay, Venita. "Extraordinary Epidemiological Quest of Dr. Burkitt." *Pediatric and Developmental Pathology* 1 (1998): 562–64.

Johnston, Christine, Jackson Orem, Fred Okuku, Mary Kalinaki, Misty Saracino, Edward Katongole-Mbidde, Merle Sande et al. "Impact of HIV Infection and Kaposi Sarcoma on Human Herpesvirus-8 Mucosal Replication and Dissemination in Uganda." *PloS One* 4, no. 1 (2009): e4222.

Kabukye, Johnblack K., Sabine Koch, Ronald Cornet, Jackson Orem, and Maria Hagglund. "User Requirements for an Electronic Medical Records System for Oncology in Developing Countries: A Case Study of Uganda." *AMIA Annual Symposium Proceedings* (2017): 1004–13.

Kaleebu, P., A. Kamali, J. Seeley, A. M. Elliott, and E. Katongole-Mbidde. "The Medical Research Council (UK)/Uganda Virus Research Institute Uganda Research Unit on AIDS — '25 Years of Research through Partnerships.'" *Tropical Medicine and International Health: TM & IH* 20, no. 2 (February 2015): E1–10.

Kaleebu, Pontiano, Wilford Kirungi, Christine Watera, Juliet Asio, Fred Lyagoba, Tom Lutalo, Anne A. Kapaata et al. "Virological Response and

Antiretroviral Drug Resistance Emerging during Antiretroviral Therapy at Three Treatment Centers in Uganda." *PloS One* 10, no. 12 (2015): e0145536.

Katabira, Elly T., Moses R. Kamya, Francis X. Mubiru, and Nathan N. Bakyaita. *HIV Infection. Diagnostic and Treatment Strategies for Health Care Workers.* Kampala: STD/AIDS Control Programme, Ministry of Health, 2000.

Katongole-Mbidde, E. "Duration of Symptoms and Histology of Hodgkin's Disease." *Lancet* 2, no. 8406 (October 6, 1984): 807–8.

———. "Management of Kaposi's Sarcoma." *Lancet* 2, no. 8297 (September 4, 1982): 563.

———. "Preparations for AIDS Vaccine Trials. Respecting Concerns of International Host Countries." *AIDS Research and Human Retroviruses* 10, no. 2 (1994): S187–89.

Katongole-Mbidde, E., C. Banura, and M. Nakakeeto. "Diagnostic Implications of Genital Kaposi's Sarcoma." *East African Medical Journal* 66, no. 8 (August 1989): 499–502.

Katongole-Mbidde, E., C. L. Olweny, B. R. Kanyerezi, and R. Owor. "Malignant Lymphoma Associated with Rheumatoid Arthritis." *East African Medical Journal* 61, no. 7 (July 1984): 544–50.

Katongole-Mbidde, E., C. L. Olweny, J. Mugerwa, and R. Owor. "Central Nervous System Involvement in Non-Hodgkin's Lymphoma (Excluding Burkitt's Lymphoma) in Ugandan Africans." *East African Medical Journal* 65, no. 12 (December 1988): 838–46.

Katongole-Mbidde, E., C. L. Olweny, D. Otim, C. F. Kiire, W. Carswell, and R. Owor. "Combination Chemotherapy and Surgery in the Treatment of Wilms' Tumour: Preliminary Communication." *East African Medical Journal* 65, no. 10 (October 1988): 692–97.

Kibudde, Solomon, Charles Kiiza Mondo, Davis Kibirige, Victoria Walusansa, and Jackson Orem. "Anthracycline Induced Cardiotoxicity in Adult Cancer Patients: A Prospective Cohort Study from a Specialized Oncology Treatment Centre in Uganda." *African Health Sciences* 19, no. 1 (March 2019): 1647–56.

Kigula-Mugambe, J. B., and F. A. Durosinmi. "Radiotherapy in Cancer Management at Mulago Hospital, Kampala, Uganda." *East African Medical Journal* 73 (1996): 611–13.

Kigula-Mugambe, J. B., and P. Wegoye. "Pattern and Experience with Cancers Treated with the Chinese GWGP80 Cobalt Unit at Mulago Hospital, Kampala." *East African Medical Journal* 77 (2000): 523–26.

Kiire, C. F., C. Gombe-Mbalawa, E. Tsega, J. Luande, L. V. Menenses, J. Okoth, C. L. Olweny, and J. Holland. "Multicentre Study of the Treatment of Primary Liver Cancer in Africa with Two Anthracycline Drugs." *Central African Journal of Medicine* 38, no. 11 (November 1992): 428–31.

Kiryabwire, J. W., M. G. Lewis, J. L. Ziegler, and I. Loefler. "Malignant Melanoma in Uganda." *East African Medical Journal* 45, no. 7 (July 1968): 498–507.

Knaul, Felicia, Julio Frenk, and Lawrence Shulman. "Closing the Cancer Divide: A Blueprint to Expand Access in Low and Middle Income Countries." SSRN Scholarly Paper. Rochester, NY: Social Science Research Network, 2011. https://papers.ssrn.com/abstract=2055430.

Krown, Susan E., Margaret Z. Borok, Thomas B. Campbell, Corey Casper, Dirk P. Dittmer, Mina C. Hosseinipour, Ronald T. Mitsuyasu, Anisa Mosam, Jackson Orem, and Warren T. Phipps. "Stage-Stratified Approach to AIDS-Related Kaposi's Sarcoma: Implications for Resource-Limited Environments." *Journal of Clinical Oncology: Official Journal of the American Society of Clinical Oncology* 32, no. 23 (August 10, 2014): 2512–13.

Kyalwazi, S. K. "Carcinoma of the Penis: A Review of 153 Patients Admitted to Mulago Hospital, Kampala, Uganda." *East African Medical Journal* 43 (1966): 415–25.

———. "Chemotherapy of Kaposi's Sarcoma: Experience with Trenimon." *East African Medical Journal* 45 (1966): 17–26.

———. "Kaposi's Sarcoma: Clinical Features, Experience in Uganda." *Antibiotic Chemotherapy* 29 (1971): 59–69.

Laker-Oketta, Miriam, Lisa Butler, Philippa Kadama-Makanga, Robert Inglis, Megan Wenger, Edward Katongole-Mbidde, Toby Maurer, Andrew Kambugu, and Jeffrey Martin. "Using Media to Promote Public Awareness of Early Detection of Kaposi's Sarcoma in Africa." *Journal of Oncology* (2020): 3254820.

Lee, T. C. "Seeing the Wood for the Trees—the Early Papers of Denis Burkitt." *Journal of the Irish Colleges of Physicians and Surgeons* 25, no. 2 (April 1996): 126–30.

Levin, C.V., B. El Gueddari, A. Meghzifene. "Radiation Therapy in Africa: Distribution and Equipment." *Radiotherapy and Oncology* 52, no. 1 (July 1999): 79–84.

Lin, Cynthia J., Edward Katongole-Mbidde, Tadeos Byekwaso, Jackson Orem, Charles S. Rabkin, and Sam M. Mbulaiteye. "Intestinal Parasites in Kaposi Sarcoma Patients in Uganda: Indication of Shared Risk Factors or Etiologic Association." *American Journal of Tropical Medicine and Hygiene* 78, no. 3 (March 2008): 409–12.

Lin, Lilie L., David S. Lakomy, Elizabeth Y. Chiao, Robert M. Strother, Meg Wirth, Ethel Cesarman, Margaret Borok et al. "Clinical Trials for Treatment and Prevention of HIV-Associated Malignancies in Sub-Saharan Africa: Building Capacity and Overcoming Barriers." *JCO Global Oncology* 6 (July 2020): 1134–46.

Lombardo, Katharine A., David G. Coffey, Alicia J. Morales, Christopher S. Carlson, Andrea M. H. Towlerton, Sarah E. Gerdts, Francis K. Nkrumah et al. "High-Throughput Sequencing of the B-Cell Receptor in African Burkitt Lymphoma Reveals Clues to Pathogenesis." *Blood Advances* 1, no. 9 (March 28, 2017): 535–44.

Low, Daniel H., Warren Phipps, Jackson Orem, Corey Casper, and Rachel A. Bender Ignacio. "Engagement in HIV Care and Access to Cancer Treatment among Patients with HIV-Associated Malignancies in Uganda." *Journal of Global Oncology* 5 (February 2019): 1–8.

Lurie, P., M. Bishaw, M. A. Chesney, M. Cooke, M. E. Fernandes, N. Hearst, E. Katongole-Mbidde, S. Koetsawang, C. P. Lindan, and J. Mandel. "Ethical, Behavioral, and Social Aspects of HIV Vaccine Trials in Developing Countries." *JAMA* 271, no. 4 (January 26, 1994): 295–301.

Lwanga, S. K., C. L. Olweny, P. M. Tukei, and K. Nishioka. "Hepatitis B Surface Antigen (HBsAg) Subtypes in Uganda. A Preliminary Report." *Tropical and Geographical Medicine* 29, no. 4 (December 1977): 381–85.

Magrath, I. T. "African Burkitt's Lymphoma. History, Biology, Clinical Features, and Treatment." *American Journal of Pediatric Hematology/Oncology* 13, no. 2 (1991): 222–46.

———. "Denis Burkitt and the African Lymphoma." *Ecancermedicalscience* 3 (2009): 159. https://doi.org/10.3332/ecancer.2009.159.

Magrath, I. T., W. Henle, R. Owor, and C. Olweny. "Antibodies to Epstein-Barr-Virus Antigens before and after the Development of Burkitt's Lymphoma in a Patient Treated for Hodgkin's Disease." *New England Journal of Medicine* 292, no. 12 (March 20, 1975): 621–23.

Magrath, I. T., J. Mugerwa, I. Bailey, C. Olweny, and Y. Kiryabwire. "Intracerebral Burkitt's Lymphoma: Pathology, Clinical Features and Treatment." *Quarterly Journal of Medicine* 43, no. 172 (October 1974): 489–508.

Magrath, I. T., J. L. Ziegler, and A. C. Templeton. "A Comparison of Clinical and Histopathologic Features of Childhood Malignant Lymphoma in Uganda." *Cancer* 33, no. 1 (January 1974): 285–94.

Master, S. P., J. F. Taylor, S. K. Kyalwazi, and J. L. Ziegler. "Immunological Studies in Kaposi's Sarcoma in Uganda." *British Medical Journal* 1, no. 5696 (March 7, 1970): 600–602.

Matrajt, Laura, Soren Gantt, Bryan T. Mayer, Elizabeth M. Krantz, Jackson Orem, Anna Wald, Lawrence Corey, Joshua T. Schiffer, and Corey Casper. "Virus and Host-Specific Differences in Oral Human Herpesvirus Shedding Kinetics among Ugandan Women and Children." *Scientific Reports* 7, no. 1 (October 12, 2017): 13105.

Mayosi, Bongani M., and Solomon R. Benatar. "Health and Health Care in South Africa—20 Years after Mandela." *New England Journal of Medicine* 371, no. 14 (October 2, 2014): 1344–53.

Mbulaiteye, Sam M., Robert J. Biggar, Paul M. Bakaki, Ruth M. Pfeiffer, Denise Whitby, Anchilla M. Owor, Edward Katongole-Mbidde, James J. Goedert, Christopher M. Ndugwa, and Eric A. Engels. "Human Herpesvirus 8 Infection and Transfusion History in Children with Sickle-Cell

Disease in Uganda." *Journal of the National Cancer Institute* 95, no. 17 (September 3, 2003): 1330–35.

Mbulaiteye, Sam, Vickie Marshall, Rachel K. Bagni, Cheng-Dian Wang, Georgina Mbisa, Paul M. Bakaki, Anchilla M. Owor et al. "Molecular Evidence for Mother-to-Child Transmission of Kaposi Sarcoma-Associated Herpesvirus in Uganda and K1 Gene Evolution within the Host." *Journal of Infectious Diseases* 193, no. 9 (May 1, 2006): 1250–57.

McGoldrick, Suzanne M., Innocent Mutyaba, Scott V. Adams, Anna Larsen, Elizabeth M. Krantz, Constance Namirembe, Peter Mooka et al. "Survival of Children with Endemic Burkitt Lymphoma in a Prospective Clinical Care Project in Uganda." *Pediatric Blood and Cancer* 66, no. 9 (September 2019): e27813. https://doi.org/10.1002/pbc.27813.

Meacham, Elizabeth, Jackson Orem, Gertrude Nakigudde, Jo Anne Zujewski, and Deepa Rao. "Exploring Stigma as a Barrier to Cancer Service Engagement with Breast Cancer Survivors in Kampala, Uganda." *Psycho-Oncology* 25, no. 10 (October 2016): 1206–11.

Menon, Manoj P., Anna Coghill, Innocent Mutyaba, Fred Okuku, Warren Phipps, John Harlan, Jackson Orem, and Corey Casper. "Whom to Treat? Factors Associated with Chemotherapy Recommendations and Outcomes among Patients with NHL at the Uganda Cancer Institute." *PloS One* 13, no. 2 (2018): e0191967. https://doi.org/10.1371/journal.pone.0191967.

Menon, Manoj P., Anna Coghill, Innocent O. Mutyaba, Warren T. Phipps, Fred M. Okuku, John M. Harlan, Jackson Orem, and Corey Casper. "Association between HIV Infection and Cancer Stage at Presentation at the Uganda Cancer Institute." *Journal of Global Oncology* 4 (September 2018): 1–9.

Minab, Rana, Wei Bu, Hanh Nguyen, Abigail Wall, Anton M. Sholukh, Meei-Li Huang, Michael Ortego et al. "Maternal Epstein-Barr Virus-Specific Antibodies and Risk of Infection in Ugandan Infants." *Journal of Infectious Diseases* 223, no. 11 (June 2021): 1897–904. https://doi.org/10.1093/infdis/jiaa654.

Molyneux, Elizabeth, Alan Davidson, Jackson Orem, Peter Hesseling, Joyce Balagadde-Kambugu, Jessie Githanga, and Trijn Israels. "The Management of Children with Kaposi Sarcoma in Resource Limited Settings." *Pediatric Blood and Cancer* 60, no. 4 (April 2013): 538–42.

Mondo, Charles Kiiza, Marcel Andrew Otim, George Akol, Robert Musoke, and Jackson Orem. "The Prevalence and Distribution of Non-Communicable Diseases and Their Risk Factors in Kasese District, Uganda." *Cardiovascular Journal of Africa* 24, no. 3 (April 2013): 52–57.

Moormann, Ann M., and José S. Lozada. "Burkitt Lymphoma in Uganda: 50 Years of Ongoing Discovery." *Pediatric Blood and Cancer* 52, no. 4 (April 2009): 433–34.

Morrow, R. H., M. C. Pike, A. Kisuule. "Survival of Burkitt's Lymphoma Patients in Mulago Hospital, Uganda." *British Medical Journal* 4 (1967): 323–27.

Morrow, R. H., M. C. Pike, P. Smith, and J. L. Ziegler. "Preliminary Epidemiological Findings of Burkitt's Lymphoma in the Mengo Districts, Uganda, 1959–1968." *Cancer Research* 34, no. 5 (May 1974): 1211–12.

Morrow, R. H., M. C. Pike, P. G. Smith, J. L. Ziegler, and A. Kisuule. "Burkitt's Lymphoma: A Time-Space Cluster of Cases in Bwamba County of Uganda." *British Medical Journal* 2, no. 5760 (May 29, 1971): 491–92.

Mugerwa, Roy D., Pontiano Kaleebu, Peter Mugyenyi, Edward Katongole-Mbidde, David L. Hom, Rose Byaruhanga, Robert A. Salata, and Jerrold J. Ellner. "First Trial of the HIV-1 Vaccine in Africa: Ugandan Experience." *BMJ: British Medical Journal* 324, no. 7331 (January 26, 2002): 226–29.

Mutebi, Miriam, Isaac Adewole, Jackson Orem, Kunuz Abdella, Olujimi Coker, Israel Kolawole, Ahmed Komen et al. "Toward Optimization of Cancer Care in Sub-Saharan Africa: Development of National Comprehensive Cancer Network Harmonized Guidelines for Sub-Saharan Africa." *JCO Global Oncology* 6 (September 2020): 1412–18.

Mutyaba, Innocent, Henry R. Wabinga, Jackson Orem, Corey Casper, and Warren Phipps. "Presentation and Outcomes of Childhood Cancer Patients at Uganda Cancer Institute." *Global Pediatric Health* 6 (2019): 2333794X19849749. https://doi.org/10.1177/2333794X19849749.

Mwanda, Walter O., Jackson Orem, Pingfu Fu, Cecilia Banura, Joweria Kakembo, Caren Auma Onyango, Anne Ness et al. "Dose-Modified Oral Chemotherapy in the Treatment of AIDS-Related Non-Hodgkin's Lymphoma in East Africa." *Journal of Clinical Oncology: Official Journal of the American Society of Clinical Oncology* 27, no. 21 (July 20, 2009): 3480–88.

Nabyonga, Juliet, and Jackson Orem. "From Knowledge to Policy: Lessons from Africa." *Science Translational Medicine* 6, no. 240 (June 11, 2014): 240ed13. https://doi.org/10.1126/scitranslmed.3008852.

Nagaiah, Govardhanan, Christy Stotler, Jackson Orem, Walter O. Mwanda, and Scot C. Remick. "Ocular Surface Squamous Neoplasia in Patients with HIV Infection in Sub-Saharan Africa." *Current Opinion in Oncology* 22, no. 5 (September 2010): 437–42.

Nakisige, Carolyn, Jessica Trawin, Sheona Mitchell-Foster, Beth A. Payne, Angeli Rawat, Nadia Mithani, Cathy Amuge et al. "Integrated Cervical Cancer Screening in Mayuge District Uganda (ASPIRE Mayuge): A Pragmatic Sequential Cluster Randomized Trial Protocol." *BMC Public Health* 20, no. 1 (January 31, 2020): 142. https://doi.org/10.1186/s12889-020-8216-9.

Nelson, Cliff L., and Norman J. Temple. "Tribute to Denis Burkitt." *Journal of Medical Biography* 2, no. 3 (August 1994): 180–83.

Newton, Robert, J. Ziegler, V. Beral, E. Mbidde, L. Carpenter, H. Wabinga, S. Mbulaiteye et al. "A Case-Control Study of Human Immunodeficiency Virus Infection and Cancer in Adults and Children Residing in

Kampala, Uganda." *International Journal of Cancer* 92, no. 5 (June 1, 2001): 622–27.

Newton, Robert, John Ziegler, Dimitra Bourboulia, Delphine Casabonne, Valerie Beral, Edward Mbidde, Lucy Carpenter et al. "The Sero-Epidemiology of Kaposi's Sarcoma-Associated Herpesvirus (KSHV/HHV-8) in Adults with Cancer in Uganda." *International Journal of Cancer* 103, no. 2 (January 10, 2003): 226–32. https://doi.org/10.1002/ijc.10817.

Niyonzima, Nixon, Henry Wannume, Sylivestor Kadhumbula, Hassan Waswa, Godfrey Osinde, Yusuf Mulumba, Tobias Tusabe, Samuel Kalungi, and Jackson Orem. "Strengthening Laboratory Diagnostic Capacity to Support Cancer Care in Uganda." *American Journal of Clinical Pathology* 156, no. 2, published ahead of print, December 10, 2020. https://doi.org/10.1093/ajcp/aqaa218.

Nkrumah, F. K., and C. L. Olweny. "Clinical Features of Burkitt's Lymphoma: The African Experience." *IARC Scientific Publications* 60 (1985): 87–95.

Obayo, Siraji, Luswa Lukwago, Jackson Orem, Ashley L. Faulx, and Christopher S. Probert. "Gastrointestinal Malignancies at Five Regional Referral Hospitals in Uganda." *African Health Sciences* 17, no. 4 (December 2017): 1051–58.

Ochieng, Joseph, Erisa Mwaka, Betty Kwagala, and Nelson Sewankambo. "Evolution of Research Ethics in a Low Resource Setting: A Case for Uganda." *Developing World Bioethics* 20, no. 1 (March 2020): 50–60.

Odonga, Alexander Mwa. *The First Fifty Years of Makerere University Medical School and the Foundation of Scientific Medical Education in East Africa.* Kampala: Makerere University Medical School, 1989.

Oeppen, R. S. "Denis Parsons Burkitt (1911–1993)." *The British Journal of Oral and Maxillofacial Surgery* 41, no. 4 (August 2003): 235.

Oettgen, H. F., D. Burkitt, and J. H. Burchenal. "Malignant Lymphoma Involving the Jaw in African Children: Treatment with Methotrexate." *Cancer* 16 (May 1963): 616–23.

Okello, Clement D., Henry Ddungu, Abrahams Omoding, Andrea M. H. Towlerton, Heather Pitorak, Katie Maggard, Sarah Ewart et al. "Capacity Building for Hematologic Malignancies in Uganda: A Comprehensive Research, Training, and Care Program through the Uganda Cancer Institute-Fred Hutchinson Cancer Research Center Collaboration." *Blood Advances* 2, no. 1 (November 30, 2018): S8–10.

Okello, Clement D., Abrahams Omoding, Henry Ddungu, Yusuf Mulumba, and Jackson Orem. "Outcomes of Treatment with CHOP and EPOCH in Patients with HIV Associated NHL in a Low Resource Setting." *BMC Cancer* 20, no. 1 (August 24, 2020): 798. https://doi.org/10.1186/s12885-020-07305-2.

Okuku, Fred, Elizabeth M. Krantz, James Kafeero, Moses R. Kamya, Jackson Orem, Corey Casper, and Warren Phipps. "Evaluation of a Predictive Staging Model for HIV-Associated Kaposi Sarcoma in Uganda."

Journal of Acquired Immune Deficiency Syndromes 74, no. 5 (April 15, 2017): 548–54.

Okuku, Fred, Abrahams Omoding, Victoria Walusansa, Martin Origa, Gerald Mutungi, and Jackson Orem. "Infection-Related Cancers in Sub-Saharan Africa: A Paradigm for Cancer Prevention and Control." *Oncology* 84, no. 2 (2013): 75–80.

Okuku, Fred, Jackson Orem, George Holoya, Chris De Boer, Cheryl L. Thompson, and Matthew M. Cooney. "Prostate Cancer Burden at the Uganda Cancer Institute." *Journal of Global Oncology* 2, no. 4 (August 2016): 181–85.

Olweny, C. L. "African Trials in Chemotherapy of Gastrointestinal Cancer." *Antibiotics and Chemotherapy* 24 (1978): 139–48.

——. "Bioethics in Developing Countries: Ethics of Scarcity and Sacrifice." *Journal of Medical Ethics* 20, no. 3 (September 1994): 169–74.

——. "Effective Communication with Cancer Patients. The Use of Analogies—a Suggested Approach." *Annals of the New York Academy of Sciences* 809 (February 20, 1997): 179–87.

——. "Ethics of Palliative Care Medicine: Palliative Care for the Rich Nations Only!" *Journal of Palliative Care* 10, no. 3 (1994): 17–22.

——. "Etiology of Endemic Burkitt's Lymphoma." *IARC Scientific Publications* 63 (1984): 647–53.

——. "Etiology of Endemic Kaposi's Sarcoma." *IARC Scientific Publications* 63 (1984): 543–48.

——. "Etiology of Hepatocellular Carcinoma in Africa." *IARC Scientific Publications* 63 (1984): 89–95.

——. "Global Inequalities in Cancer Care." *Transactions of the Royal Society of Tropical Medicine and Hygiene* 85, no. 6 (December 1991): 709–10.

——. "Goals and Rationale of Cancer Treatment." *Medical Journal of Australia* 155, no. 3 (August 5, 1991): 187–92.

——. "Lymphomas and Leukaemias. Part 1: Tropical Africa." *Clinics in Haematology* 10, no. 3 (October 1981): 873–93.

——. "Management of Kaposi's Sarcoma. Chemotherapy II." *Antibiotics and Chemotherapy* 29 (1981): 88–95.

——. "Quality of Life in Cancer Care." *Medical Journal of Australia* 158, no. 6 (March 15, 1993): 429–32.

——. "Quality of Life in Developing Countries." *Journal of Palliative Care* 8, no. 3 (1992): 25–30.

——. "The Role of Cancer Registration in Developing Countries." *IARC Scientific Publications* 66 (1985): 143–52.

——. *A Rolling Stone: An Autobiography of Charles L. M. Olweny.* Kampala: Uganda Martyrs University Research Directorate, 2014.

——. "The Uganda Cancer Institute." *Oncology* 37, no. 5 (1980): 367–70.

Olweny, C. L., I. Atine, A. Kaddu-Mukasa, E. Katongole-Mbidde, S. K. Lwanga, B. Johansson, J. Onyango, H. Host, T. Norin, and B. Willey. "Cerebrospinal Irradiation of Burkitt's Lymphoma: Failure in Preventing

Central Nervous System Relapse." *Acta Radiologica: Therapy, Physics, Biology* 16, no. 3 (June 1977): 225–31.

Olweny, C. L., I. Atine, A. Kaddu-Mukasa, R. Owor, M. Andersson-Anvret, G. Klein, W. Henle, and G. de-Thé. "Epstein-Barr Virus Genome Studies in Burkitt's and Non-Burkitt's Lymphomas in Uganda." *Journal of the National Cancer Institute* 58, no. 5 (May 1977): 1191–96.

Olweny, C. L., Margaret Borok, Ivy Gudza, Jennifer Clinch, Mary Cheang, Clem F. Kiire, Lorraine Levy, David Otim-Oyet, Joseph Nyamasve, and Harvey Schipper. "Treatment of AIDS-Associated Kaposi's Sarcoma in Zimbabwe: Results of a Randomized Quality of Life Focused Clinical Trial." *International Journal of Cancer* 113, no. 4 (February 10, 2005): 632–39.

Olweny, C. L., M. S. R. Hutt, and R. Owor. *Kaposi's Sarcoma: 2nd Symposium, Kampala, January 8–11, 1980.* Basel: Karger, 1981.

Olweny, C. L., C. A. Juttner, P. Rofe, G. Barrow, A. Esterman, R. Waltham, E. Abdi, H. Chesterman, R. Seshadri, and E. Sage. "Long-Term Effects of Cancer Treatment and Consequences of Cure: Cancer Survivors Enjoy Quality of Life Similar to Their Neighbours." *European Journal of Cancer* 29A, no. 6 (1993): 826–30.

Olweny, C. L., A. Kaddumukasa, I. Atine, R. Owor, I. Magrath, and J. L. Ziegler. "Childhood Kaposi's Sarcoma: Clinical Features and Therapy." *British Journal of Cancer* 33, no. 5 (May 1976): 555–60.

Olweny, C. L., E. Katongole-Mbidde, S. Bahendeka, D. Otim, J. Mugerwa, and S. K. Kyalwazi. "Further Experience in Treating Patients with Hepatocellular Carcinoma in Uganda." *Cancer* 46, no. 12 (December 15, 1980): 2717–22.

Olweny, C. L., E. Katongole-Mbidde, A. Kaddu-Mukasa, I. Atine, R. Owor, S. Lwanga, W. Carswell, and I. T. Magrath. "Treatment of Burkitt's Lymphoma: Randomized Clinical Trial of Single-Agent versus Combination Chemotherapy." *International Journal of Cancer* 17, no. 4 (April 15, 1976): 436–40.

Olweny, C. L., E. Katongole-Mbidde, C. Kiire, S. K. Lwanga, I. Magrath, and J. L. Ziegler. "Childhood Hodgkin's Disease in Uganda: A Ten Year Experience." *Cancer* 42, no. 2 (August 1978): 787–92.

Olweny, C. L., E. Katongole-Mbidde, D. Otim, S. K. Lwanga, I. T. Magrath, and J. L. Ziegler. "Long-Term Experience with Burkitt's Lymphoma in Uganda." *International Journal of Cancer* 26, no. 3 (1980): 261–66.

Olweny, C. L., E. K. Mbidde, J. Nkwocha, I. Magrath, and J. L. Ziegler. "Letter: Chemotherapy of Hodgkin's Disease." *Lancet* 2, no. 7893 (December 7, 1974): 1397.

Olweny, C. L., Cecilia Sepulveda, Anne Merriman, Sharon Fonn, Margaret Borok, Twalibu Ngoma, Anderson Doh, and Jan Stjernsward. "Desirable Services and Guidelines for the Treatment and Palliative Care of HIV Disease Patients with Cancer in Africa: A World Health Organization Consultation." *Journal of Palliative Care* 19, no. 3 (2003): 198–205.

Olweny, C. L., W. Sikyewunda, and D. Otim. "Further Experience with Rezoxane (ICRF 159; — NSC—129943) in Treating Kaposi's Sarcoma." *Oncology* 37, no. 3 (1980): 174–76.

Olweny, C. L., T. Toya, E. Katongole-Mbidde, J. Mugerwa, S. K. Kyalwazi, and H. Cohen. "Treatment of Hepatocellular Carcinoma with Adriamycin. Preliminary Communication." *Cancer* 36, no. 4 (October 1975): 1250–57.

Olweny, C. L., T. Toya, E. K. Mbidde, and S. K. Lwanga. "Treatment of Kaposi's Sarcoma by Combination of Actinomycin-D, Vincristine and Imidazole Carboxamide (Nsc-45388): Results of a Randomized Clinical Trial." *International Journal of Cancer* 14, no. 5 (November 15, 1974): 649–56.

Olweny, C. L., and John L. Ziegler. "Chemotherapy plus Involved-Field Radiation in Early-Stage Hodgkin's Disease." *New England Journal of Medicine* 358, no. 7 (February 14, 2008): 742; author reply 743.

———. "Treatment of Histiocytic Lymphoma in Uganda Adults." *East African Medical Journal* 48, no. 10 (October 1971): 585–91.

Olweny, C. L., J. L. Ziegler, C. W. Berard, and A. C. Templeton. "Adult Hodgkin's Disease in Uganda." *Cancer* 27, no. 6 (June 1971): 1295–1301.

Oni, Tolu, and Bongani M. Mayosi. "Mortality Trends in South Africa: Progress in the Shadow of HIV/AIDS and Apartheid." *Lancet Global Health* 4, no. 9 (September 2016): e588–e89.

Orem, Jackson. "Cancer Prevention and Control: Kaposi's Sarcoma." *Ecancermedicalscience* 13 (2019): 951. https://doi.org/10.3332/ecancer.2019.951.

Orem, Jackson, Albert Maganda, Edward Katongole Mbidde, and Elisabete Weiderpass. "Clinical Characteristics and Outcome of Children with Burkitt Lymphoma in Uganda According to HIV Infection." *Pediatric Blood and Cancer* 52, no. 4 (April 2009): 455–58.

Orem, Jackson, Billy Mayanja, Martin Okongo, and Dilys Morgan. "Strongyloides Stercoralis Hyperinfection in a Patient with AIDS in Uganda Successfully Treated with Ivermectin." *Clinical Infectious Diseases: An Official Publication of the Infectious Diseases Society of America* 37, no. 1 (July 1, 2003): 152–53. https://doi.org/10.1086/375609.

Orem, Jackson, Edward Katongole Mbidde, Bo Lambert, Silvia de Sanjose, and Elisabete Weiderpass. "Burkitt's Lymphoma in Africa, a Review of the Epidemiology and Etiology." *African Health Sciences* 7, no. 3 (September 2007): 166–75.

Orem, Jackson, Edward Katongole Mbidde, and Elisabete Weiderpass. "Current Investigations and Treatment of Burkitt's Lymphoma in Africa." *Tropical Doctor* 38, no. 1 (January 2008): 7–11.

Orem, Jackson, Yusuf Mulumba, Sara Algeri, Rino Bellocco, Fred Wabwire Mangen, Edward Katongole Mbidde, and Elisabete Weiderpass. "Clinical Characteristics, Treatment and Outcome of Childhood Burkitt's Lymphoma at the Uganda Cancer Institute." *Transactions of the Royal Society of Tropical Medicine and Hygiene* 105, no. 12 (December 2011): 717–26.

Orem, Jackson, Mwanda W. Otieno, Cecily Banura, Edward Katongole-Mbidde, John L. Johnson, Leona Ayers, Mahmoud Ghannoum et al. "Capacity Building for the Clinical Investigation of AIDS Malignancy in East Africa." *Cancer Detection and Prevention* 29, no. 2 (2005): 133–45.

Orem, Jackson, Mwanda W. Otieno, and Scot C. Remick. "AIDS-Associated Cancer in Developing Nations." *Current Opinion in Oncology* 16, no. 5 (September 2004): 468–76.

Orem, Jackson, Sven Sandin, Edward Mbidde, Fred Wabwire Mangen, Jaap Middeldorp, and Elisabete Weiderpass. "Epstein-Barr Virus Viral Load and Serology in Childhood Non-Hodgkin's Lymphoma and Chronic Inflammatory Conditions in Uganda: Implications for Disease Risk and Characteristics." *Journal of Medical Virology* 86, no. 10 (October 2014): 1796–1803.

Orem, Jackson, Sven Sandin, Caroline E. Weibull, Michael Odida, Henry Wabinga, Edward Mbidde, Fred Wabwire-Mangen, Chris Jlm Meijer, Jaap M. Middeldorp, and Elisabete Weiderpass. "Agreement between Diagnoses of Childhood Lymphoma Assigned in Uganda and by an International Reference Laboratory." *Clinical Epidemiology* 4 (2012): 339–47.

Orem, Jackson, and Henry Wabinga. "The Roles of National Cancer Research Institutions in Evolving a Comprehensive Cancer Control Program in a Developing Country: Experience from Uganda." *Oncology* 77, no. 5 (2009): 272–80.

Otieno, Mwanda W., Cecily Banura, Edward Katongole-Mbidde, John L. Johnson, Mahmoud Ghannoum, Afshin Dowlati, Rolf Renne et al. "Therapeutic Challenges of AIDS-Related Non-Hodgkin's Lymphoma in the United States and East Africa." *Journal of the National Cancer Institute* 94, no. 10 (May 15, 2002): 718–32.

Papac, Rose. "Origins of Cancer Therapy." *Yale Journal of Biology and Medicine* 74 (2001): 391–98.

Parkin, D. M., J. Ferlay, M. Hamdi-Cherif, F. Sitas, J. Thomas, H. Wabinga, and S. L. Whelan, eds. *Cancer in Africa: Epidemiology and Prevention.* Lyon: International Agency for Research on Cancer, 2003.

Parkin, D. M., H. Garcia-Giannoli, M. Raphael, A. Martin, E. Katangole-Mbidde, H. Wabinga, and J. Ziegler. "Non-Hodgkin Lymphoma in Uganda: A Case-Control Study." *AIDS* 14, no. 18 (December 22, 2000): 2929–36.

Parkin, D. M., F. Sitas, M. Chirenje, L. Stein, R. Abratt, and H. Wabinga. "Part I: Cancer in Indigenous Africans—Burden, Distribution, and Trends." *Lancet Oncology* 9, no. 7 (2008): 683–92.

Pfaller, M., J. Zhang, S. Messer, M. Tumberland, E. Mbidde, C. Jessup, M. Ghannoum. "Molecular Epidemiology and Antifungal Susceptibility of *Cryptococcus neoformans* Isolates from Ugandan AIDS Patients." *Mycology* 32 (1988): 191–99.

Phipps, Warren, Rachel Kansiime, Philip Stevenson, Jackson Orem, Corey Casper, and Rhoda A. Morrow. "Peer Mentoring at the Uganda Cancer

Institute: A Novel Model for Career Development of Clinician-Scientists in Resource-Limited Settings." *Journal of Global Oncology* 4 (September 2018): 1–11.

Phipps, Warren, Edith Nakku-Joloba, Elizabeth M. Krantz, Stacy Selke, Meei-Li Huang, Fred Kambugu, Jackson Orem, Corey Casper, Lawrence Corey, and Anna Wald. "Genital Herpes Simplex Virus Type 2 Shedding among Adults with and without HIV Infection in Uganda." *Journal of Infectious Diseases* 213, no. 3 (February 1, 2016): 439–47.

Phipps, Warren, Fred Ssewankambo, Huong Nguyen, Misty Saracino, Anna Wald, Lawrence Corey, Jackson Orem, Andrew Kambugu, and Corey Casper. "Gender Differences in Clinical Presentation and Outcomes of Epidemic Kaposi Sarcoma in Uganda." *PloS One* 5, no. 11 (November 12, 2010): e13936. https://doi.org/10.1371/journal.pone.0013936.

Pittman, K. B., C. L. Olweny, J. B. North, and P. C. Blumbergs. "Primary Central Nervous System Lymphoma. A Report of 9 Cases and Review of the Literature." *Oncology* 48, no. 3 (1991): 184–87.

Primack, A., C. L. Vogel, S. K. Kyalwazi, J. L. Ziegler, R. Simon, and P. P. Anthony. "A Staging System for Hepatocellular Carcinoma: Prognostic Factors in Ugandan Patients." *Cancer* 35, no. 5 (May 1975): 1357–64.

Purvis, S. F., E. Katongole-Mbidde, J. L. Johnson, D. G. Leonard, N. Byabazaire, C. Luckey, H. E. Schick, R. Wallis, C. A. Elmets, and C. Z. Giam. "High Incidence of Kaposi's Sarcoma-Associated Herpesvirus and Epstein-Barr Virus in Tumor Lesions and Peripheral Blood Mononuclear Cells from Patients with Kaposi's Sarcoma in Uganda." *Journal of Infectious Diseases* 175, no. 4 (April 1997): 947–50.

Rawat, Angeli, Catherine Sanders, Nadia Mithani, Catherine Amuge, Heather Pedersen, Ruth Namugosa, Beth Payne et al. "Acceptability and Preferences for Self-Collected Screening for Cervical Cancer within Health Systems in Rural Uganda: A Mixed-Methods Approach." *International Journal of Gynaecology and Obstetrics: The Official Organ of the International Federation of Gynaecology and Obstetrics* 152, no. 1(January 2021): 103–11. https://doi.org/10.1002/ijgo.13454.

Reece, P. A., I. Stafford, R. L. Abbott, C. Anderson, J. Denham, S. Freeman, R. G. Morris, P. G. Gill, and C. L. Olweny. "Two- versus 24-Hour Infusion of Cisplatin: Pharmacokinetic Considerations." *Journal of Clinical Oncology: Official Journal of the American Society of Clinical Oncology* 7, no. 2 (February 1989): 270–75.

Riley, J. P., G. A. Pestano, K. Hosford, C. Francis, J. M. Xie, P. Mugyenyi, P. Kataaha, E. Katongole-Mbidde, W. W. Anokbonggo, and J. Guyden. "Relative Reactivity of the V3 Loop PND of HIV-1 Subtypes A, B, C, D, and F with Sera from Selected Ugandan Localities." *Archives of Virology* 140, no. 8 (1995): 1393–1404.

Rochford, R., G. Feuer, J. Orem, C. Banura, E. Katongole-Mbidde, W. O. Mwanda, A. Moormann, W. J. Harrington, and S. C. Remick. "Strategies to Overcome Myelotoxic Therapy for the Treatment of Burkitt's and AIDS-Related Non-Hodgkin's Lymphoma." *East African Medical Journal* 82, no. 9 (September 2005): S155–60.

Rose, Timothy M., A. Gregory Bruce, Serge Barcy, Matt Fitzgibbon, Lisa R. Matsumoto, Minako Ikoma, Corey Casper, Jackson Orem, and Warren Phipps. "Quantitative RNAseq Analysis of Ugandan KS Tumors Reveals KSHV Gene Expression Dominated by Transcription from the LTd Downstream Latency Promoter." *PLoS Pathogens* 14, no. 12 (December 2018): e1007441. https://doi.org/10.1371/journal.ppat.1007441.

Sacks, K. L., C. Olweny, D. L. Mann, R. Simon, G. E. Johnson, D. G. Poplack, and B. G. Leventhal. "A Clinical Trial of Chemotherapy and RAJI Immunotherapy in Advanced Acute Lymphatic Leukemia." *Cancer Research* 35, no. 12 (December 1975): 3715–20.

Scheel, John R., Mahbod J. Giglou, Sophie Segel, Jackson Orem, Vivien Tsu, Moses Galukande, Jimmy Okello et al. "Breast Cancer Early Detection and Diagnostic Capacity in Uganda." *Cancer* 126, no. 10 (May 15, 2020): S2469–80.

Scheel, John R., Erika M. Nealey, Jackson Orem, Samuel Bugeza, Zeridah Muyinda, Robert O. Nathan, Peggy L. Porter, and Constance D. Lehman. "ACR BI-RADS Use in Low-Income Countries: An Analysis of Diagnostic Breast Ultrasound Practice in Uganda." *Journal of the American College of Radiology: JACR* 13, no. 2 (February 2016): 163–69.

Scheel, John R., Sue Peacock, Jackson Orem, Samuel Bugeza, Zeridah Muyinda, Peggy L. Porter, William C. Wood, Robert L. Comis, and Constance D. Lehman. "Improving Breast Ultrasound Interpretation in Uganda Using a Condensed Breast Imaging Reporting and Data System." *Academic Radiology* 23, no. 10 (October 2016): 1271–77.

Serwadda, D., and E. Katongole-Mbidde. "AIDS in Africa: Problems for Research and Researchers." *Lancet* 335, no. 8693 (April 7, 1990): 842–43.

Serwadda, D., N. K. Sewankambo, J. W. Carswell, A. C. Bayley, R.S. Tedder, R. A. Weiss, R. D. Mugerwa et al. "Slim Disease: A New Disease in Uganda and Its Association with HTLV-III Infection." *Lancet* 2 (1985): 849–52.

Sherins, R. J., C. L. Olweny, and J. L. Ziegler. "Gynecomastia and Gonadal Dysfunction in Adolescent Boys Treated with Combination Chemotherapy for Hodgkin's Disease." *New England Journal of Medicine* 299, no. 1 (July 6, 1978): 12–16.

Shulman, Lawrence N., Tharcisse Mpunga, Neo Tapela, Claire M. Wagner, Temidayo Fadelu, and Agnes Binagwaho. "Bringing Cancer Care to the Poor: Experiences from Rwanda." *Nature Reviews Cancer* 14 (2014): 815–21.

Smith, Owen. "Denis Parsons Burkitt CMG, MD, DSc, FRS, FRCS, FTCD (1911–93) Irish by Birth, Trinity by the Grace of God." *British Journal of Haematology* 156, no. 6 (March 2012): 770–76.

Song, Xiaoling, Pho Diep, Jeannette M. Schenk, Corey Casper, Jackson Orem, Zeina Makhoul, Johanna W. Lampe, and Marian L. Neuhouser. "Changes in Relative and Absolute Concentrations of Plasma Phospholipid Fatty Acids Observed in a Randomized Trial of Omega-3 Fatty Acids Supplementation in Uganda." *Prostaglandins, Leukotrienes, and Essential Fatty Acids* 114 (November 2016): 11–16.

"Special Issue: Burkitt's Lymphoma." *British Journal of Haematology* 156 (2012): 689–783.

Ssebbanja, Peter Kitonsa. *United Against AIDS: The Story of TASO.* Oxford: Strategies for Hope Trust, 2007.

Ssemwanga, Deogratius, Juliet Asio, Christine Watera, Maria Nannyonjo, Faridah Nassolo, Sandra Lunkuse, Jesus F. Salazar-Gonzalez et al. "Prevalence of Viral Load Suppression, Predictors of Virological Failure and Patterns of HIV Drug Resistance after 12 and 48 Months on First-Line Antiretroviral Therapy: A National Cross-Sectional Survey in Uganda." *Journal of Antimicrobial Chemotherapy* 75, no. 5 (May 1, 2020): 1280–89.

Story, Jon A., and David Kritchevsky. "Denis Parsons Burkitt." *Journal of Nutrition* 124 (1994): 1551–54.

Sutherland, J. C., C. L. Olweny, P. H. Levine, and M. R. Mardiney. "Epstein-Barr Virus-Immune Complexes in Postmortem Kidneys from African Patients with Burkitt's Lymphoma and American Patients with and without Lymphoma." *Journal of the National Cancer Institute* 60, no. 5 (May 1978): 941–46.

Taylor, J. F., A. C. Templeton, C. L. Vogel, J. L. Ziegler, and S. K. Kyalwazi. "Kaposi's Sarcoma in Uganda: A Clinico-Pathological Study." *International Journal of Cancer* 8, no. 1 (July 15, 1971): 122–35.

Templeton, A. C. *Tumors in a Tropical Country: A Survey of Uganda 1964–1968.* New York: Springer-Verlag, 1973.

Tornesello, Maria Lina, Benon Biryahwaho, Robert Downing, Angelo Hatzakis, Elvio Alessi, Marco Cusini, Vincenzo Ruocco et al. "Human Herpesvirus Type 8 Variants Circulating in Europe, Africa and North America in Classic, Endemic and Epidemic Kaposi's Sarcoma Lesions during Pre-AIDS and AIDS Era." *Virology* 398, no. 2 (March 15, 2010): 280–89.

Tornesello, Maria Lina, Luigi Buonaguro, Medea Cristillo, Bennon Biryahwaho, Robert Downing, Angelo Hatzakis, Elvio Alessi et al. "MDM2 and CDKN1A Gene Polymorphisms and Risk of Kaposi's Sarcoma in African and Caucasian Patients." *Biomarkers: Biochemical Indicators of Exposure, Response, and Susceptibility to Chemicals* 16, no. 1 (February 2011): 42–50.

Tumwine, Lynnette K., Rejani Lalitha, Claudio Agostinelli, Simon Luzige, Jackson Orem, Pier Paolo Piccaluga, Lawrence O. Osuwat, and Stefano A. Pileri. "Primary Effusion Lymphoma Associated with Human Herpes Virus-8 and Epstein Barr Virus in an HIV-Infected Woman from Kampala, Uganda: A Case Report." *Journal of Medical Case Reports* 5 (February 14, 2011): 60.

Tumwine, Lynnette K., Jackson Orem, Patrick Kerchan, Wilson Byarugaba, and Stefano A. Pileri. "EBV, HHV8 and HIV in B Cell Non-Hodgkin Lymphoma in Kampala, Uganda." *Infectious Agents and Cancer* 5 (June 30, 2010): 12.

Tumwine, Lynette K., Jackson Orem, and Leona W. Ayers. "EBV-Positive Grey Zone Lymphoma in an HIV Infected Man from Kampala, Uganda: Case Report." *International Journal of Medical and Pharmaceutical Case Reports* 2, no. 5 (November 15, 2014): 110–16.

Ulrickson, Matthew, Fred Okuku, Victoria Walusansa, Oliver Press, Sam Kalungi, David Wu, Fred Kambugu, Corey Casper, and Jackson Orem. "Cutaneous T-Cell Lymphoma in Sub-Saharan Africa." *Journal of the National Comprehensive Cancer Network: JNCCN* 11, no. 3 (March 1, 2013): 275–80.

Waalkes, T. P., C. W. Gehrke, W. A. Bleyer, R. W. Zumwalt, C. L. Olweny, K. C. Kuo, D. B. Lakings, and S. A. Jacobs. "Potential Biologic Markers in Burkitt's Lymphoma." *Cancer Chemotherapy Reports* 59, no. 4 (August 1975): 721–27.

Wabinga, Henry R., Sarah Nambooze, Phoebe Mary Amulen, Catherine Okello, Louise Mbus, and Donald Maxwell Parkin. "Trends in the Incidence of Cancer in Kampala, Uganda 1991–2010." *International Journal of Cancer* 135 (2014): 432–39.

Walusansa, Victoria, Fred Okuku, and Jackson Orem. "Burkitt Lymphoma in Uganda, the Legacy of Denis Burkitt and an Update on the Disease Status." *British Journal of Haematology* 156, no. 6 (March 2012): 757–60.

Ward, Robert, Saul Krugman, Joan P. Giles, A. Milton Jacobs, and Oscar Bodansky. "Infectious Hepatitis." *New England Journal of Medicine* 258, no. 9 (February 27, 1958): 407–16.

Yu, Jing Jie, Pingfu Fu, John J. Pink, Dawn Dawson, Jay Wasman, Jackson Orem, Walter O. Mwanda et al. "HPV Infection and EGFR Activation/Alteration in HIV-Infected East African Patients with Conjunctival Carcinoma." *PloS One* 5, no. 5 (May 17, 2010): e10477.

Ziegler, John L. "Early Studies of Burkitt's Tumor in Africa." *American Journal of Pediatric Hematology/Oncology* 8, no. 1 (1986): 63–65.

——. "Into and Out of Africa—Taking Over from Denis Burkitt." *British Journal of Haematology* 156, no. 6 (March 2012): 766–69.

——. "Treatment Results of 54 American Patients with Burkitt's Lymphoma Are Similar to the African Experience." *New England Journal of Medicine* 297, no. 2 (July 14, 1977): 75–80.

Ziegler, John L., L. Fass, A. Z. Bluming, I. T. Magrath, and A. C. Templeton. "Chemotherapy of Childhood Hodgkin's Disease in Uganda." *Lancet* 2, no. 7779 (September 30, 1972): 679–82.

Ziegler, John L., and E. Katongole-Mbidde. "Diminished Delayed Hypersensitivity Responses in the Legs and Feet of Patients with Endemic Kaposi's Sarcoma." *Transactions of the Royal Society of Tropical Medicine and Hygiene* 90, no. 2 (April 1996): 173–74.

———. "Kaposi's Sarcoma in Childhood: An Analysis of 100 Cases from Uganda and Relationship to HIV Infection." *International Journal of Cancer* 65, no. 2 (January 17, 1996): 200–203.

Ziegler, John L., I. T. Magrath, and C. L. Olweny. "Cure of Burkitt's Lymphoma. Ten-Year Follow-Up of 157 Ugandan Patients." *Lancet* 2, no. 8149 (November 3, 1979): 936–38.

Ziegler, John L., and Daniel G. Miller. "Lymphosarcoma Resembling the Burkitt Tumor in a Connecticut Girl." *JAMA* 198, no. 10 (1966): 1071–73.

Ziegler, John L., R. H. Morrow, L. Fass, S. K. Kyalwazi, and P. P. Carbone. "Treatment of Burkitt's Tumor with Cyclophosphamide." *Cancer* 26, no. 2 (August 1970): 474–84.

Ziegler, John L., R. H. Morrow, A. C. Templeton, C. Templeton, A. Z. Bluming, L. Fass, and S. K. Kyalwazi. "Clinical Features and Treatment of Childhood Malignant Lymphoma in Uganda." *International Journal of Cancer* 5, no. 3 (May 15, 1970): 415–25.

Ziegler, John L., Robert Newton, Dimitra Bourboulia, Delphine Casabonne, Valerie Beral, Edward Mbidde, Lucy Carpenter et al. "Risk Factors for Kaposi's Sarcoma: A Case-Control Study of HIV-Seronegative People in Uganda." *International Journal of Cancer* 103, no. 2 (January 10, 2003): 233–40.

Ziegler, John L., R. Newton, E. Katongole-Mbidde, S. Mbulataiye, K. De Cock, H. Wabinga, J. Mugerwa et al. "Risk Factors for Kaposi's Sarcoma in HIV-Positive Subjects in Uganda." *AIDS* 11, no. 13 (November 1997): 1619–26.

Ziegler, John L., T. Simonart, and R. Snoeck. "Kaposi's Sarcoma, Oncogenic Viruses, and Iron." *Journal of Clinical Virology: The Official Publication of the Pan American Society for Clinical Virology* 20, no. 3 (February 2001): 127–30.

PUBLISHED WORKS IN THE HUMANITIES AND SOCIAL SCIENCES

Abadie, Roberto. *The Professional Guinea Pig: Big Pharma and the Risky World of Human Subjects.* Durham, NC: Duke University Press, 2010.

Abdullah, Ibrahim, and Ismail Rashid. *Understanding West Africa's Ebola Epidemic: Towards a Political Economy.* London: Bloomsbury Academic, 2017.

Adas, Michael. *Domination by Design: Technological Imperatives and America's Civilizing Mission.* Cambridge, MA: Harvard University Press, 2009.

———. *Machines as the Measure of Men: Science, Technology, and Ideologies of Western Dominance.* Ithaca, NY: Cornell University Press, 1989.

Akrich, Madeleine. "The De-scription of Technical Objects." In *Shaping Technology/Building Society: Studies in Sociotechnical Change*, edited by Wiebe E. Bijker and John Law, 205–24. Cambridge, MA: MIT Press, 1992.

Allen, Tim, and Koen Vlassentoot, eds. *The Lord's Resistance Army: Myth and Reality.* London: Zed, 2010.

Allman, Jean. "Phantoms of the Archive: Kwame Nkrumah, a Nazi Pilot Named Hanna, and the Contingencies of Postcolonial History-Writing." *American Historical Review* 118 (2013): 104–29.

Anand, Nikhil. *Hydraulic City: Water and the Infrastructures of Citizenship in Mumbai.* Durham, NC: Duke University Press, 2017.

———. "Pressure: The PoliTechnics of Water Supply in Mumbai." *Cultural Anthropology* 26 (2011): 542–64.

Anand, Nikhil, Akhil Gupta, and Hannah Appel. *The Promise of Infrastructure.* Durham, NC: Duke University Press, 2018.

Anderson, Benedict. *Imagined Communities.* New York: Verso, 2006.

Anderson, David. *Histories of the Hanged.* New York: Norton, 2005.

Anderson, Warwick. *The Collectors of Lost Souls: Turning Kuru Scientists into Whitemen.* Baltimore: Johns Hopkins University Press, 2008.

———. "Introduction: Postcolonial Technoscience." *Social Studies of Science* 32, nos. 5–6 (2002): 643–58.

———. "Making Global Health History: The Postcolonial Worldliness of Biomedicine." *Social History of Medicine* 27, no. 2 (May 1, 2014): 372–84.

———. "Postcolonial History of Medicine." In *Locating Medical History: The Stories and Their Meanings,* edited by Frank Huisman and John Harley Warner, 285–306. Baltimore: Johns Hopkins University Press, 2004.

Anguria, Omongole R., ed. *Apollo Milton Obote: What Others Say.* Kampala: Fountain, 2006.

Appel, Hannah C. "Walls and White Elephants: Oil Extraction, Responsibility, and Infrastructural Violence in Equatorial Guinea." *Ethnography* 13, no. 4 (December 1, 2012): 439–65.

Arnold, David. *Colonizing the Body: State Medicine and Epidemic Disease in Nineteenth-Century India.* Berkeley: University of California Press, 1993.

———. *Everyday Technology: Machines and the Making of India's Modernity.* Chicago: University of Chicago Press, 2013.

Aronowitz, Robert. *Unnatural History: Breast Cancer and American Society.* New York: Cambridge University Press, 2007.

Asad, Talal. "Ethnographic Representation, Statistics, and Modern Power." In *From the Margins: Historical Anthropology and Its Futures,* edited by Brian Keith Axel, 66–94. Durham, NC: Duke University Press, 2002.

Asiimwe, Godfrey. "Of Extensive and Elusive Corruption in Uganda: Neo-patronage, Power, and Narrow Interests." *African Studies Review* 56, no. 2 (2013): 129–44.

———. *The Impact of Post-colonial Policy Shifts in Coffee Marketing at the Local Level in Uganda: A Case Study of Mukono District, 1962–1998.* London: Shaker, 2002.

Auyero, Javier. *Patients of the State: The Politics of Waiting in Argentina.* Durham, NC: Duke University Press, 2012.

Avirgan, Tony, and Martha Honey. *War in Uganda: The Legacy of Idi Amin.* Westport, CT: Lawrence Hill, 1982.

Banerjee, Dwaipayan. "Cancer and Secrecy in Contemporary India." *BioSocieties* 14, no. 4 (December 1, 2019): 496–511.

——. *Enduring Cancer: Life, Death, and Diagnosis in Delhi.* Durham, NC: Duke University Press, 2020.

Barrett-Gaines, Kathryn, and Lynn Khadiagala. "Finding What You Need in Uganda's Archives." *History in Africa* 27 (2000): 455–70.

Bayart, Jean-Francois. *The State in Africa: The Politics of the Belly.* Malden, MA: Polity, 2010.

Benton, Adia. "The Epidemic Will Be Militarized: Watching Outbreak as the West African Ebola Epidemic Unfolds." *Fieldsights*, October 7, 2014. https://culanth.org/fieldsights/the-epidemic-will-be-militarized-watching-outbreak-as-the-west-african-ebola-epidemic-unfolds.

——. *HIV Exceptionalism: Development through Disease in Sierra Leone.* Minneapolis: University of Minnesota Press, 2015.

——. "Whose Security? Militarization and Securitization during West Africa's Ebola Outbreak." *The Politics of Fear: Médecins sans Frontières and the West African Ebola Epidemic,* edited by Michiel Hofman and Sokhieng Au, 25–50. New York: Oxford University Press, 2017.

Berry, Sara. *Fathers Work for Their Sons.* Berkeley: University of California Press, 1985.

——. *No Condition Is Permanent.* Madison: University of Wisconsin Press, 1993.

——. "Social Institutions and Access to Resources." *Africa* 59, no. 1 (1989): 41–55.

Biehl, João Guilherme. *Will to Live: AIDS Therapies and the Politics of Survival.* Princeton, NJ: Princeton University Press, 2007.

Biehl, João Guilherme, and Adriana Petryna. *When People Come First: Critical Studies in Global Health.* Princeton, NJ: Princeton University Press, 2013.

Bijker, Wiebe E., Thomas P. Hughes, and Trevor Pinch, eds. *The Social Construction of Technological Systems: New Directions in the Sociology and History of Technology.* Cambridge, MA: MIT Press, 2012.

Biruk, Cal (Crystal). *Cooking Data: Culture and Politics in an African Research World.* Durham, NC: Duke University Press, 2018.

——. "Studying Up in Critical NGO Studies Today: Reflections on Critique and the Distribution of Interpretive Labour." *Critical African Studies* 8, no. 3 (September 1, 2016): 291–305.

Biruk, Cal (Crystal), and Ramah McKay. "Introduction." *Medicine Anthropology Theory* 6, no. 2 (May 14, 2019). https://doi.org/10.17157/mat.6.2.718.

Bledsoe, Caroline. *Contingent Lives: Fertility, Time, and Aging in West Africa.* Chicago: University of Chicago Press, 2002.

Bond, George C., and Joan Vincent. "Living on the Edge: Changing Social Structures in the Context of AIDS." In *Changing Uganda: The Dilemmas* of *Structural Adjustment and Revolutionary Change*, edited by Hölger Bernt Hansen and Michael Twaddle, 113–29. London: J. Currey, 1991.

Bourdieu, Pierre. *Outline of a Theory of Practice*. New York: Cambridge University Press, 1977.

Bowker, Gregory C., and Susan L. Star. *Sorting Things Out: Classification and Its Consequences*. Cambridge, MA: MIT Press, 1999.

Branch, Adam. *Displacing Human Rights: War and Intervention in Northern Uganda*. Oxford: Oxford University Press, 2011.

Brandt, Allan M. *The Cigarette Century: The Rise, Fall, and Deadly Persistence of the Product That Defined America*. New York: Basic Books, 2009.

——. *No Magic Bullet: A Social History of Venereal Disease in the United States since 1880* (Oxford: Oxford University Press, 1987).

Brandt, Allan M., and David C. Sloane. "Of Beds and Benches: Building the Modern American Hospital." In *The Architecture of Science*, edited by Peter Gallison and Emily Thompson, 281–305. Cambridge, MA: MIT Press, 1999.

Breckenridge, Keith. *Biometric State: The Global Politics of Identification and Surveillance in South Africa, 1850 to the Present*. Cambridge: Cambridge University Press, 2014.

Bruce-Lockhart, Katherine. "The Archival Afterlives of Prison Officers in Idi Amin's Uganda: Writing Social Histories of the Postcolonial State." *History in Africa* 45 (June 2018): 245–74.

Butt, Leslie. "The Suffering Stranger: Medical Anthropology and International Morality." *Medical Anthropology* 21, no. 1 (January 1, 2002): 1–24.

Caduff, Carlo, and Cecilia C. Van Hollen. "Cancer and the Global South." *BioSocieties* 14, no. 4 (December 1, 2019): 489–95. https://doi.org/10.1057/s41292-019-00175-3.

Chabal, Patrick. *Africa: The Politics of Suffering and Smiling*. London: Zed, 2009.

Chabal, Patrick, and John-Pascal Daloz. *Africa Works: Disorder as Political Instrument*. Bloomington: Indiana University Press, 1999.

Chalfin, Brenda. *Neoliberal Frontiers: An Ethnography of Sovereignty in West Africa*. Chicago: University of Chicago Press, 2010.

Chigudu, Simukai. *The Political Life of an Epidemic: Cholera, Crisis and Citizenship in Zimbabwe*. Cambridge: Cambridge University Press, 2020.

Cohen, David William, and E. S. Atieno Odhiambo. *Siaya: The Historical Anthropology of an African Landscape*. Oxford: J. Curry, 1989.

Comaroff, Jean. "Beyond Bare Life: Aids (Bio)Politics, and the Neoliberal Order." *Public Culture* 19, no. 1 (2007): 197–219.

Comaroff, Jean, and John L. Comaroff. *Theory from the South, or, How Euro-America Is Evolving around Africa*. Boulder, CO: Paradigm, 2012.

Conrad, Pete. *The Medicalization of Society: On the Transformation of Human Conditions into Treatable Disorders*. Baltimore: Johns Hopkins University Press, 2007.

Cook, Sir Albert Ruskin. *Uganda Memories, 1897–1940.* Kampala: Uganda Society, 1945.

Cooper, Frederick. *Africa since 1940: The Past of the Present.* New Approaches to African History. New York: Cambridge University Press, 2002.

——. *Africa in the World: Capitalism, Empire, Nation-State.* Cambridge, MA: Harvard University Press, 2014.

Cooper, Frederick, and Randall M. Packard. *International Development and the Social Sciences: Essays on the History and Politics of Knowledge.* Berkeley: University of California Press, 1997.

Cooper, Orah, and Carol Fogarty. "Soviet Economic and Military Aid to the Less Developed Countries, 1954–78." *Soviet and Eastern European Foreign Trade* 2, nos. 1–3 (1985): 54–73.

Corti, Piero, and Lucille Teasdale. *To Make a Dream Come True: Letters from Lacor Hospital Uganda.* Bergamo, Italy: Corponove Editrice, 2009.

Coser, Rose Laub. *Life in the Ward.* East Lansing: Michigan State University Press, 1962.

Crane, Johanna Tayloe. *Scrambling for Africa: AIDS, Expertise, and the Rise of American Global Health Science.* Ithaca, NY: Cornell University Press, 2013.

Crozier, Anna. *Practicing Colonial Medicine: The Colonial Medical Service in British East Africa.* London: I. B. Taurus, 2007.

Cummiskey, Julia R. "Early AIDS Research in Rakai: Ugandan Experiences and Expertise in the Creation of the African AIDS Paradigm." *International Journal of African Historical Studies* 53, no. 1 (2020): 1–26.

——. "'An Ecological Experiment on the Grand Scale': Creating an Experimental Field in Bwamba, Uganda, 1942–1950." *Isis* 111, no. 1 (March 1, 2020): 3–21.

Das, Veena. *Critical Events: An Anthropological Perspective on Contemporary India.* Oxford: Oxford University Press, 1997.

D'avignon, Robyn. "Primitive Techniques: From 'Customary' to 'Artisinal' Mining in French West Africa." *Journal of African History* 59, no. 2 (July 2018): 179–97. https://doi.org/10.1017/S0021853718000361.

——. "Spirited Geobodies: Producing Subterranean Property in Nineteenth-Century Bambuk, West Africa." *Technology and Culture* 61, no. 2 (2020): S20–48. https://doi.org/10.1353/tech.2020.0069.

Dawe, Jennifer Ann. "History of Cotton Growing in East and Central Africa: British Demand, African Supply." PhD diss., University of Edinburgh, 1993.

De Boeck, Filip. "'Poverty' and the Politics of Syncopation: Urban Examples from Kinshasa (DR Congo)." *Current Anthropology* 56, no. 11 (October 1, 2015): S146–58. https://doi.org/10.1086/682392.

De Boeck, Filip, and Sammy Baloji. *Suturing the City: Living Together in Congo's Urban Worlds.* London: Autograph, 2016.

De Boeck, Filip, and Marie-Francoise Plissart. *Kinshasa: Tales of the Invisible City.* Leuven, Belgium: Leuven University Press, 2014.

Decker, Alicia. *In Idi Amin's Shadow: Women, Gender, and Militarism in Uganda*. Athens: Ohio University Press, 2014.

de Laet, Marianne, and Annemarie Mol. "The Zimbabwe Bush Pump: Mechanics of a Fluid Technology." *Social Studies of Science* 30, no. 2 (April 2000): 225–63.

Dikeni, Sandile. *Telegraph to the Sky*. Durban: University of KwaZulu Natal Press, 2001.

Dirks, Nicholas. "Annals of the Archive: Ethnographic Notes on the Sources of History." In *From the Margins: Historical Anthropology and Its Futures*, edited by Brian Keith Axel, 47–65. Durham, NC: Duke University Press, 2002.

Djordjevic, Darja. "Pluripotent Trajectories: Public Oncology in Rwanda." *BioSocieties* 14, no. 4 (2019): 553–70. https://doi.org/10.1057/s41292-019-00160-w.

Dlamini, Jacob. *Native Nostalgia*. Auckland Park, South Africa: Jacana, 2017.

Dodge, Cole P. "Uganda—Rehabilitation, or Redefinition of Health Services?" *Social Science and Medicine* 22, no. 7 (1986): 755–61.

Dodge, Cole P., and Paul D. Wiebe, eds. *Crisis in Uganda: The Breakdown of Health Services*. New York: Pergamon, 1985.

Donovan, Kevin P. "The Rise of the Randomistas: On the Experimental Turn in International Aid." *Economy and Society* 47, no. 1 (January 2, 2018): 27–58. https://doi.org/10.1080/03085147.2018.1432153.

Doyle, Shane. *Before HIV: Sexuality, Fertility and Mortality in East Africa, 1900–1980*. Oxford: Oxford University Press, 2013.

———. *Crisis and Decline in Bunyoro*. Athens: Ohio University Press, 2006.

Droney, Damien. "Ironies of Laboratory Work during Ghana's Second Age of Optimism." *Cultural Anthropology* 29, no. 2 (2014): 363–84.

Dumit, Joseph. *Picturing Personhood: Brain Scans and Biomedical Identity*. Princeton, NJ: Princeton University Press, 2004.

Edgerton, David. "Innovation, Technology, or History: What Is the Historiography of Technology About?" *Technology and Culture* 51, no. 3 (August 15, 2010): 680–97.

———. *The Shock of the Old: Technology and Global History since 1900*. Oxford: Oxford University Press, 2006.

Edwards, Paul. "Infrastructure and Modernity: Force, Time and Social Organization in the History of Sociotechnical Systems." In *Modernity and Technology*, edited by Thomas J. Misa, Philip Brey, and Andrew Feenberg, 185–226. Cambridge, MA: MIT Press, 2003.

———. *A Vast Machine: Computer Models, Climate Data, and the Politics of Global Warming*. Cambridge, MA: MIT Press, 2010.

Ellis, Stephen. "Writing Histories of Contemporary Africa." *Journal of African History* 43, no. 1 (2002): 1–26.

Engel, Mary. "An 'Audacious and Ambitious Building': Seattle Celebrates the Opening of the New Uganda-Fred Hutch Cancer Center." *Fred Hutch*

News Service, June 4, 2015, http://www.fredhutch.org/en/news/center
-news/2015/06/an-audacious-ambitious-building.html.

Engholm, G. F., and Ali A. Mazrui. "Violent Constitutionalism in Uganda."
Government and Opposition 2, no. 4 (1967): 585–99.

Epstein, Helen. *The Invisible Cure: Why We Are Losing the Fight against
AIDS in Africa*. New York: Farrar, Straus and Giroux, 2007.

Epstein, Steven. *Impure Science: AIDS, Activism, and the Politics of Knowledge, Medicine and Society*. Berkeley: University of California Press, 1996.

———. *Inclusion: The Politics of Difference in Medical Research*. Chicago:
University of Chicago Press, 2007.

Fallers, Lloyd. *The King's Men*. London: Oxford University Press, 1964.

Fanon, Frantz. *The Wretched of the Earth*. Translated by Constance Far-
rington. New York: Grove, 1965.

———. *A Dying Colonialism*. Translated by Haakon Chevalier. New York:
Grove, 1965.

Farmer, Paul. *AIDS and Accusation*. Berkeley: University of California Press, 1992.

———. *Fevers, Feuds, and Diamonds: Ebola and the Ravages of History*. New
York: Farrar, Straus and Giroux, 2020.

———. *Infections and Inequalities: The Modern Plagues*. Berkeley: University
of California Press, 1999.

———. *Pathologies of Power: Health, Human Rights, and the New War on the
Poor*. California Series in Public Anthropology. Berkeley: University of
California Press, 2003.

Farmer, Paul, Jim Yong Kim, Arthur Kleinman, and Matthew Basilco, eds.
Reimagining Global Health: An Introduction. Berkeley: University of California Press, 2013.

Fassin, Didier. "Humanitarianism as a Politics of Life." *Public Culture* 19,
no. 3 (2007): 499–520.

Fassin, Didier. *When Bodies Remember: Experiences and Politics of AIDS in
South Africa*. Translated by Amy Jacobs and Gabrielle Varro. Berkeley:
University of California Press, 2007.

Fassin, Didier, and Mariella Pandolfi, eds. *Contemporary States of Emergency*.
Boston: Zone, 2010.

Fassin, Didier, and Helen Schneider. "The Politics of AIDS in South Africa:
Beyond the Controversies." *BMJ: British Medical Journal* 326, no. 7387
(2003): 495–97.

Faust, Drew Gilpin. *This Republic of Suffering: Death and the American Civil
War*. New York: Alfred A. Knopf, 2008.

Feierman, Steven. "A Century of Ironies in East Africa." In Philip Curtin,
Steven Feierman, Leonard Thompson, and Jan Vansina, *African History*,
352–76. London: Longman, 1995.

———. "Colonizers, Scholars and the Creation of Invisible Histories." In *Beyond the Cultural Turn: New Directions in the Study of Society and
Culture*, 182–216. Berkley: University of California Press, 1999.

———. *Peasant Intellectuals: Anthropology and History in Tanzania*. Madison: University of Wisconsin Press, 1990.

———. "Struggles for Control: The Social Roots of Health and Healing in Modern Africa." *African Studies Review* 28, no. 2/3 (1985): 73–147.

———. "When Physicians Meet: Local Medical Knowledge and Global Public Goods." In *Evidence, Ethos, and Experiment: The Anthropology and History of Medical Research in Africa*, edited by P. Wenzel Geissler and Catherine Molyneux, 171–96. New York: Berghahn, 2011.

Feierman, Steven, and John M. Janzen, eds. *The Social Basis of Health and Healing in Africa*. Berkeley: University of California Press, 1992.

Ferguson, James. *The Anti-Politics Machine: Development, Depoliticization, and Bureaucratic Power in Lesotho*. Minneapolis: University of Minnesota Press, 1994.

———. *Expectations of Modernity: Myths and Meanings of Urban Life on the Zambian Copperbelt*. Berkeley: University of California Press, 1999.

———. *Global Shadows: Africa in the Neoliberal World Order*. Durham, NC: Duke University Press, 2006.

Ferguson, James, and Akhil Gupta. "Spatializing States: Toward an Ethnography of Neoliberal Governmentality." *American Ethnologist* 29, no. 4 (2002): 981–1002.

Finnstrom, Sverker. *Living with Bad Surroundings: War, History, and Everyday Moments in Northern Uganda*. Durham, NC: Duke University Press, 2008.

———. "Wars of the Past and War in the Present: The Lord's Resistance Movement/Army in Uganda." *Africa* 76 (2006): 200–220.

Fleck, Ludwig. *Genesis and Development of a Scientific Fact*. Chicago: University of Chicago Press, 1979.

Foley, Ellen E. *Your Pocket Is What Cures You: The Politics of Health in Senegal, Studies in Medical Anthropology*. New Brunswick, NJ: Rutgers University Press, 2010.

Foster, Kira E. "Clinics, Communities, and Cost Recovery: Primary Health Care and Neoliberalism in Postapartheid South Africa." *Cultural Dynamics* 17, no. 3 (2005): 239–66.

Foucault, Michel. *The Birth of the Clinic*. New York: Pantheon, 1973.

———. *Discipline and Punish: The Birth of the Prison*. New York: Pantheon, 1977.

Fredericks, Rosalind. *Garbage Citizenship: Vital Infrastructures of Labor in Dakar, Senegal*. Durham, NC: Duke University Press, 2018.

Fred Hutch Global Oncology Brochure. Seattle: Fred Hutchinson Cancer Research Center, 2015.

Freed, Libbie. "Networks of (Colonial) Power: Roads in French Central Africa after World War I." *History and Technology* 26, no. 3 (September 1, 2010): 203–23. https://doi.org/10.1080/07341512.2010.498637.

Fullwiley, Duana. *The Encultured Gene: Sickle Cell Health Politics and Biological Difference in West Africa*. Princeton, NJ: Princeton University Press, 2011.

Furlong, Kathryn. "STS Beyond the 'Modern Infrastructure Ideal': Extending Theory by Engaging with Infrastructure Challenges in the South." *Technology in Society* 38 (2014): 139–47.

Garcia, Angela. *The Pastoral Clinic*. Berkeley: University of California Press, 2010.

Garrett, Laurie. "The Challenge of Global Health," *Foreign Affairs* 86 (2007): 14–17.

Garrey, Sasha. "Uganda's Lone Radiotherapy Machine." *Pulitzer Center Crisis Reporting*, September 4, 2014, http://pulitzercenter.org/reporting/africa -uganda-cervical-cancer-radiotherapy-cobalt.

Geissler, P. Wenzel, ed. *Para-States and Medical Science: Making African Global Health*. Durham, NC: Duke University Press, 2015.

Geissler, P. Wenzel, A. Kelly, B. Imoukhuede, and R. Pool. "'He Is Now Like a Brother, I Can Even Give Him Some Blood'—Relational Ethics and Material Exchanges in a Malaria Vaccine 'Trial Community' in the Gambia." *Social Science and Medicine* 67, no. 5 (2008): 696–707.

Geissler, P. Wenzel, Guillaume Lachenal, John Manton, Noémi Tousignant, Evgenia Arbugaeva, and Mariele Neudecker. *Traces of the Future: An Archaeology of Medical Science in Africa*. Chicago: University of Chicago Press, 2016.

Geissler, P. Wenzel, and Catherine Molyneux, eds. *Evidence, Ethos and Experiment: The Anthropology and History of Medical Research in Africa*. New York: Berghahn, 2011.

Geissler, P. Wenzel., and R. Pool. "Editorial: Popular Concerns about Medical Research Projects in Sub-Saharan Africa—a Critical Voice in Debates about Medical Research Ethics." *Tropical Medicine and International Health* 11, no. 7 (2006): 975–82.

Geissler, P. Wenzel, and Noémi Tousignant. "Capacity as History and Horizon: Infrastructure, Autonomy and Future in African Health Science and Care." *Canadian Journal of African Studies* (Revue Canadienne Des Études Africaines) 50, no. 3 (September 1, 2016): 349–59.

Giblin, James. *History of the Excluded: Making Family a Refuge from State in Twentieth-Century Tanzania*. Athens: Ohio University Press, 2005.

Gieryn, Thomas F. *Cultural Boundaries of Science: Credibility on the Line*. Chicago: University of Chicago Press, 1999.

——. "What Buildings Do." *Theory and Society* 31 (2002): 35–74.

Gingyera-Pinycwa, A. G. G. *Apolo Milton Obote and His Times*. New York: NOK, 1978.

Glemser, Bernard. *Mr. Burkitt and Africa*. Cleveland: World Publishing, 1970.

Goldstone, Brian, Juan Obarrio, and American Anthropological Association, eds. *African Futures: Essays on Crisis, Emergence, and Possibility*. Chicago: University of Chicago Press, 2016.

Good, Byron. *Medicine, Rationality, and Experience: An Anthropological Perspective*. Cambridge: Cambridge University Press, 1994.

Good, Mary-Jo DelVecchio. "Clinical Realities and Moral Dilemmas: Contrasting Perspectives from Academic Medicine in Kenya, Tanzania, and America." *Daedalus* 128, no. 4 (1999): 167.

Graboyes, Melissa. *The Experiment Must Continue: Medical Research and Ethics in East Africa, 1940–2014.* Athens: Ohio University Press, 2015.

———. "Introduction: Incorporating Medical Research into the History of Medicine in East Africa." *International Journal of African Historical Studies* 47 (2014): 379–98.

Graboyes, Melissa, and Hannah Carr. "Institutional Memory, Institutional Capacity: Narratives of Failed Biomedical Encounters in East Africa." *Canadian Journal of African Studies* (Revue Canadienne Des Études Africaines) 50, no. 3 (September 1, 2016): 361–77. https://doi.org/10.1080/00083968.2016.1266678.

Grace, Joshua. *African Motors: Technology, Gender, and the History of Development.* Durham, NC: Duke University Press, 2021.

Grady, Denise. "Uganda's Neglected Epidemic of Breast Cancer." *New York Times*, October 21, 2013. https://www.nytimes.com/2013/10/29/health/the-epidemic-uganda-is-neglecting.html.

Greene, Jeremy. *Prescribing by Numbers: Drugs and the Definition of Disease.* Baltimore: Johns Hopkins University Press, 2007.

Gupta, Akhil. *Red Tape: Bureaucracy, Structural Violence, and Poverty in India.* Durham, NC: Duke University Press, 2012.

Gusterson, Hugh. *Nuclear Rites: A Weapons Laboratory at the End of the Cold War.* Berkeley: University of California Press, 1998.

———. "Studying Up Revisited." *Political and Legal Anthropology Review* 14, no. 1 (1997): 111–43.

Guyer, Jane I. *Marginal Gains: Monetary Transactions in Atlantic Africa.* Chicago: University of Chicago Press, 2004.

Guyer, Jane I., and Samuel M. Eno Belinga. "Wealth in People as Wealth in Knowledge:, Accumulation and Composition in Equatorial Africa." *Journal of African History* 36 (1995): 91–120.

Hamdy, Sherine. *Our Bodies Belong to God: Organ Transplants, Islam, and the Struggle for Human Dignity in Egypt.* Berkeley: University of California Press, 2012.

Hansen, Hölger Bernt. "Uganda in the 1970s: A Decade of Paradoxes and Ambiguities." *Journal of Eastern African Studies* 7, no. 1 (2003): 83–103.

Hansen, Hölger Bernt, and Michael Twaddle, eds. *Changing Uganda: The Dilemmas of Structural Adjustment and Revolutionary Change*, Eastern African Studies. London: J. Currey, 1991.

———, eds. *Uganda Now: Between Decay and Development.* London: J. Currey, 1988.

Hanson, Holly Elizabeth. *Landed Obligation: The Practice of Power in Buganda.* Portsmouth, NH: Heinemann, 2003.

Hart, Jennifer. *Ghana on the Go.* Bloomington: Indiana University Press, 2016.

Harvey, David. *Spaces of Global Capitalism*. London: Verso, 2006.

Hayden, Cori. *When Nature Goes Public: The Making and Unmaking of Bioprospecting in Mexico*. Princeton, NJ: Princeton University Press, 2003.

Headrick, Daniel R. *The Tools of Empire: Technology and European Imperialism in the Nineteenth Century*. New York: Oxford University Press, 1981.

Heaton, Matthew M. *Black Skin, White Coats: Nigerian Psychiatrists, Decolonization, and the Globalization of Psychiatry*. Athens: Ohio University Press, 2013.

Hecht, Gabrielle. *Being Nuclear: Africans and the Global Uranium Trade*. Cambridge, MA: MIT Press, 2012.

———. "Interscalar Vehicles for an African Anthropocene: On Waste, Temporality, and Violence." *Cultural Anthropology* 33, no. 1 (2018): 109–41.

———. *The Radiance of France*. Cambridge, MA: MIT Press, 2009.

Ho, Karen. *Liquidated: An Ethnography of Wall Street*. Durham, NC: Duke University Press, 2009.

Hodges, Sarah. "The Global Menace." *Social History of Medicine* 25, no. 3 (August 1, 2012): 719–28. https://doi.org/10.1093/shm/hkr166.

Hundle, Anneeth Kaur. "Exceptions to the Expulsion: Violence, Security and Community among Ugandan Asians, 1972–79." *Journal of Eastern African Studies* 7, no. 1 (February 1, 2013): 164–82.

Hunt, Nancy Rose. *A Colonial Lexicon: Of Birth Ritual, Medicalization, and Mobility in the Congo*. Durham, NC: Duke University Press, 1999.

———. "Le Bebe en Brousse: European Women, African Birth Spacing, and Colonial Intervention in Breast Feeding in the Belgian Congo." *International Journal of African Historical Studies* 21, no. 3 (1988): 401–32.

———. *Suturing New Medical Histories of Africa*. Münster: LIT Verlag, 2013.

Hunter, Mark. *Love in the Time of AIDS: Inequality, Gender, and Rights in South Africa*. Bloomington: Indiana University Press, 2010.

Hutchinson, Sharon. *Nuer Dilemmas: Coping with Money, War, and the State*. Berkeley: University of California Press, 1996.

Iliffe, John. *The African AIDS Epidemic: A History*. Athens: Ohio University Press, 2005.

———. *East African Doctors: A History of the Modern Profession*. Kampala: Fountain, 2002.

Ingham, Kenneth. *Obote: A Political Biography*. London: Routledge, 2014.

International Atomic Energy Agency. *Disposal of Radioactive Waste*. IAEA Safety Standards. Vienna: IAEA, 2011.

International Civil Aviation Agency. *Refusing Radioactive Material Shipments for Transfer by Air*. Information Paper no. 20. February 2013. https://www.icao.int/safety/DangerousGoods/Working%20Group%20of%20the%20Whole/IP08%20Att.pdf#search=Refusing%20Radioactive%20Material%20Shipments%20for%20Transfer%20by%20Air.

Jackson, Steven J. "Rethinking Repair." In *Media Technologies: Essays on Communication, Materiality, and Society*, edited by Tarleton Gillespie,

Pablo J. Boczkowski, and Kirsten A. Foot, 221–39. Cambridge, MA: MIT Press, 2014.

Jain, S. Løchlann. "Cancer Butch." *Cultural Anthropology* 22, no. 4 (2007): 501–38.

——. *Malignant: How Cancer Becomes Us*. Berkeley: University of California Press, 2013.

Janzen, John M., and William Arkinstall. *The Quest for Therapy in Lower Zaire*, Comparative Studies of Health Systems and Medical Care. Berkeley: University of California Press, 1978.

Jones, Ben. *Beyond the State in Rural Uganda*. Edinburgh: Edinburgh University Press, 2009.

Kaleeba, Noerine. *We Miss You All: AIDS in the Family*. Kampala: AIDS Support Organization, 1991.

Kasasira, Ridel. "WikiLeaks: America Feared Theft of Nuclear Material from Mulago." *Daily Monitor*, September 11, 2011. https://www.monitor.co.ug/uganda/news/national/wikileaks-america-feared-theft-of-nuclear-material-from-mulago-1499818.

Kasozi, A. B. K., Nakanyike Musisi, and James Mukooza Sejjengo. *The Social Origins of Violence in Uganda, 1964–1985*. Montreal: McGill-Queen's University Press, 1994.

Kaufman, Sharon. *And a Time to Die: How American Hospitals Shape the End of Life*. Chicago: University of Chicago Press, 2005.

——. *Ordinary Medicine: Extraordinary Treatments, Longer Lives, and Where to Draw the Line*. Durham, NC: Duke University Press, 2015.

Keating, Peter, and Alberto Cambrosio. *Cancer on Trial: Oncology as a New Style of Practice*. Chicago: University of Chicago Press, 2012.

Kenworthy, Nora, Lynn M. Thomas, and Johanna Crane. "Introduction." *Medicine Anthropology Theory* 5, no. 2 (May 15, 2018). https://doi.org/10.17157/mat.5.1.613.

Kirksey, Eben. "Caring as Chemo-Ethnographic Method." Member Voices, *Fieldsights*, November 20, 2017. https://culanth.org/fieldsights/caring-as-chemo-ethnographic-method.

Kiwanuka, Maria. *The Public Procurement and Disposal of Public Assets (Contracts) Regulations 2014*. Statutory Instruments Supplement no. 3. Entebbe, Uganda: UPPC, 2014. https://www.ppda.go.ug/download/regulations/regulations/central_government_regulations/2014/PPDA-Regs-2014.pdf.

Klaits, Frederick. *Death in a Church of Life: Moral Passion during Botswana's Time of AIDS*. Berkeley: University of California Press, 2010.

Kodesh, Neil. *Beyond the Royal Gaze*. Charlottesville: University of Virginia Press, 2010.

Krueger, Gretchen. *Hope and Suffering: Children, Cancer, and the Paradox of Experimental Medicine*. Baltimore: Johns Hopkins University Press, 2008.

Kuhanen, Jan. "The Historiography of HIV and AIDS in Uganda." *History in Africa* 35, no. 1 (January 14, 2009): 301–25.

Kutcher, Gerald. *Contested Medicine: Cancer Research and the Military*. Chicago: University of Chicago Press, 2009.

Kyemba, Henry. *A State of Blood: The Inside Story of Idi Amin*. New York: Ace, 1977.

Lalani, Z. *Uganda Asian Expulsion: 90 Days and Beyond through the Eyes of the International Press*. Bloomington: Indiana University Press, 1997.

Landau, Paul. "Explaining Surgical Evangelism in Colonial Southern Africa: Teeth, Pain and Faith." *Journal of African History* 37, no. 2 (1996): 261–81.

Langwick, Stacey Ann. "Articulate(d) Bodies: Traditional Medicine in a Tanzanian Hospital." *American Ethnologist* 35, no. 3 (August 21, 2008): 428–39.

———. *Bodies, Politics, and African Healing: The Matter of Maladies in Tanzania*. Bloomington: Indiana University Press, 2011.

Larkin, Brian. "The Politics and Poetics of Infrastructure." *Annual Review of Anthropology* 42, no. 1 (2013): 327–43.

———. *Signal and Noise: Media, Infrastructure, and Urban Culture in Nigeria*. Durham, NC: Duke University Press, 2008.

Laszlo, John. *The Cure of Childhood Leukemia: Into the Age of Miracles*. New Brunswick, NJ: Rutgers University Press, 1996.

Latour, Bruno. *Science in Action: How to Follow Scientists and Engineers through Society*. Milton Keynes, UK: Open University Press, 1987.

Latour, Bruno, and Steve Woolgar. *Laboratory Life: The Social Construction of Scientific Facts*, Sage Library of Social Research 80. Beverly Hills: SAGE, 1979.

Leopold, Mark. *Idi Amin: The Story of Africa's Icon of Evil*. New Haven, CT: Yale University Press, 2020.

———. *Inside West Nile: Violence, History and Representation on an African Frontier*, World Anthropology. Oxford: J. Currey, 2005.

Levi, Primo. *The Drowned and the Saved*. New York: Vintage, 1989.

Lindemann, Stefan. "Just Another Change of Guard? Broad-Based Politics and Civil War in Museveni's Uganda." *African Affairs* 110 (2011): 387–416.

Livingston, Julie. *Debility and the Moral Imagination in Botswana*, African Systems of Thought. Bloomington: Indiana University Press, 2005.

———. *Improvising Medicine: An African Oncology Ward in an Emerging Cancer Epidemic*. Durham, NC: Duke University Press, 2012.

———. "Pregnant Children and Half-Dead Adults: Modern Living and the Quickening Life Cycle in Botswana." *Bulletin of the History of Medicine* 77, no. 1 (March 20, 2003): 133–62.

Livingstone, David N. *Putting Science in Its Place: Geographies of Scientific Knowledge*. Chicago: University of Chicago Press, 2003.

Lock, Margaret, and Vinh-Kim Nguyen. *An Anthropology of Biomedicine*. Malden, MA: Wiley-Blackwell, 2010.

Lorde, Audre. *The Cancer Journals*. New York: Penguin, 2020.

Lonsdale, John, and Bruce Berman. *Unhappy Valley*. Athens: Ohio University Press, 1992.

Löwy, Ilana. *Preventive Strikes: Women, Precancer, and Prophylactic Surgery.* Baltimore: Johns Hopkins University Press, 2010.

Lubega, Henry. "Dr. Olweny Went on Leave but Never Returned to Office." *Daily Monitor,* October 6, 2013, http://www.monitor.co.ug/Magazines /PeoplePower/Dr-Olweny-went-on-leave-but-never-returned-to-office/- /689844/2019912/-/6x35nw/-/index.html.

Lyons, Maryinez. *The Colonial Disease: A Social History of Sleeping Sickness in Northern Zaire, 1900–1940.* New York: Cambridge University Press, 1992.

MacGaffey, Janet. *The Real Economy of Zaire: The Contribution of Smuggling and Other Unofficial Activities to National Wealth.* London: J. Currey, 1991.

MacLeish, Kenneth. *Making War at Fort Hood.* Princeton, NJ: Princeton University Press, 2013.

Magara, James. *Uganda Jubilee Handbook 2012: Commemorate. Celebrate. Contemplate.* Kampala: New Life, 2012.

Mamdani, Mahmood. *From Citizen to Refugee: Uganda Asians Come to Britain.* Cape Town: Pambazuka, 2011.

———. *Politics and Class Formation in Uganda.* Kampala: Fountain, 2001.

———. "The Ugandan Asian Expulsion: Twenty Years After." *Journal of Refugee Studies* 6, no. 3 (January 1, 1993): 265–73.

Marks, Harry M. *The Progress of Experiment: Science and Therapeutic Reform in the United States, 1900–1990,* Cambridge History of Medicine. New York: Cambridge University Press, 1997.

Marks, Shula. "What Is Colonial about Colonial Medicine? And What Has Happened to Imperialism and Health?" *Social History of Medicine* 10, no. 2 (August 1, 1997): 205–19.

Martin, David. *General Amin.* London: Faber and Faber, 1974.

Martin, Emily. "The End of the Body?" *American Ethnologist* 19, no. 1 (1992): 121–40.

———. *Flexible Bodies: Tracking Immunity in American Culture—From the Days of Polio to the Age of AIDS.* Boston: Beacon, 1994.

Masco, Joseph. *The Nuclear Borderlands: The Manhattan Project in Post–Cold War New Mexico.* Princeton, NJ: Princeton University Press, 2006.

Mauss, Marcel. *The Gift.* 1950. New York: Norton, 2000.

———. "Techniques of the Body." *Economy and Society* 2, no. 1 (1973): 70–88.

Mavhunga, Clapperton Chakanetsa. *Transient Workspaces: Technologies of Everyday Innovation in Zimbabwe.* Cambridge, MA: MIT Press, 2014.

Mazrui, Ali A. "Between Development and Decay: Anarchy, Tyranny and Progress under Idi Amin." *Third World Quarterly* 2, no. 1 (1980): 44–58.

———. "The Blood of Experience: The Failed State and Political Collapse in Africa." *World Policy Journal* 12, no. 1 (1995): 28–34.

———. "Leadership in Africa: Obote of Uganda." *International Journal* 25, no. 3 (1970): 538–64. https://doi.org/10.2307/40200856.

Mbembe, J. A. *On the Postcolony*. Studies on the History of Society and Culture. Berkeley: University of California Press, 2001.

McKay, Ramah. *Medicine in the Meantime: The Work of Care in Mozambique*. Durham, NC: Duke University Press, 2017.

Mendenhall, Emily. "Syndemics: A New Path for Global Health Research." *Lancet* 389, no. 10072 (2017): 889–91.

——. *Syndemic Suffering: Social Distress, Depression, and Diabetes Among Mexican Immigrant Women*. London: Routledge, 2016.

Mendenhall, Emily, and Shane A. Norris. "When HIV Is Ordinary and Diabetes New: Remaking Suffering in a South African Township." *Global Public Health* 10, no. 4 (2015): 449–62.

Mendenhall, Emily, Gregory Barnabas Omondi, Edna Bosire, Gitonga Isaiah, Abednego Musau, David Ndetei, and Victoria Mutiso. "Stress, Diabetes, and Infection: Syndemic Suffering at an Urban Kenyan Hospital." *Social Science and Medicine* 146 (2015): 11–20.

Miescher, Stephan F. "Building the City of the Future: Visions and Experiences of Modernity in Ghana's Akosombo Township." *Journal of African History* 53 (2012): 367–90.

Mika, Marissa. "Cytotoxic: Notes on Chemotherapy at the Lymphoma Treatment Center, Uganda Cancer Institute, Kampala." *BioSocieties* 14, no. 4 (December 1, 2019): 573–82.

——. "Fifty Years of Creativity, Crisis, and Cancer in Uganda." *Canadian Journal of African Studies* (Revue Canadienne Des Études Africaines) 50, no. 3 (September 1, 2016): 395–413.

——. "The Half-Life of Radiotherapy and Other Transferred Technologies." *Technology and Culture* 61, no. 2 (2020): S135–57.

Mitchell, Timothy. *Rule of Experts: Egypt, Techno-politics, Modernity*. Berkeley: University of California Press, 2002.

Mkhwanazi, Nolwazi. "Medical Anthropology in Africa: The Trouble with a Single Story." *Medical Anthropology* 35, no. 2 (March 3, 2016): 193–202.

Mol, Annemarie. *The Logic of Care: Health and the Problem of Patient Choice*. London: Routledge, 2008.

Molyneux, C. S., and P. W. Geissler. "Editorial: Ethics and Ethnography in Medical Research in Africa." *Social Science and Medicine* 67, no. 5 (2008): 685–95.

Moorman, Marissa Jean. *Powerful Frequencies: Radio, State Power, and the Cold War in Angola, 1931–2002*. Athens: Ohio University Press, 2019.

Moran-Thomas, Amy. *Traveling with Sugar: Chronicles of a Global Epidemic*. Berkeley: University of California Press, 2019.

Moss, A. "AIDS in the 'Gay' Areas of San Francisco." *Lancet* 1 (1983): 923–24.

Mueller, Lucas M. "Cancer in the Tropics: Geographical Pathology and the Formation of Cancer Epidemiology." *BioSocieties* 14, no. 4 (December 1, 2019): 512–28. https://doi.org/10.1057/s41292-019-00152-w.

Mukherjee, Siddhartha. *The Emperor of All Maladies: A Biography of Cancer*. New York: Scribner, 2010.

Mulemi, Benson. "Cancer Crisis and Treatment Ambiguity in Kenya." In *Anthropologies of Cancer in Transnational Worlds*, edited by Holly F. Mathews, Nancy J. Burke, and Eirini Kampriani, 156–76. New York: Routledge, 2015.

———. *Coping with Cancer and Adversity: Hospital Ethnography in Kenya*. Leiden: African Studies Center, 2010.

———. "Technologies of Hope: Managing Cancer in a Kenyan Hospital." In *Making and Unmaking Public Health in Africa: Ethnographic and Historical Perspectives*, edited by Ruth Prince and Rebecca Marsland, 162–86. Athens: Ohio University Press, 2013.

———. "Therapeutic Eclecticism and Cancer Care in a Kenyan Hospital Ward." In *African Medical Pluralism*, edited by William C. Olsen and Carolyn Sargent, 207–26. Bloomington: Indiana University Press, 2017.

Murphy, Michelle. *Sick Building Syndrome and the Problem of Uncertainty: Environmental Politics, Technoscience, and Women Workers*. Durham, NC: Duke University Press, 2006.

Mutongi, Kenda. *Matatu: A History of Popular Transportation in Nairobi*. Chicago: University of Chicago Press, 2017.

———. "Thugs or Entrepreneurs: Perceptions of *Matatu* Operations in Nairobi, 1970 to the Present." *Africa* 76 (2006): 549–68.

———. *Worries of the Heart*. Chicago: University of Chicago Press, 2007.

Mwanguhya, Charles. "Uganda: Faire Thee Well Dr. Okullo Epak." *Daily Monitor* May 2, 2007.

Nader, Laura. "Up the Anthropologist—Perspectives Gained from Studying Up." In *Reinventing Anthropology*, edited by Dell Hymes, 284–311. New York: Vintage, 1974.

Nakatudde, Olive. "PAC Grills Mulago Officials Over the Delayed Purchase of a Cobalt Machine." Uganda Radio Network, February 3, 2014. https://ugandaradionetwork.com/story/pac-grills-mulago-officials-over-the-delayed-purchase-of-a-cobalt-machine.

Namutebi, Joyce, and John Odkyek. "Oyam South MP Okullo Epak Dead." *New Vision*, April 25, 2007.

Nayenga, Peter. "The Overthrowing of Idi Amin: An Analysis of the War." *Africa Today* 31 (1984): 69–91.

Nguyen, Vinh-Kim. "Government-by-Exception: Enrolment and Experimentality in Mass HIV Treatment Programmes in Africa." *Society and Health* 7 (2009): 196–217.

———. *The Republic of Therapy: Triage and Sovereignty in West Africa's Time of AIDS*. Durham, NC: Duke University Press, 2010.

Nixon, Rob. *Slow Violence and the Environmentalism of the Poor*. Cambridge, MA: Harvard University Press, 2011.

Nsubuga, Godfrey. *The Person of Dr. Milton Obote: A Classic Personality Study*. Kampala: Nissi, 2012.

Ogot, Bethwell A., and William Robert Ochieng. *Decolonization and Independence in Kenya, 1940–93*. Athens: Ohio University Press, 1995.

Okeke, Iruka N. "African Biomedical Scientists and the Promises of 'Big Science.'" *Canadian Journal of African Studies* (Revue Canadienne Des Études Africaines) 50, no. 3 (September 1, 2016): 455–78. https://doi.org/10.1080/00083968.2016.1266677.

——. *Divining without Seeds: The Case for Strengthening Laboratory Medicine in Africa.* Ithaca, NY: Cornell University Press, 2011.

——. "Partnerships for Now?" *Medicine Anthropology Theory* 5, no. 2 (May 15, 2018). https://doi.org/10.17157/mat.5.2.531.

Oloka-Onyango, J. "'New-Breed' Leadership, Conflict, and Reconstruction in the Great Lakes Region of Africa: A Sociopolitical Biography of Uganda's Yoweri Kaguta Museveni." *Africa Today* 50 (2004): 29–52.

Ong, Aihwa, and Stephen J. Collier, eds. *Global Assemblages: Technology, Politics, and Ethics as Anthropological Problems.* Malden, MA: Blackwell, 2005.

Osseo-Asare, Abena Dove Agyepoma. *Bitter Roots the Search for Healing Plants in Africa.* Chicago: University of Chicago Press, 2014.

Packard, Randall M. *Global Health: A History of Interventions into the Lives of Other Peoples.* Baltimore: Johns Hopkins University Press, 2016.

——. *The Making of a Tropical Disease: A Short History of Malaria.* Johns Hopkins Biographies of Disease. Baltimore: Johns Hopkins University Press, 2007.

——. *White Plague, Black Labor: Tuberculosis and the Political Economy of Health and Disease in South Africa.* Berkeley: University of California Press, 1989.

Park, Emma. "'Human ATMs': M-Pesa and the Expropriation of Affective Work in Safaricom's Kenya." *Africa: The Journal of the International African Institute* 90, no. 5 (2020): 914–33.

Parle, Julie, and Vanessa Noble. "New Directions and Challenges in Histories of Health, Healing and Medicine in South Africa." *Medical History* 58, no. 2 (April 2014): 147–65. https://doi.org/10.1017/mdh.2014.1.

Peterson, Derek. *Creative Writing: Translation, Bookkeeping, and the Work of Imagination in Colonial Kenya.* Portsmouth, NH: Heinemann, 2004.

——. *Ethnic Patriotism and the East African Revival.* Cambridge: Cambridge University Press, 2012.

——. "Uganda's History from the Margins." *History in Africa* 40, no. 1 (November 2013): S23–25.

Peterson, Derek R., and Edgar C. Taylor. "Rethinking the State in Idi Amin's Uganda: The Politics of Exhortation." *Journal of Eastern African Studies* 7 (2013): 58–82.

Peterson, Kristin. *Speculative Markets: Drug Circuits and Derivative Life in Nigeria.* Durham, NC: Duke University Press, 2014.

——. "AIDS Policies for Markets and Warriors: Dispossession, Capital, and Pharmaceuticals in Nigeria." In *Medicine, Mobility, and Power in Global Africa: Transnational Health and Healing,* edited by Hansjorg Dilger,

Abdoulaye Kane, and Stacey Langwick, 138–62. Bloomington: Indiana University Press, 2012.

Petryna, Adriana. *Life Exposed: Biological Citizens after Chernobyl*, In-Formation Series. Princeton, NJ: Princeton University Press, 2002.

———. *When Experiments Travel: Clinical Trials and the Global Search for Human Subjects*. Princeton, NJ: Princeton University Press, 2009.

Petryna, Adriana, Andrew Lakoff, and Arthur Kleinman, eds. *Global Pharmaceuticals: Ethics, Markets, Practices*. Durham, NC: Duke University Press, 2006.

Pfeiffer, James, and Rachel Chapman. "Anthropological Perspectives on Structural Adjustment and Public Health." *Annual Review of Anthropology* 39 (2010): 149–65.

Piot, Charles. *Nostalgia for the Future: West Africa after the Cold War*. Chicago: University of Chicago Press, 2010.

Pratt, Mary Louise. *Imperial Eyes: Travel Writing and Transculturation*. London: Routledge, 2003.

Prestholdt, Jeremy. *Domesticating the World: African Consumerism and the Genealogies of Globalization*. Berkeley: University of California Press, 2008.

Prince, Ruth Jane, and Rebecca Marsland, eds. *Making and Unmaking Public Health in Africa: Ethnographic and Historical Perspectives*. Athens: Ohio University Press, 2014.

Pringle, Yolana. "Neurasthenia at Mengo Hospital, Uganda: A Case Study in Psychiatry and a Diagnosis, 1906–50." *Journal of Imperial and Commonwealth History* 44, no. 2 (March 3, 2016): 241–62.

Proctor, Robert. *Cancer Wars: How Politics Shapes What We Know and Don't Know about Cancer*. New York: Basic Books, 1995.

Puri, Sunita. *That Good Night: Life and Medicine in the Eleventh Hour*. New York: Viking, 2019.

Radin, Joanna. *Life on Ice: A History of New Uses for Cold Blood*. Chicago: University of Chicago Press, 2017.

Redfield, Peter. "The Half-Life of Empire in Outer Space." *Social Studies of Science* 32, nos. 5–6 (2002): 791–825.

———. "A Less Modest Witness: Collective Advocacy and Motivated Truth in a Medical Humanitarian Movement." *American Ethnologist* 33, no. 1 (February 2006): 3–26.

———. *Life in Crisis: The Ethical Journey of Doctors without Borders*. Berkeley: University of California Press, 2013.

Renne, Elisha P. *The Politics of Polio in Northern Nigeria*. Bloomington: Indiana University Press, 2010.

Reverby, Susan. *Examining Tuskegee: The Infamous Syphilis Study and Its Legacy*. Baltimore: Johns Hopkins University Press, 2013.

Reverby, Susan, and David Rosner. "Beyond the Great Doctors." In *Health Care in America: Essays in Social History*, edited by Susan Reverby and David Rosner, 3–16. Philadelphia: Temple University Press, 1979.

———. "Beyond the Great Doctors Revisited." In *Locating Medical History*, edited by Frank Huisman and John Harley Warner, 167–93. Baltimore: Johns Hopkins University Press, 2004.

Reynolds, L. A., and E. M. Tansye, eds. *British Contributions to Medical Research and Education in Africa after the Second World War.* Wellcome Witnesses to Twentieth Century Medicine 10. London: Wellcome Trust Centre for the History of Medicine at UCL, 2001.

Rice, Andrew. *The Teeth May Smile but the Heart Does Not Forget: Murder and Memory in Uganda.* New York: Picador, 2010.

Riles, Annelise. *The Network Inside Out.* Ann Arbor: University of Michigan Press, 2000.

Risse, Guenter B. *Mending Bodies, Saving Souls: A History of Hospitals.* New York: Oxford University Press, 1999.

Rodgers, Dennis, and Bruce O'Neill. "Infrastructural Violence: Introduction to the Special Issue." *Ethnography* 13, no. 4 (December 1, 2012): 401–12.

Roitman, Janet. *Fiscal Disobedience: An Anthropology of Economic Regulation in Central Africa.* Princeton, NJ: Princeton University Press, 2005.

Rose, Nikolas S. *The Politics of Life Itself: Biomedicine, Power, and Subjectivity in the Twenty-First Century.* Princeton, NJ: Princeton University Press, 2007.

Rosenberg, Charles E. *The Care of Strangers: The Rise of America's Hospital System.* Baltimore: Johns Hopkins University Press, 1995.

———. *The Cholera Years.* Chicago: University of Chicago Press, 1987.

———. "Pathologies of Progress: The Idea of Civilization as Risk." *Bulletin of the History of Medicine* 72, no. 4 (Winter 1998): 714–30.

———. "The Therapeutic Revolution: Medicine, Meaning and Social Change in Nineteenth-Century America." *Perspectives in Biology and Medicine* 20, no. 4 (1977): 485–506.

Rottenburg, Richard. "Social and Public Experiments and New Figurations of Science and Politics in Postcolonial Africa." *Postcolonial Studies* 12, no. 4 (2009): 423–40.

Saunders, Barry. *CT Suite: The Work of Diagnosis in the Age of Noninvasive Cutting.* Durham, NC: Duke University Press, 2008.

Savage, L. "Former African Cancer Research Powerhouse Makes Plans for a Return to Greatness." *Journal of the National Cancer Institute* 99, no. 15 (August 1, 2007): 1144–45, 1151.

Scheper-Hughes, Nancy, and Margaret Lock. "The Mindful Body: A Prolegomenon to Future Work in Medical Anthropology." *Medical Anthropology Quarterly* 1 (1987): 1–36.

Schmidt, Elizabeth. *Foreign Intervention in Africa.* Cambridge: Cambridge University Press, 2013.

Schoenbrun, David. *A Green Place: A Good Place.* Portsmouth, NH: Heineman, 1998.

Schultheis, Michael J. "The Ugandan Economy and General Amin, 1971–1974." *Studies in Comparative International Development* 10, no. 3 (September 1, 1975): 3–34.

Schumaker, Lyn. *Africanizing Anthropology: Fieldwork, Networks, and the Making of Cultural Knowledge in Central Africa.* Durham, NC: Duke University Press, 2001.

———. "History of Medicine in Sub-Saharan Africa." In *The Oxford Handbook of the History of Medicine,* edited by Mark Jackson, 275–79. Oxford: Oxford University Press, 2011.

Scott, James C. *Seeing Like a State: How Certain Schemes to Improve the Human Condition Have Failed.* Yale Agrarian Studies. New Haven, CT: Yale University Press, 1998.

Seth, Suman. "Putting Knowledge in Its Place: Science, Colonialism, and the Postcolonial." *Postcolonial Studies* 12, no. 4 (2009): 373–88.

Shapin, Steven, and Simon Schaffer. *Leviathan and the Air Pump: Hobbes, Boyle, and the Experimental Life.* Princeton, NJ: Princeton University Press, 1989.

Shaw, Timothy M. "Uganda under Amin: The Costs of Confronting Dependence." *Africa Today* 20, no. 2 (1973): 32–45.

Simone, Abdou Maliq. "People as Infrastructure: Intersecting Fragments in Johannesburg." *Public Culture* 16, no. 3 (2004): 407–29.

Sitas, F., D. M. Parkin, M. Chirenje, L. Stein, R. Abratt, and H. Wabinga. "Part II: Cancer in Indigenous Africans—Causes and Control." *Lancet Oncology* 9, no. 8 (2008): 786–95.

Sivaramakrishnan, Kavita. "An Irritable State: The Contingent Politics of Science and Suffering in Anti-Cancer Campaigns in South India (1940–1960)." *BioSocieties* 14, no. 4 (December 1, 2019): 529–52.

———. *As the World Ages: Rethinking a Demographic Crisis.* Cambridge, MA: Harvard University Press, 2018.

Smith, Daniel Jordan. *A Culture of Corruption: Everyday Deception and Popular Discontent in Nigeria.* Princeton, NJ: Princeton University Press, 2008.

Sontag, Susan. *Illness as Metaphor and AIDS and Its Metaphors.* New York: Picador, 2001.

Southall, Aidan W., and Peter C. W. Gutkind. *Townsmen in the Making: Kampala and Its Suburbs.* Kampala: East African Institute of Social Research, 1957.

Star, Susan Leigh. "The Ethnography of Infrastructure." *American Behavioral Scientist* 43, no. 3 (November 1, 1999): 377–91.

Stevens, Rosemary. *In Sickness and in Wealth: American Hospitals in the Twentieth Century.* Baltimore: Johns Hopkins University Press, 1999.

Stoler, Ann Laura, ed. *Imperial Debris: On Ruins and Ruination.* Durham, NC: Duke University Press, 2013.

Strathern, Marilyn, "Cutting the Network" *Journal of the Royal Anthropological Institute* 2, no. 3 (September 1996): 517–35.

Street, Alice. *Biomedicine in an Unstable Place: Infrastructure and Personhood in a Papua New Guinean Hospital.* Durham, NC: Duke University Press, 2014.

Stultiens, Andrea. "Ebifananyi: A Study of Photographs in Uganda in and through an Artistic Practice." PhD diss., Leiden University, 2018. https://openaccess.leidenuniv.nl/handle/1887/67951.

——. *The Photographer: Deo Kyakulagira* (Edam, The Netherlands: YDoc, 2012).

Stultiens, Andrea, and Marissa Mika. *Staying Alive: Documenting the Uganda Cancer Institute.* Stockholm: Paradox, 2017.

Summers, Carol. "Radical Rudeness: Ugandan Social Critiques in the 1940s." *Journal of Social History* 39 (2006): 741–70.

Tappan, Jennifer. "Blood Work and 'Rumors' of Blood: Nutritional Research and Insurrection in Buganda, 1935–1970." *International Journal of African Historical Studies* 47, no. 3 (September 2014): 473–94.

——. *The Riddle of Malnutrition: The Long Arc of Biomedical and Public Health Interventions in Uganda.* Athens: Ohio University Press, 2017.

——. "The True Fiasco: The Treatment and Prevention of Sever Acute Malnutrition in Uganda 1950–1974." In *Global Health in Africa: Historical Perspectives on Culture, Epidemiology, and Disease Control,* edited by Tamara Giles Vernick and James Webb Jr., 92–113. Athens: Ohio University Press, 2013.

Taylor, Edgar C. "Affective Registers of Postcolonial Crisis: The Kampala Tank Hill Party." *Africa* 89, no. 3 (2019): 541–61.

——. "Asians and Africans in Ugandan Urban Life, 1959–1972." PhD diss., University of Michigan, 2016.

——. "Risk and Labor in the Archives: Archival Futures in Uganda." *Africa* (forthcoming).

Taylor, Janelle S. "What the Word 'Partnership' Conjoins, and What It Does." *Medicine Anthropology Theory* 5, no. 2 (May 15, 2018). https://doi.org/10.17157/mat.5.2.526.

Thiong'o, Ngugi wa. *Something Torn and New: An African Renaissance.* New York: Basic Books, 2009.

Thomas, Lynn M. *Politics of the Womb: Women, Reproduction, and the State in Kenya.* Berkeley: University of California Press, 2003.

Tilley, Helen. *Africa as a Living Laboratory.* Chicago: University of Chicago Press, 2011.

Tokaty, A. B. "Soviet Rocket Technology." *Technology and Culture* 4, no. 4 (1963): 515–28.

Tousignant, Noémi. *Edges of Exposure: Toxicology and the Problem of Capacity in Postcolonial Senegal.* Durham, NC: Duke University Press, 2018.

Tripp, Aili Mari. *Museveni's Uganda: Paradoxes of Power in a Hybrid Regime.* Boulder, CO: Rienner, 2010.

Trouillot, Michel-Rolph. *Silencing the Past: Power and the Production of History.* Boston: Beacon, 1995.

Turshen, Meredith. *Privatizing Health Services in Africa.* New Brunswick, NJ: Rutgers University Press, 1999.

Twaddle, Michael. *Expulsion of a Minority: Essays on Ugandan Asians.* London: Athlone Press for the Institute of Commonwealth Studies, 1975.

van der Geest, Sjaak, and Kaja Finkler. "Hospital Ethnography: Introduction." *Social Science and Medicine* 59, no. 10 (November 2004): 1995–2001.

Vansina, Jan. *Paths in the Rainforest.* Madison: University of Wisconsin Press, 1990.

Varmus, Harold. "Medical Research Centers in Mali and Uganda: Overcoming Obstacles to Building Scientific Capacity and Promoting Global Health." *Science and Diplomacy* 3 (2014).

Vaughan, Megan. "Conceptualising Metabolic Disorder in Southern Africa: Biology, History and Global Health." *BioSocieties* 14, no. 1 (April 1, 2019): 123–42.

——. *Curing Their Ills: Colonial Power and African Illness.* Cambridge, UK: Polity, 1991.

——. "Healing and Curing: Issues in the Social History and Anthropology of Medicine in Africa." *Social History of Medicine* 7, no. 2 (August 1, 1994): 283–95.

Vaughan, Megan, Kafui Adjaye-Gbewonyo, and Marissa Mika, eds. *Epidemiological Change and Chronic Disease in Sub-Saharan Africa: Social and Historical Perspectives.* London: UCL Press, 2021.

Vogel, Morris J., and Charles E. Rosenberg. *The Therapeutic Revolution: Essays in the Social History of American Medicine.* Philadelphia: University of Pennsylvania Press, 1979.

von Schnitzler, Antina. *Democracy's Infrastructure: Techno-politics and Protest after Apartheid.* Princeton, NJ: Princeton University Press, 2016.

Wailoo, Keith. *Drawing Blood: Technology and Disease Identity in Twentieth-Century America.* Henry E. Sigerist Series in the History of Medicine. Baltimore: Johns Hopkins University Press, 1997.

——. *How Cancer Crossed the Color Line.* Oxford: Oxford University Press, 2011.

Wallman, Sandra. *Kampala Women Getting By.* Athens: Ohio University Press, 1996.

Warner, John Harley. *The Therapeutic Perspective: Medical Practice, Knowledge, and Identity in America.* Princeton, NJ: Princeton University Press, 2014.

Webel, Mari K. *The Politics of Disease Control: Sleeping Sickness in Eastern Africa, 1890–1920.* Athens: Ohio University Press, 2019.

Weibe, Paul D., and Cole P. Dodge. *Beyond Crisis Development Issues in Uganda.* Kampala: Makerere Institute of Social Research, 1987.

Wendland, Claire L. *A Heart for the Work: Journeys through an African Medical School.* Chicago: University of Chicago Press, 2010.

——. "Opening Up the Black Box: Looking for a More Capacious Version of Capacity in Global Health Partnerships." *Canadian Journal of African*

Studies (Revue Canadienne Des Études Africaines) 50, no. 3 (September 1, 2016): 415–35. https://doi.org/10.1080/00083968.2016.1266675.

White, Luise. *The Comforts of Home: Prostitution in Colonial Nairobi*. Chicago: University of Chicago Press, 1990.

———. *Speaking with Vampires: Rumor and History in Colonial Africa*. Berkeley: University of California Press, 2000.

———. "'They Could Make Their Victims Dull': Genders and Genres, Fantasies and Cures in Colonial Southern Uganda." *American Historical Review* 100, no. 5 (1995): 1379–1402.

Whyte, Susan Reynolds, ed. *Second Chances: Surviving AIDS in Uganda*. Durham, NC: Duke University Press, 2014.

Whyte, Susan Reynolds, Sjaak van der Geest, and Anita Hardon. *Social Lives of Medicines, Cambridge Studies in Medical Anthropology*. New York: Cambridge University Press, 2002.

Whyte, Susan Reynolds, Michael Whyte, and Betty Kyaddondo. "Health Workers Entangled: Confidentiality and Certification." In *Morality, Hope and Grief: Anthropologies of AIDS*, edited by Hansjorg Dilger and Ute Luig, 80–101. New York: Berghahn, 2010.

Yarrow, Thomas. "Remains of the Future: Rethinking the Space and Time of Ruination through the Volta Resettlement Project, Ghana." *Cultural Anthropology* 32, no. 4 (2017): 566–91. https://doi.org/10.14506/ca32.4.06.

Yates-Doerr, Emily. *The Weight of Obesity*. Berkeley: University of California Press, 2015.

Zeller, Diane. "The Establishment of Western Medicine in Buganda." PhD diss., Columbia University, 1971.

Index

breast cancer, 4, 14, 18, 113, 116, 117, 143, 151, 195n8, 203n60

British colonial medical establishment, 29, 33, 44, 45

British Empire Cancer Campaign, 7, 8, 31, 42, 45, 150

British Journal of Cancer, 34

British Journal of Surgery, 33

British Medical Journal, 31

Buganda, 1, 20, 45, 49, 56; riots, 32

"bunker, the," 23, 115, 120, 122, 124, 128, 129. *See also* radiotherapy

Burchenal, Joseph, 37, 38

Burkitt, Denis, 25–28, 32–41, 44–46, 48, 53, 54, 55, 58

Burkitt's lymphoma, 7, 9, 10, 17, 26, 102, 104, 107; distribution of, 49, 50; emergency, 4; Epstein Barr virus, potential links to, 18; and Lasker Foundation award, 61; Lymphoma Treatment Center, 42–45, 50, 52, 59; patients, 102, 104, 110, 111, 112, 131, 148, 151, 161; research, 27, 32–37, 44, 48, 53–59, 61, 63, 70, 78, 93, 95, 99, 101, 147, 149, 150, 160; survival and follow-up, 38, 39, 40, 41, 53–59, 62, 63, 70, 71–76, 93, 142, 151; United States, 40

Busia, 54, 109

cancer and its metaphors, 96

Cancer Chemotherapy National Service Center, 107

cancer-corporate care nexus, 14

cancer drugs, 94, 107, 143. *See also* chemotherapy

cancer in Africa, 17–19, 140

"Cancer in Africa" conference, 40

"Cancer in an African Community, 1897–1956," 32

cancer incidence, 18, 30, 140

cancer registration, 18, 25, 26, 31, 69, 131, 140, 203n60

cancer research: and care, 19, 27, 41, 53, 63; collaborations and partnerships, 9, 123, 135, 146; infrastructure and systems, 8, 43, 44, 45, 102, 139, 149; at Makerere Medical School, 27, 32, 41, 42, 46, 98; as technology transfer, 13; in Uganda, 17, 26, 27, 45, 140, 146; at the Uganda Cancer Institute, 10, 53, 60, 78, 98, 138, 145, 146, 149, 150. *See also* Burkitt's lymphoma

Cancer Research Committee (Makerere), 26, 33

Canon, Rumanzi, 22

capacity, 12, 66, 82, 100, 122, 130, 132, 133, 134, 142, 196n16

Carbone, Paul, 37, 39, 40, 66

care: for cancer, 8–10, 14–15, 19, 27, 42–45, 94–96, 101–2, 105, 128, 134, 139, 141, 147, 149–50, 160–61, 168; for families, 49–53; for late-stage cancers, 111; palliative, 7, 11, 94, 96, 103, 115–16, 132, 139; for patient hopes, 116; for Uganda as a nation, 69

caretakers, 2–6, 9, 11, 21, 27, 44–45, 49, 51, 53, 73, 96, 111, 112, 117, 147, 161–64

Carswell, Wilson, 136

Casper, Corey, 131, 132, 134, 139, 140, 146

Catholics, 6, 128

central nervous system relapse, 78, 115, 168, 195

cervical cancer, 18, 115, 116, 131, 142

chemotherapy: "armamentarium," 95, 103; austerity, 113–14; Burkitt's lymphoma treatment, 27, 32, 38–41, 61–63, 66, 118; clinical trials, 7, 9, 17, 44, 51, 63, 66, 78, 94, 130, 166; costs, 94, 98, 112; curative potential, 11, 59, 61, 66, 111, 112; experimentation and care, 15, 26, 76; *keemo*, 114; palliation and salvage, 132, 154, 157; poison, 37; preparation and administration, 3, 5, 6, 14, 21, 43, 52, 64, 66, 68, 80, 93, 104–5, 109–10, 113–14, 148, 162, 164, 167; *saba saba*, 96, 102–6; side effects, 38, 51, 102–6, 135, 155; supplies, 76, 81, 95, 97, 98, 103, 110, 165; Uganda Cancer Institute as research center for, 17, 40, 42, 95, 137, 138, 150, 166; weapons research, 106–8

CIA operatives, 60

civil servants, 46, 62, 65, 78, 80

civil war, 10, 22, 95, 96, 98, 119, 127, 129. *See also* violence

cleanliness round, 113, 145

Clifford, Peter, 37, 40

clinical deserts, 12

clinical trials, 7, 9, 14, 17, 40–44, 53, 59, 63, 66, 77, 94, 95, 101, 138, 166

clothing for patients, 51, 158, 163

coffins, 112, 154, 159, 160

cohort: Burkitt's lymphoma, 62, 63, 69–76; cancer chemotherapist, 61; HIV

patients, 138, 139, 140; infection-
    related cancers, 142; Kaposi's sar-
    coma, 140; Ugandan physicians, 140
collaborations and partnerships: build-
    ings, 149–52; with Fred Hutch,
    131, 139–50; half-life of research
    partnerships, 129–30; inequality in,
    149–52; international, 7, 8, 9, 10, 13,
    104, 122, 131–39, 142–50, 167; with In-
    ternational Atomic Energy Agency,
    115, 119, 120–23; material remains of,
    129–30, 131, 151–52; public/private,
    20; research partnerships, 8, 9, 10,
    97, 101, 129–34, 167; with World
    Health Organization, 140
colonial: conquest, 15–16; development
    and developmentalism, 9, 15, 45
Colonial Medical Research Council, 26
Colonial Medical Service, 27, 28, 46
Comis, Robert, 59, 194n57
consent, informed, 21, 99, 104, 136, 149
Cook, Albert, 31
cooking and food preparation, 14, 44,
    49, 51, 64, 76, 78, 149, 157, 158, 160,
    165–67
Cooper, Fred, 13
"Cornell medicine," 52
Coutinho, Alex, 135–36, 195n57
Crane, Johanna, 133
creativity, 13, 82; creativity and crisis, 10,
    24, 116, 134
cyclophosphamide, 13, 38, 39, 61, 105,
    107, 110, 112
cytotoxic agents, cytotoxic drugs, 9, 21,
    37, 38, 54, 66, 76, 82, 98, 114, 136.
    See also chemotherapy

Davies, A. G., 25
Davies, J. N. P., 25, 26, 27, 28, 29, 30, 31,
    32, 33, 34, 36, 41
decolonization, 45, 46
de Laet, Marianne, 123
diagnosis, 32, 55, 109, 112, 117, 118, 155,
    156, 157
dictator, dictatorship, 9, 97. See also
    Amin, Idi
diseases of civilization, 16, 30
disgust, 4, 167
disintegrating state, 62, 63, 121, 177
"doing everything," 112
"doing research," 145, 151
"doing something" for patients, 119
Donka: X-ray of an African Hospital, 109

Dr. M, 102–8
drugs. See chemotherapy; cytotoxic
    agents, cytotoxic drugs
dry ice, 79, 131
Dr. Z, 116, 119, 120, 121, 122, 124, 125, 127,
    128
durable, durability, 8, 75, 133, 134
durable remission, 61, 95, 104, 107

East African disease ecology, 29
East African doctors, 17
East African economic community, 67
East African Medical Journal, 26, 30
Ebola: impact on radiotherapy, 127–29;
    West African epidemic of 2013–15, 12
economic war, 61, 64, 65, 66
Edinburgh, 27, 30, 47, 100
Edwards, Paul, 15
electricity, 15, 64, 71, 77, 78, 123, 125, 131
Electricity Board, 77
empiso mukaaga, 114
Emuron, 75
Endicott, Kenneth, 107
end-of-life care, 109, 112, 118. See also
    care; palliative care
Engel, Mary, 145
enkadde and enkadde nnyo, 123
Entebbe Airport, 42, 76
environmental health and environmen-
    tal health factors, 12, 29, 33, 35
Epak, Yefusa Okullo, 132
essential drug list, 82
ethics, 27, 44; of Africanization, 47; of
    quality care, 82; of training, 47;
    of Ugandanization, 65 (see also
    Africanization)
Ethiopia, 107
ethnographic fieldwork, 21, 23, 47, 58,
    113, 151, 166
experimental infrastructure, 10, 15, 41,
    43, 60, 64, 120, 134, 148, 151, 165. See
    also infrastructure
experiments, 8, 10, 12, 16, 24, 26, 53, 61,
    108, 138, 148, 149, 174
expertise, 10, 15, 26, 38, 47, 108, 120, 150,
    170
experts, 17, 68, 69, 122, 168
extraction, 9, 11, 12, 16

"face sheets," 49, 55, 153
families, 3, 9, 14, 27, 39, 44, 45, 48, 49,
    50–57, 60, 64, 71–76, 81, 94, 96, 103–
    4, 109, 112, 114, 144, 160, 165

transport, 2, 44, 72, 74, 98, 100, 112, 126, 155, 156, 161
trauma, 111; of war, 121
travel, 10, 35, 71, 72, 74, 100, 156
treatment of entire families, 14, 50
triage, 4, 12, 53, 94, 101, 102, 150, 157, 160, 203
Tripp, Aili, 19, 176
tropical medicine, 27, 28
tuberculosis, 30, 128, 141, 164
tumor regression, 38, 51, 52, 106
tumor safari, 34, 35, 36, 37, 38, 53
typhoid fever, 30, 59, 65

Uganda Cancer Institute (UCI): African cancer care, 17–19; Amin's impact on, 62–65, 80–82; after austerity, 113–14, 131–34, 149–52; austerity's impact on, 108–13; Burkitt's lymphoma patient follow-up in 1970s at, 69–76; establishment of, 42–45; ethnographic and historical research at, 21–24; everyday life at, 1–6, 49–53, 153–68; as experimental infrastructure, 15–16; Fred Hutch collaboration, 131–34, 139–45; and global oncology, 139–40; grand opening of Lymphoma Treatment Center, 46–49; historical overview, 7–10; and HIV-related Kaposi's sarcoma research, 135–39; Lasker Foundation award, 61–62; meanings of, 59–60; as microcosm of Uganda, 19–20; as a museum, 99–102; National Cancer Institute relations with, 8, 17, 37, 40–46, 53, 61–63, 66–67, 76, 81, 95–99, 107, 131, 150; patient recruitment at, 53–59; and radiotherapy department relations, 120; research in 1970s at, 76–80; survival in 1970s, 65–69, 93–94; survival from the 1980s to the 2000s, 94–99; UCI–Fred Hutch Cancer Center, 145–52
Ugandanization, 9, 65, 67
Uganda Virus Research Institute, 35
uncertainty, 65, 68, 73, 81, 117, 121
United Kingdom, 17, 22, 26, 27, 28, 30, 32, 38, 46, 70, 80, 98, 100
University of California San Francisco, 101, 137, 139, 140
University of Edinburgh, 27, 30, 47, 100
urbanization, 17, 29

US goodwill, 67, 133
US National Nuclear Security Administration, 127

VAMP, 37, 38
Vaughan, Megan, 17
veins, 102, 105, 153
verandah, 35, 154, 155, 158, 161, 162, 168
vernacular, 14, 96, 177
Victoria Falls, 35
Vietnam War, 45
village chiefs, 37, 39
villages, 14, 31, 39, 51, 53, 57, 71–76, 145, 154, 158, 160, 165, 166
vincristine, 37, 61, 105, 110, 137, 144
violence: cancer and metaphorical violence, 96, 104–6; chemotherapy administration, 113–14; epidemics, 17; fear of, 71–73; *saba saba*, 104–5; state, 19, 20, 65, 68, 77, 81; structural, 108–9; violent technologies, 96, 106–8; war of liberation, 95–96, 102, 105, 106, 108, 120–21
viruses: Epstein-Barr, 18, 69, 70, 142; etiology of cancer and viruses, 11; hepatitis B and C, 18; human herpes, 8, 18; human papillomavirus, 18, 142; insect vector, 35
visible, visibility, 15, 17, 18, 27, 32, 39, 62, 132, 142, 148, 168
Vogel, Charles, 53, 60, 67, 68, 99, 100, 137
Volberding, Paul, 138
Volkswagen Beetle, 55, 56, 71, 74
vomiting, 3, 6, 19, 103, 106, 135, 163

Wabinga, Henry, 140
Walusansa, Victoria, 22
Wandegeya, 1, 30, 155, 156
war, 10, 20–23, 27–30, 45, 46, 61, 64–66, 81, 93–98, 100–108, 113, 114, 119–21, 125–29, 135, 147
ward rounds, 4, 5, 52, 68, 80, 101, 135, 145, 153–61
War on Terror, 119, 125
water supply, 62, 125, 177
WikiLeaks, 127
Williams, Ted, 34
World Bank, 95
World Health Organization, 54, 65, 96, 100, 137, 140, 141
World War II, 27, 28, 45, 103, 106, 107
Wright, Denis, 40